T0263991

# Autoimmune Endocrine Disorders

*Guest Editor*

SIMON H.S. PEARCE, MD

# ENDOCRINOLOGY AND METABOLISM CLINICS OF NORTH AMERICA

www.endo.theclinics.com

*Consulting Editor*
DEREK LEROITH, MD, PhD

June 2009 • Volume 38 • Number 2

SAUNDERS an imprint of ELSEVIER, Inc.

**W.B. SAUNDERS COMPANY**
*A Division of Elsevier Inc.*

1600 John F. Kennedy Boulevard • Suite 1800 • Philadelphia, Pennsylvania 19103-2899

http://www.theclinics.com

ENDOCRINOLOGY AND METABOLISM CLINICS OF NORTH AMERICA Volume 38, Number 2
June 2009 ISSN 0889-8529, ISBN-13: 978-1-4377-0471-6, ISBN-10: 1-4377-0471-9

Editor: Rachel Glover
Developmental Editor: Donald Mumford

© 2009 Elsevier ■ **All rights reserved.**

This journal and the individual contributions contained in it are protected under copyright by Elsevier, and the following terms and conditions apply to their use:

**Photocopying**
Single photocopies of single articles may be made for personal use as allowed by national copyright laws. Permission of the Publisher and payment of a fee is required for all other photocopying, including multiple or systematic copying, copying for advertising or promotional purposes, resale, and all forms of document delivery. Special rates are available for educational institutions that wish to make photocopies for non-profit educational classroom use. For information on how to seek permission visit www.elsevier.com/permissions or call: (+44) 1865 843830 (UK)/(+1) 215 239 3804 (USA).

**Derivative Works**
Subscribers may reproduce tables of contents or prepare lists of articles including abstracts for internal circulation within their institutions. Permission of the Publisher is required for resale or distribution outside the institution. Permission of the Publisher is required for all other derivative works, including compilations and translations (please consult www.elsevier.com/permissions).

**Electronic Storage or Usage**
Permission of the Publisher is required to store or use electronically any material contained in this journal, including any article or part of an article (please consult www.elsevier.com/permissions). Except as outlined above, no part of this publication may be reproduced, stored in a retrieval system or transmitted in any form or by any means, electronic, mechanical, photocopying, recording or otherwise, without prior written permission of the Publisher.

**Notice**
No responsibility is assumed by the Publisher for any injury and/or damage to persons or property as a matter of products liability, negligence or otherwise, or from any use or operation of any methods, products, instructions or ideas contained in the material herein. Because of rapid advances in the medical sciences, in particular, independent verification of diagnoses and drug dosages should be made.

Although all advertising material is expected to conform to ethical (medical) standards, inclusion in this publication does not constitute a guarantee or endorsement of the quality or value of such product or of the claims made of it by its manufacturer.

*Endocrinology and Metabolism Clinics of North America* (ISSN 0889-8529) is published quarterly by Elsevier Inc., 360 Park Avenue South, New York, NY 10010-1710. Months of issue are March, June, September, and December. Business and Editorial Offices: 1600 John F. Kennedy Boulevard, Suite 1800, Philadelphia, PA 19103-2899. Customer Service Office: 11830 Westline Industrial Drive, St. Louis, MO 63146. Periodicals postage paid at New York, NY and additional mailing offices. Subscription prices are USD 242.00 per year for US individuals, USD 408.00 per year for US institutions, USD 124.00 per year for US students and residents, USD 304.00 per year for Canadian individuals, USD 500.00 per year for Canadian institutions, USD 352.00 per year for international individuals, USD 500.00 per year for international institutions, and USD 184.00 per year for international and Canadian and foreign students/residents. To receive student/resident rate, orders must be accompanied by name of affiliated institution, date of term, and the signature of program/residency coordinator on institution letterhead. Orders will be billed at individual rate until proof of status is received. Foreign air speed delivery is included in all *Clinics* subscription prices. All prices are subject to change without notice. **POSTMASTER:** Send address changes to *Endocrinology and Metabolism Clinics of North America*, Elsevier Periodicals Customer Service, 11830 Westline Industrial Drive, St. Louis, MO 63146. **Customer Service: 1-800-654-2452 (U.S. and Canada). From outside of the US and Canada: 1-314-453-7041. Fax: 1-314-453-5170. For print support, e-mail: journalscustomerservice-usa@elsevier.com. For online support, e-mail: journals onlinesupport-usa@elsevier.com.**

*Reprints.* For copies of 100 or more, of articles in this publication, please contact the Commercial Rights Department, Elsevier Inc., 360 Park Avenue South, New York, NY 10010-1710; phone: (+1) 212-633-3813; fax: (+1) 212-462-1935; e-mail: reprints@elsevier.com.

*Endocrinology and Metabolism Clinics of North America* is covered in *MEDLINE/PubMed (Index Medicus)*, *EMBASE/Excerpta Medica, Current Contents/Clinical Medicine, Current Contents/Life Sciences, Science Citation Index, ISI/BIOMED, BIOSIS,* and *Chemical Abstracts.*

Printed and bound by CPI Group (UK) Ltd, Croydon, CR0 4YY
Transferred to Digital Print 2011

# Contributors

## CONSULTING EDITOR

**DEREK LEROITH, MD, PhD**
Chief, Division of Endocrinology, Metabolism, and Bone Diseases, Mount Sinai School of Medicine, New York, New York

## GUEST EDITOR

**SIMON H.S. PEARCE, MD**
Professor, Institute of Human Genetics, University of Newcastle, International Center for Life, Central Parkway, Newcastle upon Tyne, United Kingdom

## AUTHORS

**WIEBKE ARLT, MD, DSc, FRCP**
Professor of Medicine, MRC Senior Clinical Fellow, Division of Medical Sciences, Institute of Biomedical Research, University of Birmingham, Birmingham, United Kingdom

**J. PAUL BANGA, PhD**
Professor of Endocrine Immunology, Department of Diabetes and Endocrinology, King's College London School of Medicine, Denmark Hill Campus, The Rayne Institute, London, United Kingdom

**EDWARD M. BROWN, MD**
Professor of Medicine, Division of Endocrinology, Diabetes and Hypertension, Department of Medicine, Brigham and Women's Hospital, Boston, Massachusetts

**TALAL A. CHATILA, MD, MSc**
Professor of Pediatrics; and Chief, Division of Immunology, Allergy and Rheumatology, Department of Pediatrics, The David Geffen School of Medicine, University of California, Los Angeles, California

**TIM D. CHEETHAM, MB, ChB, MD, MRCP, MRCPCH**
Senior Lecturer in Paediatric Endocrinology, Institute of Human Genetics, University of Newcastle, Newcastle upon Tyne, United Kingdom

**SELÇUK DAĞDELEN, MD**
Clinical Research Fellow, Department of Diabetes and Endocrinology, King's College London School of Medicine, Denmark Hill Campus, The Rayne Institute, London, United Kingdom; and Instructor, Department of Endocrinology and Metabolism, Hacettepe University, School of Medicine, Ankara, Turkey

**TERRY F. DAVIES, MD**
Thyroid Research Unit, Mount Sinai School of Medicine and the James J. Peters VA Medical Center, New York, New York

**JANE DICKINSON, MBChB, FRCP, FRCOphth**
Consultant Ophthalmologist, Department of Ophthalmology, Newcastle upon Tyne
Hospitals NHS Trust, Newcastle upon Tyne, United Kingdom

**LASZLO HEGEDÜS, MD, DMSc**
Professor of Medicine and Endocrinology, Department of Endocrinology and Metabolism,
Odense University Hospital, University of Southern Denmark, Odense, Denmark

**KEVAN C. HEROLD, MD**
Professor, Department of Immunobiology, Yale University; and Department of Internal
Medicine, Yale University, New Haven, Connecticut

**GEORG A. HOLLÄNDER, MD**
Professor of Molecular Medicine in Pediatrics, Laboratory of Pediatric Immunology,
Department of Biomedicine, University of Basel and The University Children's Hospital
(UKBB), Basel, Switzerland

**EYSTEIN S. HUSEBYE, MD, PhD**
Professor, Section of Endocrinology, Institute of Medicine, University of Bergen, Norway;
and Department of Medicine, Haukeland University Hospital, Bergen, Norway

**YI-CHI M. KONG, PhD**
Professor, Department of Immunology and Microbiology, Wayne State University School
of Medicine, Detroit, Michigan

**RAUF LATIF, PhD**
Thyroid Research Unit, Mount Sinai School of Medicine and the James J. Peters VA
Medical Center, New York, New York

**KRISTIAN LØVÅS, MD, PhD**
Section of Endocrinology, Institute of Medicine, University of Bergen, Norway;
and Department of Medicine, Haukeland University Hospital, Bergen, Norway

**TONY R. MERRIMAN, PhD**
Associate Professor, Department of Biochemistry, University of Otago, Dunedin,
New Zealand

**SYED A. MORSHED, PhD**
Thyroid Research Unit, Mount Sinai School of Medicine and the James J. Peters VA
Medical Center, New York, New York

**GRETEL NUSSPAUMER, PhD**
Postdoctoral Fellow, Laboratory of Pediatric Immunology, Department of Biomedicine,
University of Basel and The University Children's Hospital (UKBB), Basel, Switzerland

**CATHERINE J. OWEN, MBBS, MRCP, MRCPCH, PhD**
Specialist Registrar Paediatric Endocrinology, Institute of Human Genetics, University
of Newcastle, Newcastle upon Tyne, United Kingdom

**SIMON H.S. PEARCE, MD**
Professor, Institute of Human Genetics, University of Newcastle, International Center
for Life, Central Parkway, Newcastle upon Tyne, United Kingdom

**PETROS PERROS, MBBS, MD, FRCP**
Consultant Endocrinologist, Department of Endocrinology, Newcastle upon Tyne
Hospitals NHS Trust, Newcastle upon Tyne, United Kingdom

**NICOLE REISCH, MD**
Marie Curie Intra-European Fellow, Division of Medical Sciences, Institute of Biomedical
Research, University of Birmingham, Birmingham, United Kingdom

**NORIKO SHIKAMA, PhD**
Postdoctoral Fellow, Laboratory of Pediatric Immunology, Department of Biomedicine,
University of Basel and The University Children's Hospital (UKBB), Basel, Switzerland

**FRANK WALDRON-LYNCH, MD, PhD**
Department of Internal Medicine, Yale University, New Haven, Connecticut

**MONE ZAIDI, MD**
Thyroid Research Unit and the Mount Sinai Bone Program, Mount Sinai School
of Medicine, New York, New York

# Contents

CD4 + CD25 + regulatory T (TR) lymphocytes are essential to the maintenance of immunologic tolerance in the host. The discovery of Foxp3 as a transcription factor essential to the differentiation of TR ushered in detailed studies of the molecular mechanisms of TR cell development, peripheral homeostasis, and effector functions. In humans, loss of function mutations in genes that regulate T-cell development and function have been associated with TR cell deficiency or dysfunction and syndromes of autoimmunity and immune dysregulation. Augmentation of TR cells by immunotherapy and pharmacologic agents is a promising strategy for the treatment of allergic and autoimmune diseases.

Autoimmune polyendocrine syndrome type-1 clinically manifests as the triad of hypoparathyroidism, primary adrenocortical insufficiency, and chronic mucocutaneous candidiasis. Mutations in the gene that encodes the autoimmune regulator protein, AIRE, have been identified as the cause of the autoimmune polyendocrine syndrome type-1. The loss of immunologic tolerance to tissue-restricted antigens consequent to an absence of AIRE expression in the thymus results in the thymic export of autoreactive T cells that initiate autoimmunity. In this article, we discuss the role of AIRE in autoimmune polyendocrine syndrome type-1 and identify issues that still need to be addressed to fully understand the molecular pathophysiology of this complex syndrome.

The search for the susceptibility alleles for the complex genetic conditions of type 1 diabetes and autoimmune thyroid diseases has gained momentum in recent years. Studies have revealed several novel disease susceptibility alleles of relevance to both conditions, which brings the total number of genetic variants contributing to type 1 diabetes to ten. Additional genetic loci remain to be discovered, particularly in the autoimmune thyroid diseases. In the future, the density and coverage of single nucleotide polymorphisms available for high throughput genotyping will improve, and detailed analysis of the role of copy number variants in these diseases will shed new light on the pathogenesis of these common endocrinopathies.

Refinements in our understanding of the pathogenic mechanisms of Type 1 diabetes from studies of animal models and clinical observation have led to new clinical trials to prevent disease progression and restore the loss of β-cells that defines the disease. Antigen-specific agents have shown initial promise and non–antigen-specific agents now have improved safety compared with older agents. In addition, preclinical studies with other agents have shown efficacy. Ultimately, a combination of immunologic and cellular therapies may be needed to restore metabolic control. Agents that augment recovery of dysfunctional β-cells, and other compounds that may be able to induce β-cell replication, are logical additions once immune tolerance is achieved.

The thyroid-stimulating hormone receptor (TSHR) has a central role in thyrocyte function and is also one of the major autoantigens for the autoimmune thyroid diseases. We review the post-translational processing, multimerization, and intramolecular cleavage of TSHR, all of which may modulate its signal transduction. The recent characterization of monoclonal antibodies to the TSHR, including stimulating, blocking, and neutral antibodies, have also revealed unique biologic insights into receptor activation and the variety of these TSHR antibodies may help explain the multiple clinical phenotypes seen in autoimmune thyroid diseases. Knowledge of the structure/function relationship of the TSHR is beginning to provide a greater understanding of thyroid physiology and thyroid autoimmunity.

Graves' disease affects only humans. Although it is a treatable illness, medical therapy with antithyroid drugs is imperfect, showing high rates of recurrence. Furthermore, the etiology and treatment of the associated ophthalmopathy still represent problematic issues. Animal models could contribute to the solution of such problems by providing a better understanding of the underlying pathogenesis and could be used for evaluating novel therapeutic strategies. This article discusses the pursuit of a better experimental model for hyperthyroid Graves' disease and outlines how this research has clarified the immunology of the disease.

Currently there are three well-established treatment options for hyperthyroid Graves' disease (GD): antithyroid drug therapy with thionamides (ATD), radioactive iodine treatment with $^{131}$I, and thyroid surgery. This article reviews the current evidence so the reader can evaluate advantages and disadvantages of these treatment modalities. Surgery is rarely used, except for patients who have a large goiter or ophthalmopathy. Fewer than 50% of patients treated with ATD remain in long-term remission. Therefore, radioactive iodine is used increasingly. No data as yet support the routine use of biologic therapies (eg, rituximab). Prospective, randomized studies comparing available and any novel therapeutic options for GD are needed. The focus of these studies should include, but not be limited to, cost and quality of life.

Thyroid-associated orbitopathy is the most frequent and troublesome nonthyroidal complication of Graves' disease. It is mandatory to determine whether sight-threatening orbitopathy is present, as this requires prompt and aggressive treatment. Therapies for non–sight-threatening disease range from supportive measures only to medical therapies for active eye disease and surgical rehabilitation for burnt-out disease. Intravenous steroids and orbital radiotherapy are the mainstays of medical therapy. Rehabilitative surgery is frequently a staged process that may involve sequentially: orbital decompression, strabismus surgery, and eyelid procedures. Smoking cessation is recommended at all disease stages. Treatment within a multidisciplinary team consisting of both endocrinologists and ophthalmologists may lead to optimal patient outcomes.

Autoimmune Addison's disease and autoimmune ovarian insufficiency are caused by selective targeting by T and B lymphocytes to the steroidogenic apparatus in these organs. Autoantibodies toward 21-hydroxylase are a clinically useful marker for autoimmune Addison's disease. Autoantibodies to 21-hydroxylase are found in premature ovarian insufficiency, but others also can be present, notably antibodies against side-chain cleavage enzyme. The autoimmune response primarily targets the theca cells, yielding elevated concentrations of inhibin, which is emerging as a useful diagnostic marker for autoimmune etiology of ovarian insufficiency. Little is known about its immunogenetics, but in contrast to Addison's disease, several experimental models of autoimmune premature ovarian insufficiency are available for study.

Despite treatment with glucocorticoids and mineralocorticoids, the ability to work and quality of life of patients who have adrenal insufficiency remains low. There are no helpful objective measures of optimal glucocorticoid replacement, so this is best achieved by careful clinical assessment. Adequacy of mineralocorticoid replacement may be judged by assessing postural change in blood pressure, serum electrolytes, and plasma renin activity. Novel delayed-release and sustained-release formulations of hydrocortisone seem to more closely mimic diurnal serum cortisol rhythms than conventional hydrocortisone tablets. Such preparations are currently being evaluated and may play a role in management of patients who have adrenal insufficiency.

**THE CLINICS ARE NOW AVAILABLE ONLINE!**

Access your subscription at:
**www.theclinics.com**

# Foreword

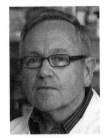

Derek LeRoith, MD, PhD
*Consulting Editor*

This issue of *Endocrinology and Metabolism Clinics* focuses on clinical and molecular advances in autoimmune endocrine conditions.

In the opening article, Talal Chatila describes the role of the thymus-derived natural regulatory T lymphocytes, which are important for immunological tolerance. Recent studies have determined the lineage markers and differentiation pathways of natural regulatory T lymphocytes and that mutations in *FOXP3*, the key transcriptional regulator in these cells, leads to autoimmune diseases, such as neonatal type 1 diabetes and other endocrinopathies. Modulation of these regulatory T lymphocytes may prove to be useful in treating certain food allergies and autoimmune diseases.

Noriko Shikama, Gretel Nusspaumer, and Georg Holländer discuss the mechanisms involved in the autoimmune polyendocrinopathy syndrome type 1. Mutations in the gene encoding the autoimmune regulator protein (AIRE) prevents the thymus from expressing many nonthymic self-antigens that would normally cause deletion of developing T lymphocytes. Thus, these auto-reactive T lymphocytes are exported and can induce the autoimmune process. The result is a syndrome consisting of mucocutaneous candidiasis, hypoparathyroidism, and adrenocortical insufficiency. The authors also describe in detail the AIRE gene; its structure, function, and regulation; and its role in the thymus.

Autoimmune thyroid disease, including Graves' and autoimmune hypothyroidism, as well as autoimmune type 1 diabetes (TID), are genetic disorders that share common loci, but also have their own specific genetic loci. Simon Pearce and Tony Merriman describe the relationship of the human leukocyte antigen alleles, encoded within the major histocompatibility complex (MHC), as an example of a shared susceptibility locus. Other examples include the lymphoid tyrosine phosphatase, cytotoxic T-lymphocyte antigen-4, CD25, and the interferon-induced helicase-1 gene locus. Meanwhile, loci specific for autoimmune thyroid disease include those for the thyrotropin receptor, Fc receptor–like S, and CD40 genes. For type 1 diabetes, the insulin gene is an excellent example. The authors conclude that in type 1 diabetes, while numerous non-MHC loci have been found, they each probably only contribute a small percentage towards the genetic susceptibility to the disease.

Endocrinol Metab Clin N Am 38 (2009) xiii–xv
doi:10.1016/j.ecl.2009.02.001
0889-8529/09/$ – see front matter © 2009 Published by Elsevier Inc.

endo.theclinics.com

Frank Waldron-Lynch and Kevan Herold in their article describe the exciting new developments in type 1 diabetes that relate to the immunopathogenesis of this classic autoimmune disorder and that have led to immunomodulatory therapeutic trials. Following preclinical trials that were quite successful, human trials followed using insulin, Diapep277, and GAD65 as antigen therapy. Meanwhile, non–antigen-specific immunomodulation was tried using nicotinamide, immunosuppressive therapies, and anti-CD20 and anti-CD3 monoclonal antibodies. While these therapies are yet to be useful, they have paved the way for future attempts at "curing" type 1 diabetes.

In the article by Rauf Latif, Syed Morshed, Mone Zaidi, and Terry Davies, we are introduced to some new concepts regarding the thyrotropin receptor. While the thyrotropin receptor is known to control thyroid maturation and function, it has also been shown to be expressed in extrathyroidal tissue, including adipocytes and bone cells. In adipocytes, the thyrotropin receptor may stimulate human orbital fibroblasts to differentiate and further stimulate adipogenesis. Thyrotropin may inhibit osteoclastogenesis and activate osteoblastogenesis and may therefore be antiresorptive and anabolic in bone. Recently identified human thyrotropin receptor monoclonal antibodies have also revealed additional detail about the structure–function correlates of the receptor.

In their article, Selçuk Dağdelen, Yi-chi Kong, and Paul Banga point out the need for experimental animal models of hyperthyroid Graves' disease. Such models would help us better understand the underlying pathophysiology of hyperthyroid Graves' disease and point the way to better therapies, given that there are variations in the disease presentation and that the disorder often recurs. The authors describe the earlier animal models, including the Shimojo model that induced anti–thyrotropin receptor antibodies, models developed by DNA injection using the thyrotropin receptor gene, models developed by the adenovirus method, and, more recently, models developed by passive transfer of thyrotropin receptor monoclonal antibodies with thyroid stimulating antibody activity. While the road has been long and steep, the more recent models are showing promise in enabling investigators to study the mechanisms involved in the autoimmunity and the presentations, including, for example, Graves' ophthalmopathy.

Two articles deal with management of Graves' hyperthyroidism and thyroid-associated orbitopathy. Laszlo Hegedüs discusses the standard management of hyperthyroidism, including antithyroid medication, radioactive ablation therapy, and surgery, and the pros and cons of each. The novel use of monoclonal antibody therapy in Graves' disease is also described. Jane Dickinson and Petros Perros discuss the perennially difficult clinical problem of orbitopathy, its diverse presentation, and when and how to treat. These two articles are important clinical therapeutic components of this issue.

Adrenal insufficiency has a number of causes, but a common cause in westernized countries is autoimmune adrenalitis. While Addison's disease is often associated with type 1 diabetes and thyroid disease, it may also be associated with gonadal failure secondary to this autoimmune process that affects many endocrine glands. As discussed by Eystein Husebye and Kristian Løvås, some autoantibodies, such as 21-hydroxylase, are useful in the diagnosis of autoimmune Addison's disease. In the case of ovarian failure, antibodies to side-chain cleavage enzyme and 17-hydoxylase may also be useful. Recently interest has increased about the role of vitamin D deficiency and autoimmune disorders and whether replacement therapy may reduce the burden of these disorders.

Treating adrenal insufficiency and avoiding adrenal crises can be quite challenging. These days patients also have legitimate expectations for a good quality of life and a full sense of well-being. Nicole Reisch and Wiebke Arlt discuss the use of glucorti-coid therapy and the considerations for the use of mineralocorticoid therapy. They also suggest that dehydroepiandrosterone replacement may in fact be quite useful to increase the energy level and libido in women with adrenal insufficiency.

Autoimmune polyglandular syndromes are very diverse, with many varieties of both major components and minor manifestations. Catherine Owen and Tim Cheetham describe in detail the various syndromes, their manifestations, the diagnostic criteria, and the prognosis. In addition, they appropriately stress that early detection, correct diagnosis, and early intervention can preclude many of the complications that occur with these syndromes.

Autoimmune hypoparathyroidism may be an isolated disorder or a component of the autoimmune polyglandular syndromes. Edward Brown discusses the calcium-sensing receptor (which his group discovered) and its role in controlling whole-body calcium homeostasis. Soon after the calcium-sensing receptor was characterized, autoantibodies to this important receptor were discovered in cases of hypoparathy-roidism. These antibodies may activate or inhibit the receptor. Activation of the receptor causes hypoparathyroidism, whereas inhibitory antibodies result in hyper-parathyroidism. Mutations of the calcium-sensing receptor are associated with familial hypocalciuric hypercalcemia.

This timely issue on autoimmune endocrine disorders brings to the reader the latest in our understanding of the pathogenesis of the diseases, the complexity of their presentations, and the management of each condition. I believe it will be extremely informative to the endocrinologist and wish to thank Professor Pearce and the authors for their marvelous contributions.

Derek LeRoith, MD, PhD
Division of Endocrinology, Metabolism, and Bone Diseases
Mount Sinai School of Medicine
One Gustave L. Levy Place
Box 1055, Altran 4-36
New York, NY 10029, USA

E-mail address:
derek.leroith@mssm.edu (D. LeRoith)

# Preface

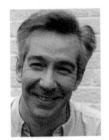

Simon H.S. Pearce, MD
*Guest Editor*

Autoimmune disorders are among the most frequently encountered conditions in endocrine practice. Despite this, and disregarding minor developments in drug delivery, treatment has remained effectively unchanged for more than 50 years for thyroid disorders and even longer for autoimmune diabetes. This situation might be acceptable if the existing treatments were perfect and if patient quality of life and satisfaction were high; however, this is clearly not the case. In particular, people who have autoimmune diabetes, Addison's disease, and thyroid eye disease are left with chronic and morbid conditions, manageable only to a certain extent. Thus far, the promises of the 1980s and 1990s from the emerging fields of molecular immunology and molecular genetics have failed (by any objective measure) to deliver improved healthcare for individuals who have autoimmune endocrinopathy. Nevertheless, the evidence-based approach to therapeutics and detailed evaluation of the outcome of existing treatment regimens have led to some advances in care delivery. Pragmatic reviews by leading international experts outline the clinical state of the art in several articles in this volume.

Work at numerous molecular laboratories has led to substantial leaps in our understanding of the basic mechanisms of autoimmune disease. Contributions to this knowledge have come from the study of the rare monogenic human autoimmune conditions, identification of disease loci in the genetically complex conditions, a detailed understanding of the structural biology of several of the key autoantigens, and an amazing capacity to replicate disease in genetically manipulated mouse models. With this background, I feel optimistic that the therapeutic paradigm is shifting and that we are in a strong position to deliver new treatments for autoimmunity in the next decade. I am particularly excited by the use of novel immunotherapeutic agents in type 1 diabetes and in Graves' disease (in man and in mouse), which are outlined within this volume. I hope the studies described (and to a substantial degree executed) by these pioneering clinical investigators represent the tip of the therapeutic iceberg, and that a flood of similar treatment regimens will mean that a revolution in autoimmune disease management is just around the corner. I know our patients have waited long enough.

Endocrinol Metab Clin N Am 38 (2009) xvii–xviii
doi:10.1016/j.ecl.2009.01.013
0889-8529/09/$ – see front matter © 2009 Published by Elsevier Inc.

**endo.theclinics.com**

This is the first bound volume to which I have contributed as an editor, and I wish to thank Derek LeRoith and Rachel Glover for their guidance on this project. I also thank my mentors in endocrinology, Pat Kendall Taylor and Raj Thakker; my parents (both physicians), as mentors in medicine and in life; and my wife and children for their constant support.

Simon H.S. Pearce, MD
Newcastle University
Institute of Human Genetics, International Centre for Life
Central Parkway
Newcastle upon Tyne, GB NE1 3BZ, UK

E-mail address:
s.h.s.pearce@ncl.ac.uk (S.H.S. Pearce)

# Regulatory T Cells: Key Players in Tolerance and Autoimmunity

Talal A. Chatila, MD, MSc

---

**KEYWORDS**

- Regulatory T cells • Foxp3 • Tolerance
- Autoimmunity • IPEX • CD25

---

Regulatory T ($T_R$) cells represent a distinct T-cell lineage that has a key role in tolerance to self-antigens and the prevention of autoimmune disease, as well as the inappropriate immune responses involved in allergic disease.[1–3] $T_R$ cells are characterized by a set of phenotypic and functional attributes that distinguish them from conventional T cells. They are predominantly $CD4^+CD25^+$, T-cell receptor (TCR) ab[+]. $T_R$ cells are anergic and do not produce interleukin-2 (IL-2).[4] When activated, they suppress the proliferation and cytokine production of conventional $CD4^+CD25^-$ T cells as well as that of $CD8^+$ T cells and established Th1 and Th2 cells.[5–8] $CD4^+CD25^+$ $T_R$ cells produce transforming growth factor beta (TGF-β) and IL-10, two cytokines endowed with immunosuppressive functions that have critical functions in $T_R$ cell biology.

Most peripheral $T_R$ cells are programmed in the thymus and are known as natural $T_R$ ($nT_R$) cells.[3] Other $T_R$ cells known as induced or adaptive ($iT_R$) cells are derived de novo from a naïve $CD4^+$ precursor pool in peripheral lymphoid tissues following antigenic stimulation in the presence of TGF-β and IL-2. Intense effort has gone into defining the molecular events that guide $T_R$ cells through development and lineage commitment, and those that enable the acquisition and maintenance of $T_R$ cell phenotypic and functional attributes. The recent advances made in elucidating those pathways are reviewed herein.

## FOXP3: A CRITICAL FACTOR FOR $T_R$ CELL STABILITY AND FUNCTION

Although $T_R$ cells are characterized by the expression of a distinctive combination of surface antigens including CD25, CTLA-4, and GITR, the cardinal hallmark of a $T_R$ cell

---

Work for this article was supported by National Institutes of Health grants R01AI065617 and R21AI80002.

Division of Immunology, Allergy and Rheumatology, Department of Pediatrics, The David Geffen School of Medicine, University of California, MDCC 12-430, 10833 Le Conte Avenue, Los Angeles, CA 90095-1752, USA

E-mail address: tchatila@mednet.ucla.edu

Endocrinol Metab Clin N Am 38 (2009) 265–272
doi:10.1016/j.ecl.2009.01.002
0889-8529/09/$ – see front matter
© 2009 Elsevier Inc. All rights reserved.

is the forkhead family transcription factor forkhead box p3 (Foxp3), which is indispensable to their suppressive activity, phenotype stability, and survival in the periphery.[3]

Foxp3 was initially thought to function as a transcriptional repressor[9]; however, it has become clear that it may function as either a transcriptional activator or repressor depending on the context.[10,11] The transcriptional functions of Foxp3 are enabled by the capacity of its different domains to interact with distinct sets of regulatory proteins to form large macromolecular transcriptional complexes. An N-terminal domain mediates transcriptional activation and repression; zinc finger and leucine zipper domains mediate homo- and hetero-oligomerization of Foxp3 with related members of the Foxp family; and a carboxyl terminal forkhead domain mediates binding to specific DNA response elements. Foxp3 also includes residues that contribute to the physical association of Foxp3 with other transcription factors, including the nuclear factor of activated T cells (NFAT) and Runx1/AMl1, both of which contribute to the transcriptional program and suppressive functions of $T_R$ cells.[12,13] An isoform of Foxp3 is expressed that lacks an N-terminal domain 33 amino acid peptide that is encoded by exon 2. This isoform is ineffective in conferring regulatory function upon expression in conventional T cells ($T_{conv}$).[14]

## $NT_R$ VERSUS $IT_R$ AND TR-1 CELLS

$Foxp3^+$ $T_R$ cells are unique among the effector T-cell subsets in that they are comprised of two developmentally distinct populations—$nT_R$ cells, which develop in the thymus, and adaptive or induced $iT_R$ cells, which are induced de novo in the periphery from $T_{conv}$ cells. The two populations display a close affinity in their regulatory function and phenotype but are not identical. The phenotypic and genetic attributes of $nT_R$ cells are "hard-wired," with most them persisting even in the absence of Foxp3. This persistence is a reflection of an irreversible commitment to the $T_R$ cell lineage that occurs in the course of thymic selection and maturation of $nT_R$ cells. In contrast, $iT_R$ cells are "plastic," developing upon antigenic stimulation of $T_{conv}$ cells in the presence of TGF-$\beta$ and IL-2 (**Fig. 1**).[15–18] Foxp3, whose expression in $iT_R$ cells is induced by the action of TGF-$\beta$ and T-cell receptor signaling, is required for the suppressive functions of $iT_R$ cells, similar to the situation of their $nT_R$ cell counterparts (D. Haribhai, T.A. Chatila, and C.B. Williams, unpublished observations, 2009). $iT_R$ cells have been demonstrated to develop during induction of oral tolerance to an allergen and may have an important role in tolerance induction in immunotherapy[19,20]; however, their phenotype is less stable than that of $nT_R$ cells. Whereas the Foxp3 locus is stably hypomethylated in $nT_R$ cells, it is weakly so in adaptive $iT_R$ cells.[21] The suppressive function and Foxp3 expression levels of the latter may accordingly decline over time.

In addition to the $Foxp3^+$ $iT_R$ cells, another class of $T_R$ cells is the $Foxp3^-IL-10^+$ T regulatory type 1 (Tr-1) cells, derived by the ex vivo activation of naïve $CD4^+$ T cells in the presence of IL-10 or by IL-10–conditioned dendritic cells.[22] Previous studies attempting to track these cells in vivo have been impeded by the lack of clear markers that could distinguish Tr-1 cells from $Foxp3^+$ $nT_R$ and $iT_R$ cells, which also express IL-10, especially after activation. Recent studies have overcome this limitation by using IL-10 locus-tagged mice, revealing $Foxp3^-$ Tr-1–like cells to be particularly abundant in the small and large intestine, where they have an essential role in down-regulating the inflammatory response triggered by the commensal flora.[23–25] $Foxp3^-$ Tr-1–like cells share with $Foxp3^+$ $iT_R$ cells a requirement for TGF-$\beta$ for their in vivo differentiation, but it remains unclear whether Tr-1 cells branch off from a common differentiation pathway with $Foxp3^+$ $iT_R$ cells or arise by a separate pathway. Whereas earlier studies

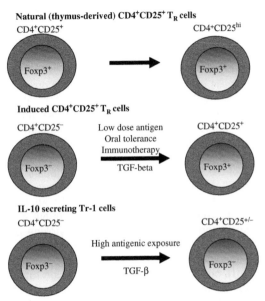

**Fig. 1.** Natural and induced $T_R$ cell populations. (*Upper panel*) Natural (thymic) CD4$^+$CD25$^+$ $T_R$ cells develop in the thymus and are exported to the periphery where they constitutively express Foxp3. (*Middle panel*) CD4$^+$CD25$^-$Foxp3$^-$ cells can be induced to differentiate into CD4$^+$CD25$^+$Foxp3$^+$ $T_R$ cells under special conditions, including low antigen exposure, oral tolerance, and immunotherapy. Induction in vitro can be achieved by stimulation in the presence of TGF-beta. (*Lower panel*) IL-10 secreting Tr-1 and related $T_R$ are Foxp3$^-$ and are induced in vivo in a TGF-beta–dependent manner, usually in the context of high antigenic exposure, such as in the gastrointestinal tract and in chronic infection.

have implicated Tr-1 in mucosal tolerance, the precise contributions of Foxp3$^+$ $T_R$ cells and Foxp3$^-$ Tr-1 cells to induced tolerance remains to be carefully analyzed with the newer analytical tools now available.

## BREAKDOWN OF TOLERANCE AND AUTOIMMUNITY DUE TO FOXP3 DEFICIENCY

Loss of function mutations in the gene for Foxp3 underlie the lymphoproliferative disease of the Scurfy mouse and the homologous autoimmune lymphoproliferative disorder in man, termed *immune dysregulation polyendocrinopathy enteropathy X-linked syndrome* (IPEX). In humans, loss of function *FOXP3* mutations result in the IPEX syndrome.[1,26] The hallmark of IPEX is immune dysregulation due to the lack of functional $T_R$ cells. It typically presents in a male infant with enteropathy, autoimmune endocrinopathy, immune-mediated cytopenias, and dermatitis. There is also allergic dysregulation that manifests in particular as food allergy, eosinophilia, and elevated IgE levels.[27,28] The autoimmune endocrinopathy is characterized by early onset type 1 diabetes, frequently beginning in the first year of life. Thyroiditis resulting in either hyper- or hypothyroidism is also common. Some of the allergic dysregulation in IPEX results from the presence in circulation of $T_R$ cell precursors that secrete large amounts of Th2 cytokines, especially IL-4, whereas it is tempting to speculate that the food allergy is a manifestation of $iT_R$ cell deficiency.[29–31] Foxp3 deficiency in mice, whether due to natural or induced mutations, gives rise to a fatal autoimmune and inflammatory disorder called Scurfy that has many of the features of IPEX.[32] In both mice and humans, female carriers are asymptomatic, consistent with X-linked recessive inheritance.

The immunopathology of Foxp3 deficiency results from unchecked T-cell activation due to the lack of regulatory restraint by CD4$^+$CD25$^+$ T$_R$ cells.[33,34] The fact that Foxp3 is essential for T$_R$ cell function is supported by the observation that forced expression of Foxp3 in effector T cells endows them with regulatory properties and some, but not all, of the phenotypic markers of regulatory T cells.[35,36] Also, adoptive transfer of CD4$^+$CD25$^+$ T$_R$ cells rescues Scurfy mice from disease, and Foxp3-transduced CD4$^+$CD25$^-$ T cells suppress wasting and colitis induced by the transfer of CD4$^+$CD25$^-$ T cells into RAG-deficient mice.[35,37]

Foxp3 deficiency is permissive to the development in the thymus of T$_R$ cell precursors that share many of the phenotypic and genetic attributes of T$_R$ cells; however, unlike Foxp3-sufficient T$_R$ cells, Foxp3-deficient T$_R$ cell precursors fail to mediate suppression.[29,31] Once in the periphery, they acquire the attributes of an activated cytotoxic cell phenotype. They express high levels of mRNA encoding granzymes, some killer cell markers, and a mixed Th1 and Th2 cytokine profile. In particular, they secrete large amounts of IL-4 and other Th2 cytokines, which may account for much of the allergic dysregulation associated with Foxp3 deficiency.[27,29,31] Circulating Foxp3-deficient T$_R$ cell precursors also exhibit a high rate of apoptotic death, possibly due to suboptimal responses to growth factors such as IL-2. The continued requirement for Foxp3 expression to maintain the phenotype of mature T$_R$ cells in the periphery was demonstrated in experiments in which the acute inactivation of the locus for Foxp3 rapidly led to the loss of T$_R$ cell regulatory function. Acute Foxp3 deficiency also alters the transcriptional program of T$_R$ cells in a manner reminiscent of Foxp3-deficient T$_R$ cell precursors.[38]

## OTHER HERITABLE DISORDERS OF T$_R$ CELLS

IPEX-like syndromes in humans and mice also arise from mutations along the IL-2 signaling pathway, including loss of function mutations in the IL-2 receptor alpha chain (CD25) and the IL-2–responsive transcription factor STAT5b, the latter with an associated phenotype of resistance to growth hormone.[39–41] CD25 deficiency has been associated with early onset of type 1 diabetes in humans, consistent with the phenotype observed in IPEX syndrome due to Foxp3 mutations. More broadly, the CD25 and IL-2 gene loci have been associated with type 1 diabetes in humans (see the article by authors elsewhere in this issue) and mice, respectively, indicating the essential function of this pathway in maintaining tolerance to islet beta cells (**Fig. 2**).[42,43]

## T$_R$ CELL–DIRECTED THERAPIES IN AUTOIMMUNITY

Manipulation of T$_R$ cells is an attractive strategy for immunotherapy, as suggested by adoptive transfer of T$_R$ cells to treat experimental autoimmune diseases.[44,45] Similar treatment strategies are being developed in humans, in whom it is envisaged that cellular therapy with antigen-specific T$_R$ cells may allow the development of long-term immune modulation without the problem of general immunosuppression and systemic toxicity.[46,47] Other approaches include the derivation for therapeutic use of human cell lines that stably express ectopic Foxp3, which converts both naïve and antigen-specific memory CD4$^+$ T cells into cells with T$_R$ cell–like properties.[48] T$_R$ cell therapy may also be rendered more effective by combining it with immunomodulatory drugs that spare T$_R$ cells while targeting conventional T cells. One such drug is rapamycin, an inhibitor of the mTor pathway, which has an important role in T-cell proliferation and survival. The mTor pathway is relatively inactive in T$_R$ cells, which

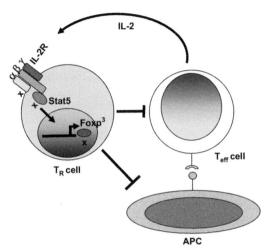

**Fig. 2.** Genetic lesions resulting in $T_R$ cell deficiency/dysfunction and autoimmunity. Activation of effector T ($T_{eff}$) cells by antigen-presenting cells (APC) triggers $T_{eff}$ cell activation and IL-2 production. Signaling by the IL-2/IL-2 receptor (IL-2R)/STAT5 pathway is essential for the competency of $T_R$ cells and helps maintain high level expression of Foxp3. It enables the suppression by $T_R$ cells of both APC and $T_{eff}$ cell function. X denotes genetic defects associated with IPEX (Foxp3) and IPEX-like syndromes (IL-2Ra chain and STAT5b).

employ an alternative IL-2 receptor-coupled STAT5 pathway to mediate cell growth and proliferation.[49,50] A second approach is to use histone deacetylase inhibitors, which promote the development of Foxp3$^+$ i$T_R$ cells.[51]

## SUMMARY

Impressive progress has been made in elucidating molecular mechanisms underlying $T_R$ cell development and differentiation. The stage is now set to tackle some important outstanding issues in the field. These issues include the nature of the molecular circuitry governing the early development of n$T_R$ cells in the thymus, the mechanisms underlying suppressive function of $T_R$ cells, the respective roles of n$T_R$ and i$T_R$ cells in dominant tolerance, and the nature of the molecular pathways mediating their nonredundant functions. The striking allergic dysregulation and food allergy associated with the IPEX syndrome indicates a fundamental role for $T_R$ cells in tolerance to allergens, especially foods. Pharmacologic interventions that aim to bolster $T_R$ cell development and function, alone or together with immunotherapy, offer the potential for novel therapeutic strategies in the treatment of allergic and autoimmune diseases.

## REFERENCES

1. Chatila TA. Role of regulatory T cells in human diseases. J Allergy Clin Immunol 2005;116:949–59.
2. Bacchetta R, Gambineri E, Roncarolo MG. Role of regulatory T cells and FOXP3 in human diseases. J Allergy Clin Immunol 2007;120:227–35.
3. Zheng Y, Rudensky AY. Foxp3 in control of the regulatory T cell lineage. Nat Immunol 2007;8:457–62.
4. Shevach EM. CD4$^+$CD25$^+$ suppressor T cells: more questions than answers. Nat Rev Immunol 2002;2:389–400.

5. Thornton AM, Shevach EM. CD4+CD25+ immunoregulatory T cells suppress polyclonal T cell activation in vitro by inhibiting interleukin 2 production. J Exp Med 1998;188:287–96.

6. Xu D, Liu H, Komai-Koma M, et al. CD4+CD25+ regulatory T cells suppress differentiation and functions of Th1 and Th2 cells, *Leishmania major* infection, and colitis in mice. J Immunol 2003;170:394–9.

7. Stassen M, Jonuleit H, Muller C, et al. Differential regulatory capacity of CD25+ T regulatory cells and preactivated CD25+ T regulatory cells on development, functional activation, and proliferation of Th2 cells. J Immunol 2004;173:267–74.

8. Suvas S, Kumaraguru U, Pack CD, et al. CD4+CD25+ T cells regulate virus-specific primary and memory CD8+ T cell responses. J Exp Med 2003;198:889–901.

9. Schubert LA, Jeffery E, Zhang Y, et al. Scurfin (FOXP3) acts as a repressor of transcription and regulates T cell activation. J Biol Chem 2001;276:37672–9.

10. Marson A, Kretschmer K, Frampton GM, et al. Foxp3 occupancy and regulation of key target genes during T-cell stimulation. Nature 2007;445:931–5.

11. Zheng Y, Josefowicz SZ, Kas A, et al. Genome-wide analysis of Foxp3 target genes in developing and mature regulatory T cells. Nature 2007;445:936–40.

12. Ono M, Yaguchi H, Ohkura N, et al. Foxp3 controls regulatory T-cell function by interacting with AML1/Runx1. Nature 2007;446:685–9.

13. Wu Y, Borde M, Heissmeyer V, et al. FOXP3 controls regulatory T cell function through cooperation with NFAT. Cell 2006;126:375–87.

14. Allan SE, Passerini L, Bacchetta R, et al. The role of 2 FOXP3 isoforms in the generation of human CD4+ Tregs. J Clin Invest 2005;115:3276–84.

15. Chen W, Jin W, Hardegen N, et al. Conversion of peripheral CD4+CD25− naive T cells to CD4+CD25+ regulatory T cells by TGF-beta induction of transcription factor Foxp3. J Exp Med 2003;198:1875–86.

16. Fantini MC, Becker C, Monteleone G, et al. Cutting edge: TGF-beta induces a regulatory phenotype in CD4+CD25− T cells through Foxp3 induction and down-regulation of Smad7. J Immunol 2004;172:5149–53.

17. Zheng SG, Wang J, Wang P, et al. IL-2 is essential for TGF-beta to convert naive CD4+CD25− cells to CD25+Foxp3+ regulatory T cells and for expansion of these cells. J Immunol 2007;178:2018–27.

18. Davidson TS, DiPaolo RJ, Andersson J, et al. Cutting edge: IL-2 is essential for TGF-beta-mediated induction of Foxp3+ T regulatory cells. J Immunol 2007; 178:4022–6.

19. Mucida D, Kutchukhidze N, Erazo A, et al. Oral tolerance in the absence of naturally occurring Tregs. J Clin Invest 2005;115:1923–33.

20. Apostolou I, von Boehmer H. In vivo instruction of suppressor commitment in naive T cells. J Exp Med 2004;199:1401–8.

21. Floess S, Freyer J, Siewert C, et al. Epigenetic control of the Foxp3 locus in regulatory T cells. PLoS Biol 2007;5:e38.

22. O'Garra A, Vieira PL, Vieira P, et al. IL-10-producing and naturally occurring CD4+ Tregs: limiting collateral damage. J Clin Invest 2004;114:1372–8.

23. Calado DP, Paixao T, Holmberg D, et al. Stochastic monoallelic expression of IL-10 in T cells. J Immunol 2006;177:5358–64.

24. Kamanaka M, Kim ST, Wan YY, et al. Expression of interleukin-10 in intestinal lymphocytes detected by an interleukin-10 reporter knockin tiger mouse. Immunity 2006;25:941–52.

25. Maynard CL, Harrington LE, Janowski KM, et al. Regulatory T cells expressing interleukin 10 develop from Foxp3+ and Foxp3− precursor cells in the absence of interleukin 10. Nat Immunol 2007;8:931–41.

26. Torgerson TR, Ochs HD. Immune dysregulation, polyendocrinopathy, enteropathy, X-linked: forkhead box protein 3 mutations and lack of regulatory T cells. J Allergy Clin Immunol 2007;120:744–50.
27. Chatila TA, Blaeser F, Ho N, et al. JM2, encoding a forkhead-related protein, is mutated in X-linked autoimmunity-allergic dysregulation syndrome. J Clin Invest 2000;106:R75–81.
28. Torgerson TR, Linane A, Moes N, et al. Severe food allergy as a variant of IPEX syndrome caused by a deletion in a noncoding region of the FOXP3 gene. Gastroenterology 2007;132:1705–17.
29. Gavin MA, Rasmussen JP, Fontenot JD, et al. Foxp3-dependent programme of regulatory T-cell differentiation. Nature 2007;445:771–5.
30. Gavin MA, Torgerson TR, Houston E, et al. Single-cell analysis of normal and FOXP3-mutant human T cells: FOXP3 expression without regulatory T cell development. Proc Natl Acad Sci U S A 2006;103:6659–64.
31. Lin W, Haribhai D, Relland LM, et al. Regulatory T cell development in the absence of functional Foxp3. Nat Immunol 2007;8:359–68.
32. Lin W, Truong N, Grossman WJ, et al. Allergic dysregulation and hyperimmunoglobulinemia E in Foxp3 mutant mice. J Allergy Clin Immunol 2005;116:1106–15.
33. Clark LB, Appleby MW, Brunkow ME, et al. Cellular and molecular characterization of the scurfy mouse mutant. J Immunol 1999;162:2546–54.
34. Blair PJ, Bultman SJ, Haas JC, et al. CD4$^+$CD8$^-$ T cells are the effector cells in disease pathogenesis in the scurfy (sf) mouse. J Immunol 1994;153:3764–74.
35. Fontenot JD, Gavin MA, Rudensky AY. Foxp3 programs the development and function of CD4$^+$CD25$^+$ regulatory T cells. Nat Immunol 2003;4:330–6.
36. Hori S, Nomura T, Sakaguchi S. Control of regulatory T cell development by the transcription factor Foxp3. Science 2003;299:1057–61.
37. Khattri R, Cox T, Yasayko SA, et al. An essential role for Scurfin in CD4$^+$CD25$^+$ T regulatory cells. Nat Immunol 2003;4:337–42.
38. Williams LM, Rudensky AY. Maintenance of the Foxp3-dependent developmental program in mature regulatory T cells requires continued expression of Foxp3. Nat Immunol 2007;8:277–84.
39. Caudy AA, Reddy ST, Chatila T, et al. CD25 deficiency causes an immune dysregulation, polyendocrinopathy, enteropathy, X-linked-like syndrome, and defective IL-10 expression from CD4 lymphocytes. J Allergy Clin Immunol 2007;119:482–7.
40. Cohen AC, Nadeau KC, Tu W, et al. Cutting edge: decreased accumulation and regulatory function of CD4$^+$CD25$^{high}$ T cells in human STAT5b deficiency. J Immunol 2006;177:2770–4.
41. Malek TR. The biology of interleukin-2. Annu Rev Immunol 2008;26:453–79.
42. Vella A, Cooper JD, Lowe CE, et al. Localization of a type 1 diabetes locus in the IL2RA/CD25 region by use of tag single-nucleotide polymorphisms. Am J Hum Genet 2005;76:773–9.
43. Yamanouchi J, Rainbow D, Serra P, et al. Interleukin-2 gene variation impairs regulatory T cell function and causes autoimmunity. Nat Genet 2007;39:329–37.
44. Wing K, Fehervari Z, Sakaguchi S. Emerging possibilities in the development and function of regulatory T cells. Int Immunol 2006;18:991–1000.
45. Verbsky JW. Therapeutic use of T regulatory cells. Curr Opin Rheumatol 2007;19:252–8.
46. Roncarolo MG, Battaglia M. Regulatory T-cell immunotherapy for tolerance to self antigens and alloantigens in humans. Nat Rev Immunol 2007;7:585–98.
47. Tang Q, Bluestone JA. Regulatory T-cell physiology and application to treat autoimmunity. Immunol Rev 2006;212:217–37.

48. Allan SE, Alstad AN, Merindol N, et al. Generation of potent and stable human CD4(+) T regulatory cells by activation-independent expression of FOXP3. Mol Ther 2008;16:194–202.
49. Battaglia M, Stabilini A, Roncarolo MG. Rapamycin selectively expands CD4$^+$CD25$^+$Foxp3$^+$ regulatory T cells. Blood 2005;105:4743–8.
50. Zeiser R, Leveson-Gower DB, Zambricki EA, et al. Differential impact of mTOR inhibition on CD4$^+$CD25$^+$Foxp3$^+$ regulatory T cells as compared to conventional CD4$^+$ T cells. Blood 2008;111:453–63.
51. Tao R, de Zoeten EF, Ozkaynak E, et al. Deacetylase inhibition promotes the generation and function of regulatory T cells. Nat Med 2007;13:1299–307.

# Clearing the AIRE: On the Pathophysiological Basis of the Autoimmune Polyendocrinopathy Syndrome Type-1

Noriko Shikama, PhD, Gretel Nusspaumer, PhD,
Georg A. Holländer, MD*

**KEYWORDS**

- APS-1 • AIRE • Autoimmunity • Negative selection
- Transcription • Tissue-restricted antigens

*"Our air[e] up here is good for the disease - I mean good against the disease… but it is also good for the disease." Slightly adapted from "The Magic Mountain" by Thomas Mann, 1924*

Autoimmunity is caused by an inappropriate immune response directed against self-components of the host. This aberrant reactivity typically results in tissue damage, which leads to partial or complete loss of organ function. Although each individual autoimmune disease is relatively rare, combined, the diseases affect 1 in 20 individuals in developed countries,[1] where they cause a third of all premature deaths among people of working age. The current list of autoimmune disorders contains more than 80 distinct disease entities that vary in phenotype, age of first clinical presentation, gender distribution, and natural course.[2] This enormous clinical diversity reflects the complex molecular and cellular mechanisms responsible for the establishment and maintenance of immunologic tolerance. Consequently, autoimmunity implies a failure of the regulatory mechanisms that normally prevent such destructive responses.

This work was supported by the Swiss National Foundation grant 3100-68310.02, by a grant from European Community 6th Framework Program Euro-Thymaide and Euraps, by NIH grant ROI-A1057477-01. Noriko Shikama and Gretel Nusspaumer contributed equally to this article.

Laboratory of Pediatric Immunology, Department of Biomedicine, University of Basel and The University Children's Hospital (UKBB), Mattenstrasse 28, 4058 Basel, Switzerland
* Corresponding author.
*E-mail address:* georg-a.hollaender@unibas.ch (G.A. Holländer).

Endocrinol Metab Clin N Am 38 (2009) 273–288
doi:10.1016/j.ecl.2009.01.011
0889-8529/09/$ – see front matter © 2009 Elsevier Inc. All rights reserved.

endo.theclinics.com

Breakdown of immunologic tolerance seems to be the result of a complex interplay between genetic polymorphisms that predispose an individual to develop common autoimmune disorders and several environmental factors, such as hormones, infections, and therapeutic agents.[3] Although many of these genetic and environmental influences highlight a central role of T cells, the precise molecular underpinning that allows autoimmunity to occur is still largely unknown. In contrast to autoimmune diseases determined by multiple genes, monogenic defects that cause autoimmunity are rare "experiments of nature" but provide a unique opportunity to dissect in detail the pathogenic mechanisms. In this context, autoimmune polyendocrine syndrome type-1 (APS-1) constitutes a particularly informative example of a monogenic autoimmune disease.[4–6] Caused by mutations in the gene that encodes for the autoimmune regulator protein (*AIRE*), APS-1 has provided a novel understanding of how the thymus gains the ability to express nonthymic self-antigens required for the deletion of developing T cells with an autoreactive specificity. In the absence of functional *AIRE*, the thymus fails to express a normal repertoire of up to several thousand peripheral (ie, nonthymic) tissue antigens, which consequently results in the maturation and export of autoreactive T cells.[7–9] This article summarizes the unique role of *AIRE* in thymic function and the pathogenesis of APS-1.

## CLINICAL PRESENTATION OF AUTOIMMUNE POLYENDOCRINE SYNDROME TYPE-1

The typical clinical presentation of APS-1 (also known as autoimmune polyendocrinopathy-candidiasis-ectodermal dystrophy [APECED]; online mendelian inheritance in man [OMIM] #240,300) was first described in 1946.[10] APS-1 is characterized by severe autoimmunity to different endocrine organs and chronic candidiasis, both of which become clinically apparent in the pediatric age group. As a rare autosomal recessive disorder, the general incidence of APS-1 is not easily determined because the syndrome is infrequent in certain countries (such as the United States) but displays a high prevalence in specific ethnic populations. For example, a high frequency of APS-1 has been observed among Finns (1:25,000), Sardinians (1:14,400), and Iranian Jews (1:9000).[5] The female to male ratio of patients affected by APS-1 reveals a slight female preponderance.[11]

The clinical diagnosis of APS-1 is based on the presence of at least two of the three major clinical manifestations: chronic mucocutaneous candidiasis, primary hypoparathyroidism, and primary adrenocortical insufficiency (Addison's disease) (see the article by Owen and Cheetham elsewhere in this issue). For most ethnic populations (with the notable exception of Iranian Jews), *Candida albicans* infections are the most common pathology of APS-1.[4,12] This type of fungal disease typically affects the skin, the nails, and the oral, esophageal, and vaginal mucosa and ranges from local to widespread severe infections. Because patients who have APS-1 generate a normal humoral immune response to *Candida* antigens, they are spared from disseminated candidiasis. T cells from individuals who have APS-1 display a selective deficiency in their response to *Candida* antigens that confers an increased susceptibility to this pathogen.

Hypoparathyroidism is typically the first endocrine disease to occur. It manifests in children at an average age of 8 years and affects as many as 90% of patients who have APS-1.[11] NALP5 seems to be a parathyroid-specific autoantigen (see the article by Brown elsewhere in this issue).[13] The detection of antibodies against this autoantigen seems to be diagnostic for hypoparathyroidism in the context of APS-1. Adrenocortical insufficiency is usually the third disease to appear, and it affects 60% to 100% of patients who have APS-1, with an average age at onset of 12 years.[11] Antibodies against steroid 21-hydroxylase, steroid 17a-hydroxylase, and P450 side-chain cleavage can be detected in patients who have APS-1 with adrenocortical insufficiency.[5,14,15] Autoimmune endocrinopathies other than the aforementioned are also recognized in patients who have APS-1, including (with decreasing frequency) premature ovarian failure, type 1 diabetes mellitus, primary testicular failure, autoimmune thyroiditis, and hypophysitis.[5,16]

Autoimmune-mediated pathologies of the gastrointestinal tract feature prominently in patients who have APS-1: pernicious anemia, hepatitis, chronic atrophic gastritis, and constipation or diarrhea that may be linked to the destruction of gastrointestinal endocrine cells.[5] Malabsorption occurs in a third to a quarter of all patients who have APS-1 and seems to be related to pancreatic insufficiency, villous atrophy, and bacterial overgrowth. The ectodermal manifestations of the syndrome include dental enamel hypoplasia, keratopathy, vitiligo, alopecia, nail pitting, and tympanic membrane calcification.[5]

Finally, hyposplenism/asplenism occurs relatively frequently in patients who have APS-1 and may be caused by a progressive autoimmune-mediated destruction or vascular insult involving the spleen.[5] The consequent loss of splenic function may constitute a potentially life-threatening complication because the immune response to encapsulated bacteria may be compromised in these patients. Children may present initially with a minor clinical manifestation (eg, malabsorption) before a single major feature of APS-1 (typically chronic mucocutaneous candidiasis) becomes apparent and eventually the full clinical picture evolves.[17]

The remarkably diverse phenotype of APS-1 and the striking clinical variation even between siblings with an identical mutation in the *AIRE* gene cannot be explained easily by a defective *AIRE* function alone.[18] It is likely that other loci, such as the major histocompatibility antigens (major histocompatibility complex and human leukocyte antigen) may, in addition to environmental factors, modify the monogenic trait of APS-1.[19,20] The same human leukocyte antigen haplotypes that are associated in patients who have APS-1 and Addison's disease, alopecia, and diabetes are also preferentially found in patients who do not have APS-1 and suffer from these disorders.[21] The possibility that disease-modifying genes change target organ involvement and affect disease severity is further suggested by observations in *AIRE*-deficient (knockout) mice, in which the genetic background influences the phenotype.[22,23] Linkage studies in humans have not yet been performed to identify novel modifier loci, however, but there is expectation that they may be identical to genes involved in the polygenic development of other, more common immune diseases.[24,25]

**THE AIRE GENE**

*AIRE*, as the molecular cause of APS-1, was identified in 1997 by two separate groups using positional cloning in Finnish patients who had APS-1 and their families, taking advantage of the high frequency of the disease in this population.[26,27] The gene maps to human chromosome 21q22.3, identifying a locus relevant for autoimmunity that lies outside the human leukocyte antigen region on chromosome 6. The direct molecular control of *AIRE* transcription remains elusive, although several binding sites for known transcription factors have been mapped to the *AIRE* promoter.[28] The *AIRE* gene is approximately 13 kb in length, is composed of 14 exons, and encodes for a polypeptide of 545 amino acids, which may have several isoforms because of alternative splicing. The AIRE protein displays several predicted and elsewhere functionally characterized domains that are typical for chromatin-associated transcriptional regulators (**Fig. 1**).[9,26,27,29] The homogeneously staining region at the amino-terminal end

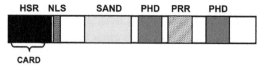

**Fig. 1.** Schematic representation of the human AIRE protein structure. HSR, homogeneously staining region at amino acids 1–106; CARD, caspase recruitment domain at amino acids 8–96; NLS, nuclear localization signal at amino acids 113–133; SAND domain (named after Sp100, AIRE, NucP41/75, DEAF-1) at amino acids 181–280; PHD, plant homeodomain type zinc-finger at amino acids 299–340 and 434–475; PRR, proline-rich region at amino acids 350–407.

of the molecule is a domain required for the homomultimerization. Within this sequence, a previously undescribed caspase recruitment domain recently was localized that is needed for the transactivation activity of *AIRE*.[30]

The SAND domain, which in other proteins confers DNA binding activity, constitutes an additional, previously defined motif.[31,32] In comparison to other transcription factors, the critical DNA interacting residues within the SAND domain are altered in *AIRE*, questioning the precise role of this sequence for the molecule's function.[32] *AIRE* also contains two plant homeodomain (PHD) zinc-finger motifs that are located in the middle of the molecule and toward its carboxy-terminal end. PHD domains are restricted to nuclear transcriptional regulators, including coactivators and chromatin-modeling proteins of the polycomb and trithorax groups.[33] In addition to the contested E3 ubiquitin ligase activity,[34,35] the first PHD domain has been shown to preferably bind to histone H3 that is unmethylated at lysine 4 (H3K4me0), which suggests a role for *AIRE* in chromatin remodeling (see later discussion).[36]

Specific E3 ligases have been shown to function as key regulators of immune tolerance, however, and mutations to E3 ligases can lead to the development of autoimmune disease.[37] The two PHD domains are separated by a proline-rich region that may, by analogy to other proteins, be involved in protein-protein interactions. Independent of these structural features, the functional characteristics of *AIRE* suggest that it acts in a different fashion from sequence-specific transcription factors. *AIRE* influences the expression of a significant fraction of the total genome (see later discussion), which renders it unlikely that *AIRE* binds directly to the promoter or enhancer regions of coordinately regulated genes. *AIRE* mutations in patients who have APS-1 are often of limited value in identifying the function of specific domains, because the observed mutations commonly result in truncated proteins or no protein at all.[9,38,39] The similarities with other proteins that contain a PHD or a SAND domain (eg, the SP100 family of transcriptional coactivators) suggest a role for *AIRE* in chromatin-dependent transcriptional regulation, possibly by modifying the nuclear sublocalization of chromosomal regions.

The *AIRE* mutations in patients who have APS-1 mainly cluster in three regions that display a high degree of evolutionary conservation. Approximately two thirds are confined to homogeneously staining region, and most of the remaining mutations are preferentially situated in the SAND domain and in the first PHD domain.[9,40] Specific mutations vary among the different ethnicities and occasionally can identify a homogeneous population by revealing a potential founder effect. Only one defective allele has been noted in as many as 9% of patients in a larger APS-1 cohort, which may be because of the generation of a dominant interfering form of the *AIRE* protein.[9,41] A mutation in the SAND domain that acts as a dominant negative form of *AIRE* and impairs the access of the wild-type molecule to sites of transcription has been described.[42] Six percent of patients who have APS-1 do not carry mutations in the open reading frame of the *AIRE* gene,[4] which suggests that mutations in the noncoding region may affect *AIRE* expression (eg, secondary to RNA instability). Alternatively, a mutation in a gene other than *AIRE* may produce a defect that phenocopies the loss of *AIRE* expression, because such a gene product could interact with *AIRE* to affect target gene expression.

## THE THYMIC EXPRESSION OF AIRE

*AIRE* is primarily expressed by medullary thymic epithelial cells (mTECs) positioned at the corticomedullary junction and in the depths of the medulla.[43–46] TECs constitute the most abundant cell type within the thymic stroma and are indispensable for T-cell differentiation and selection.[47] The *AIRE*-positive mTEC typically represent postmitotic cells that display the characteristic features of competent antigen-presenting cells (eg, the expression of MHC class II, CD40, CD80, PD-L1).[46,48,49] *AIRE* is detected in these cells as punctate structures in the nucleus. This spatial organization and *AIRE*'s interaction with different nuclear proteins, including the global transcription cofactor CBP (histone acetyltransferase, cyclic AMP-response element binding protein-binding protein)[29,50] suggest that *AIRE* may regulate gene expression by recruiting components of the transcription complex to specific regions of the genome via interactions with the nuclear matrix.[51,52] The observation that RANK-mediated activation of the NF-kB2 pathway in mTEC induces *AIRE* expression and the translocation and nuclear accumulation of CBP also can be taken as circumstantial evidence for a model in which *AIRE* cooperates with other transcription factors to effect gene transcription.[30]

The ability of mTEC to express a broad range of antigens (including antigens from extrathymic tissues; see later discussion) has been explained by two different models. The "terminal differentiation" model proposes that the capacity to express tissue restricted-antigens (TRA) is achieved with the maturation to a postmitotic, mature cell stage,[53] whereas the "developmental model" asserts that immature mTECs are still multipotent and use several transcriptional programs in parallel to allow expression of a broad array of antigens.[54] In the first model, *AIRE* becomes transcriptionally active as mTECs differentiate, whereas in the second model *AIRE* is expected to affect thymic epithelial cell differentiation. The data from studies identifying prospective *AIRE*-positive mTEC using specific cell surface markers[48] and from investigations demonstrating a low proliferative activity of *AIRE*-positive mTEC[49] currently favor the "terminal differentiation" model, although further studies are still required to fully resolve this issue.

## THE ROLE OF AIRE IN THYMIC FUNCTION

The thymus achieves two interrelated functions essential for the adaptive immune system: the life-long generation of new T cells and the production of T cells that express an antigen receptor repertoire tolerant to harmless self-antigens but reactive to injurious foreign antigens. Because the repertoire of T-cell antigen receptor (TCR) specificities is randomly generated during development, immature thymocytes have to pass a checkpoint at which the chosen TCR is scrutinized for its utility. This process has been termed "negative thymic selection," and it strives to prevent potentially harmful (ie, autoreactive) T cells from further differentiation, should they recognize their cognate antigen with high avidity. Mature mTECs (and bone marrow derived dendritic cells and macrophages) have been recognized in their capacity as potent antigen-presenting cells to effect negative selection within the thymic microenvironment.[7,55] An important prerequisite for negative thymic selection by mTECs is their ability to express and present a broad array of self-antigens.[7] This range of antigens should represent not only ubiquitously expressed proteins but also antigens from most, if not all, of the peripheral tissues. mTEC function is challenged with the extraordinary task of displaying a collection of self-peptides that mirrors the spectrum of antigens usually present only elsewhere in the body.

The thymic expression of TRA is undeniably a physiologic property of mTEC that only recently was fully recognized. **Table 1** provides a list of TRA that previously were identified as targets in APS-1 and other autoimmune disorders. Termed "promiscuous gene expression," the capacity to express TRA is highly conserved between mice and humans,[56] and it displays several features that render it distinct from the control of cell lineage–specific gene expression.[7] The promiscuously expressed genes tend to localize in the genome in clusters[56–58] and are expressed in mTEC at lower concentrations when compared with the corresponding peripheral tissues.[45,59] Typically, TRA expression neither complies with the temporal regulation observed in the pre- and postnatal development of particular cell lineages nor follows a gender-specific expression pattern.[7,58] These special features allow the TCR repertoire to be shaped in a fashion that is independent of time-controlled developmental changes in gene expression, such as those observed with the onset of puberty.

The availability of a mouse model of APS-1 has greatly facilitated the recognition of the role of *AIRE* in the context of TRA expression and negative thymic selection (**Fig. 2**). *AIRE* knockout mice display several autoimmune manifestations that mimic the features of human APS-1, including mononuclear cell infiltrations of several organs and the presence of autoantibodies directed against different tissues.[60–62] The number of organs affected and the degree of autoimmunity depend on the genetic background of the mouse strain but increase with age.[22,23] This observation relates to the accumulating evidence that subtle variations in the intrathymic expression levels of self-antigen affect the threshold of central tolerance.[7,45] Microarray-based gene expression analysis that compares the transcriptome of mTEC isolated from either *AIRE*-deficient or wild-type mice identified a large number of genes whose expression is clearly *AIRE* dependent because their transcripts are either missing or markedly decreased in the mutant.[57,58,60] Although it would be interesting to detail the gene expression profile in mTECs of patients who have APS-1, such data are currently not available, and insights into *AIRE*-dependent TRA expression in human have to be extrapolated from the mouse model and the profile of autoantibodies directed at tissues targeted in patients who have APS-1.[5,11]

Consistent with a role of *AIRE* in controlling the expression of some TRA are observations in experimental systems demonstrating that the overexpression of *AIRE* in vitro results in an increase in promiscuous gene expression.[30,63] Conversely, TRA transcription cannot be detected under conditions in which a mutant form of *AIRE* is expressed that unfolds its amino-terminal caspase recruitment domain and consequently loses its transactivation potential secondary to the probable disruption of protein-protein interactions.[30] Not all TRA are under the transcriptional control of *AIRE*, however, which suggests that factors other than *AIRE* contribute also to promiscuous gene expression.[57,58,60]

Despite several features in common with other nuclear proteins and transcription factors, the molecular mechanisms by which *AIRE* promotes the expression of TRA remain unclear but may include transcriptional regulation via epigenetic modifications.[7,58] Posttranslational modifications, including the methylation, acetylation, and phosphorylation of histone tails (known as histone code or histone marks), are crucial for regulating chromatin structure, gene transcription, and the epigenetic state of the cell.[64] For instance, methylation at lysine 4 of histone H3 (H3K4me) marks a site of active transcription. Recent studies demonstrated that *AIRE* preferentially binds to histone H3 unmethylated at lysine 4 (H3K4me0) in the nucleosomal context.[36] In view of this binding specificity, a novel model was proposed as to how *AIRE* may control TRA expression. In this context, TRA promoters contain high levels of H3K4me0 to which *AIRE* binds once it is expressed in mature mTECs. This interaction of *AIRE* with H3K4me0 is then believed to recruit transcription factors such as CBP to the TRA promoters.[36,50,65,66] As a result, these genes are transcriptionally de-repressed and promiscuous gene expression is initiated. Aberrant thymic negative selection caused by the absence of *AIRE* is credited with the continued repression of TRA. Although this model is attractive for explaining *AIRE*'s function at a molecular level, it needs further experimental validation.

Direct evidence for a decisive role of AIRE in negative thymic selection has come from experimental models in which TCR transgenic mice express the cognate antigen in an *AIRE*-dependent fashion.[45,67] Under these and comparable conditions,[68] a direct gene dosage effect between the level of antigen expression, the degree of autoreactive T-cell deletion, and the incidence of autoimmunity has been observed, which underscores the need for a precise regulation of TRA required for the induction and maintenance of thymic tolerance.

In addition to its role in promiscuous gene expression, *AIRE* also seems to directly regulate genes that are important for other thymic epithelial cell functions, including the expression of transcription factors, chemokines, and proteins involved in peptide processing and presentation.[69,70] The lack of *AIRE* expression in mature mTECs of patients who have APS-1 may be associated with alterations in the phenotype and architectural organization of these cells (T. Barthlott, PhD, and G.A. Holländer, MD, unpublished data, 2006),[71] although subtle changes in the thymic microenvironment were observed in some but not other studies.[60–62]

Negative thymic selection is not entirely efficient and inadvertently permits the emigration of some autoreactive T cells with low affinity TCRs for self-antigens. To avoid the occurrence of autoimmunity, additional mechanisms are in place to secure the induction and maintenance of self-tolerance within the thymus and the periphery. One of these mechanisms is the thymic generation of regulatory T cells ($T_{reg}$), a specialized subpopulation of cells that controls self-reactive T cells and maintains immune system homeostasis and tolerance to self-antigens (see the article by Chatila elsewhere in this issue).[72] Paradoxically, the positive selection of $T_{reg}$ requires a high affinity interaction of their TCR with the corresponding ligand expressed by thymic stromal cells.[73] In this context it is noteworthy that mTECs have been demonstrated to induce or facilitate the production TRA-specific $T_{reg}$,[74] although other intrathymic stromal cells, such as thymic dendritic cells and cortical TECs, have been shown to select $T_{reg}$.[75,76] Engaging an ostensibly common pathway, the generation of $T_{reg}$ also depends on the expression of the costimulatory molecule CD40, which is typically expressed on the cell surface of mature mTECs and dendritic cells.[77] Because the signals required to yield $T_{reg}$ are seemingly uncoupled from a specific thymic cell source, the relative contribution of TECs and dendritic cells in fostering the generation of $T_{reg}$ needs to be resolved.

Several observations have questioned but not completely excluded a role of *AIRE* in the positive selection of $T_{reg}$, however. In fact, the absolute number, relative frequency, and suppressive function of $T_{reg}$ are unaffected in *AIRE* deficient mice, and experiments that engrafted *AIRE*-deficient and wild-ype thymic tissue into the same mouse demonstrated that these recipients still develop autoimmunity.[62,69] Besides, mice rendered double-deficient for *AIRE* and *Foxp3* (the transcription factor

**Table 1**
Thymic expression of autoantigens relevant to autoimmune polyendocrine syndrome type-1 and other known autoimmune diseases

| | Autoantigen | Organ | Disease | Thymic Expression | AIRE Dependent Expression[a] | Reference |
|---|---|---|---|---|---|---|
| APS-1 | Insulin | Pancreas | Type 1 diabetes | Yes | Yes | 20,56,60,83 |
| | Glutamic acid decarboxylase 65 (GAD65) | | | – | – | 14,15,20 |
| | IA-2 (tyrosine phosphatase-like protein) | | | Yes | Yes | 14,15,20,56,83 |
| | Thyroid peroxidase (TPO) | Thyroid | Thyroiditis | Yes | Yes[b] | 15,56 |
| | Thyroglobin (TG) | | | Yes | No[b] | 15,56 |
| | NALP5 | Parathyroid | Hypoparathyroidism | Yes | Yes[b] | 13 |
| | Cyp11a1/P450 scc (SCC) | Adrenal gland and gonads | Addison's disease and hypogonadism | Yes | – | 14,15,84 |
| | Cyp17a1/P450 c17a (17α-OH) | | | – | – | 14,15,84,85 |
| | Cyp21A/P450 c21 (21-OH) | Adrenal gland | Addison's disease | – | – | 14,15,86 |
| | SOX9 | Skin | Vitiligo | Yes[b] | – | 87 |
| | SOX10 | | | – | – | 87 |
| | Tyrosine hydroxylase (TH) | Skin | Alopecia | – | – | 14,88 |
| | Histidine decarboxylase (HDC) | Intestine | Gastrointestinal dysfunction | Yes | – | 56,89 |
| | Tryptophan hydroxylase (TPH) | | Malabsorption | Yes | Yes | 14,70,90 |
| | Cyp1A2/P450 1A2 | Liver | Autoimmune hepatitis | Yes | Yes | 14,60,91 |
| | Cyp2A6/P450 2A6 | | | – | – | 92 |
| | Aromatic L-amino acid decarboxylase (AADC) | Liver Skin | Autoimmune hepatitis Vitiligo | – | – | 14,93 |

| others | | | | | |
|---|---|---|---|---|---|
| Myelin oligodendrocyte glycoprotein (MOG) | Brain | Multiple sclerosis | Yes | Yes | 56 |
| Myelin basic protein (MBP) | | | Yes | – | 56 |
| Myelin proteolipid protein (PLP/DM20) | | | Yes | No | 56,83 |
| Glutamic acid decarboxylase 67 (GAD67) | Pancreas | Type 1 diabetes | Yes | No | 56,60,83 |
| H+K+ ATPase α | Stomach | Autoimmune gastritis | Yes | Yes | 56,83 |
| Ret S-Ag (retinal S-antigen) | Eye | Uveitis | Yes | Yes | 56,83 |
| Interphotoreceptor retinoid-binding protein (IRBP) | | | Yes | Yes | 56,68 |
| Nicotinic acetylcholine receptor α-subunit (CHRNA1) | Muscle | Myasthenia gravis | Yes | Yes | 83,94 |

[a] AIRE-dependent expression is determined either in mice (microarray or RT-PCR analysis by comparing AIRE wild-type versus AIRE knockout) or in humans (correlation of the expression levels between TRA and AIRE). Some data are taken from publicly available datasets.[58,60]

[b] G. Nusspaumer, PhD, N. Shikama, PhD, T. Zalac, BSc, G. A. Holländer, MD, unpublished data, 2006.

– Not determined.

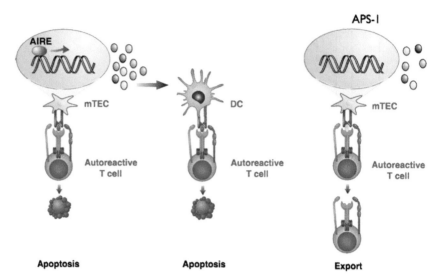

**Fig. 2.** AIRE plays an essential role in intrathymic negative selection to eliminate autoreactive thymocytes. mTEC present peptide:MHC complexes to induce apoptosis in thymocytes that express a TCR with high affinity for self-peptides. (*Left panel*) In mTEC, AIRE promotes the expression of TRA, which assures the negative selection of thymocytes with a high affinity TCR specific for an AIRE-regulated TRA. Experimental evidence also suggests that some TRA are shed, taken up by dendritic cells (DC) and subsequently cross-presented to effect negative selection of autoreactive thymocytes. (*Right panel*) The lack of functional AIRE in mTEC of patiets who have APS-1 precludes the thymic expression and presentation of some (ie, AIRE-controlled) of the TRA. This results in a loss of the negative selection of thymocytes with high affinity for such TRAs. After the postselection maturation in the thymus, autoreactive T cells are exported to peripheral lymphoid tissues.

essential for $T_{reg}$ function) display a more severe autoimmune phenotype when compared with mice with a single defect for either gene,[78] which favors a mechanism of disease in the APS-1 model that is independent of $T_{reg}$.

## EXTRATHYMIC AIRE EXPRESSION AND ITS FUNCTION

*AIRE* expression also has been noted in tissues other than the thymus but not in many of the typical APS-1 target organs, including the adrenal cortex, the thyroid gland, and the pancreas.[44] Low levels of *AIRE* have been detected in immature and mature lymphoid cells and cells of the monocytic/dendritic lineage.[44,79] The specific role of *AIRE*, if any, continues to be unknown for these cells, however, because TRA expression cannot be detected and the transfer of bone marrow cells from *AIRE*-deficient donors into wild-type recipients is insufficient to break tolerance and provoke autoimmunity.[60,80] *AIRE* transcripts also have been noticed in lymph node stromal cells,[43,81] which suggests that the purging of the peripheral T-cell repertoire of self-reactive cells may be controlled by peripheral *AIRE* expression. The scope of TRA expression in these stromal cells remains ill-defined, not least because *AIRE*-dependent TRA such as insulin could not be detected in these cells.[81]

AIRE expression has been noted in the gonads, particularly in the germ cells of the testis (N. Shikama, PhD, and G. A. Holländer, MD, unpublished data, 2006).[82] Although expressed sporadically in spermatogonia and spermatocytes, AIRE protein does not affect TRA expression in these cells. Lack of AIRE expression in the testis results in a reduction of the scheduled apoptotic wave typically observed during spermatogenesis, however, although it does not affect the morphology or further differentiation of germ cells.[82] It has been tempting to speculate that AIRE may play a role in a checkpoint designed to keep the germline stable.

## SUMMARY

The identification of AIRE not only has offered a unique opportunity to gain valuable insight into the pathophysiology of APS-1 but also has granted a better understanding of the molecular mechanism whereby the thymus achieves promiscuous gene expression for the induction of self-tolerance. Several important questions in relation to *AIRE* and its function in APS-1 remain unanswered. For instance, the precise molecular mechanism by which *AIRE* regulates the expression and efficient presentation of TRA is still incompletely understood, as are the mechanisms for promiscuous expression of non-*AIRE*–regulated genes in mTEC. The possible influences of *AIRE* on the development and survival of mTEC are also unresolved. The controversy of whether *AIRE* expression serves an extrathymic function in the establishment of T-cell tolerance needs to be settled, and an explanation must be found as to why patients who have APS-1 are particularly susceptible to *Candida* but not other infections. Finally, it is important to detail the cellular and molecular mechanisms that account for the APS-1 disease features that are unrelated to the endocrine and fungal pathologies. Answers to these issues are obviously of pressing clinical relevance.

## REFERENCES

1. Jacobson DL, Gange SJ, Rose NR, et al. Epidemiology and estimated population burden of selected autoimmune diseases in the United States. Clin Immunol Immunopathol 1997;84(3):223–43.
2. Karopka T, Fluck J, Mevissen HT, et al. The Autoimmune Disease Database: a dynamically compiled literature-derived database. BMC Bioinformatics 2006; 7:325–41.
3. Rosen FS, Mackay I. The immunology series comes to an end. N Engl J Med 2001;345(18):1343–4.
4. Vogel A, Strassburg CP, Obermayer-Straub P, et al. The genetic background of autoimmune polyendocrinopathy-candidiasis-ectodermal dystrophy and its autoimmune disease components. J Mol Med 2002;80(4):201–11.
5. Betterle C, Zanchetta R. Update on autoimmune polyendocrine syndromes (APS). Acta Biomed 2003;74(1):9–33.
6. Eisenbarth GS, Gottlieb PA. Autoimmune polyendocrine syndromes. N Engl J Med 2004;350(20):2068–79.
7. Kyewski B, Klein L. A central role for central tolerance. Annu Rev Immunol 2006; 24:571–606.
8. Mathis D, Benoist C. A decade of AIRE. Nat Rev Immunol 2007;7(8):645–50.
9. Peterson P, Peltonen L. Autoimmune polyendocrinopathy syndrome type 1 (APS1) and AIRE gene: new views on molecular basis of autoimmunity. J Autoimmun 2005;25(Suppl):49–55.
10. Leonard F. Chronic idiopathic hypoparathyroidism with superimposed Addison's disease in a child. J Clin Endocrinol 1946;6:493–506.
11. Betterle C, Greggio NA, Volpato M. Clinical review 93: autoimmune polyglandular syndrome type 1. J Clin Endocrinol Metab 1998;83(4):1049–55.

12. Ahonen P, Myllarniemi S, Sipila I, et al. Clinical variation of autoimmune polyendocrinopathy-candidiasis-ectodermal dystrophy (APECED) in a series of 68 patients. N Engl J Med 1990;322(26):1829–36.

13. Alimohammadi M, Bjorklund P, Hallgren A, et al. Autoimmune polyendocrine syndrome type 1 and NALP5, a parathyroid autoantigen. N Engl J Med 2008; 358(10):1018–28.

14. Soderbergh A, Myhre AG, Ekwall O, et al. Prevalence and clinical associations of 10 defined autoantibodies in autoimmune polyendocrine syndrome type I. J Clin Endocrinol Metab 2004;89(2):557–62.

15. Perniola R, Falorni A, Clemente MG, et al. Organ-specific and non-organ-specific autoantibodies in children and young adults with autoimmune polyendocrinopathy-candidiasis-ectodermal dystrophy (APECED). Eur J Endocrinol 2000; 143(4):497–503.

16. Neufeld M, Maclaren NK, Blizzard RM. Two types of autoimmune Addison's disease associated with different polyglandular autoimmune (PGA) syndromes. Medicine (Baltimore) 1981;60(5):355–62.

17. Myhre AG, Halonen M, Eskelin P, et al. Autoimmune polyendocrine syndrome type 1 (APS I) in Norway. Clin Endocrinol (Oxf) 2001;54(2):211–7.

18. Ishii T, Suzuki Y, Ando N, et al. Novel mutations of the autoimmune regulator gene in two siblings with autoimmune polyendocrinopathy-candidiasis-ectodermal dystrophy. J Clin Endocrinol Metab 2000;85(8):2922–6.

19. Sidransky E. Heterozygosity for a Mendelian disorder as a risk factor for complex disease. Clin Genet 2006;70(4):275–82.

20. Gylling M, Tuomi T, Bjorses P, et al. SS-cell autoantibodies, human leukocyte antigen II alleles, and type 1 diabetes in autoimmune polyendocrinopathy-candidiasis-ectodermal dystrophy. J Clin Endocrinol Metab 2000;85(12):4434–40.

21. Halonen M, Eskelin P, Myhre AG, et al. AIRE mutations and human leukocyte antigen genotypes as determinants of the autoimmune polyendocrinopathy-candidiasis-ectodermal dystrophy phenotype. J Clin Endocrinol Metab 2002; 87(6):2568–74.

22. Jiang W, Anderson MS, Bronson R, et al. Modifier loci condition autoimmunity provoked by AIRE deficiency. J Exp Med 2005;202(6):805–15.

23. Niki S, Oshikawa K, Mouri Y, et al. Alteration of intra-pancreatic target-organ specificity by abrogation of AIRE in NOD mice. J Clin Invest 2006;116(5): 1292–301.

24. Liston A. There and back again: autoimmune polyendocrinopathy syndrome type I and the AIRE knockout mouse. Drug Discov Today Dis Models 2006;3(1):33–40.

25. Adamson KA, Cheetham TD, Kendall-Taylor P, et al. The role of the IDDM2 locus in the susceptibility of UK APS1 subjects to type 1 diabetes mellitus. Int J Immunogenet 2007;34(1):17–21.

26. Finnish-German APECED Consortium. An autoimmune disease, APECED, caused by mutations in a novel gene featuring two PHD-type zinc-finger domains. Nat Genet 1997;17(4):399–403.

27. Nagamine K, Peterson P, Scott HS, et al. Positional cloning of the APECED gene. Nat Genet 1997;17(4):393–8.

28. Murumagi A, Vahamurto P, Peterson P. Characterization of regulatory elements and methylation pattern of the autoimmune regulator (AIRE) promoter. J Biol Chem 2003;278(22):19784–90.

29. Gibson TJ, Ramu C, Gemund C, et al. The APECED polyglandular autoimmune syndrome protein, AIRE-1, contains the SAND domain and is probably a transcription factor. Trends Biochem Sci 1998;23(7):242–4.

30. Ferguson BJ, Alexander C, Rossi SW, et al. AIRE's CARD revealed, a new structure for central tolerance provokes transcriptional plasticity. J Biol Chem 2008; 283(3):1723–31.
31. Michelson RJ, Collard MW, Ziemba AJ, et al. Nuclear DEAF-1-related (NUDR) protein contains a novel DNA binding domain and represses transcription of the heterogeneous nuclear ribonucleoprotein A2/B1 promoter. J Biol Chem 1999;274(43):30510–9.
32. Bottomley MJ, Collard MW, Huggenvik JI, et al. The SAND domain structure defines a novel DNA-binding fold in transcriptional regulation. Nat Struct Biol 2001;8(7):626–33.
33. Aasland R, Gibson TJ, Stewart AF. The PHD finger: implications for chromatin-mediated transcriptional regulation. Trends Biochem Sci 1995;20(2):56–9.
34. Uchida D, Hatakeyama S, Matsushima A, et al. AIRE functions as an E3 ubiquitin ligase. J Exp Med 2004;199(2):167–72.
35. Bottomley MJ, Stier G, Pennacchini D, et al. NMR structure of the first PHD finger of autoimmune regulator protein (AIRE1). Insights into autoimmune polyendocrinopathy-candidiasis-ectodermal dystrophy (APECED) disease. J Biol Chem 2005; 280(12):11505–12.
36. Org T, Chignola F, Hetenyi C, et al. The autoimmune regulator PHD finger binds to non-methylated histone H3K4 to activate gene expression. EMBO Rep 2008;9(4): 370–6.
37. Lin AE, Mak TW. The role of E3 ligases in autoimmunity and the regulation of autoreactive T cells. Curr Opin Immunol 2007;19(6):665–73.
38. Pitkanen J, Peterson P. Autoimmune regulator: from loss of function to autoimmunity. Genes Immun 2003;4(1):12–21.
39. Heino M, Peterson P, Kudoh J, et al. APECED mutations in the autoimmune regulator (AIRE) gene. Hum Mutat 2001;18(3):205–11.
40. Su MA, Anderson MS. AIRE: an update. Curr Opin Immunol 2004;16(6):746–52.
41. Ilmarinen T, Eskelin P, Halonen M, et al. Functional analysis of SAND mutations in AIRE supports dominant inheritance of the G228W mutation. Hum Mutat 2005; 26(4):322–31.
42. Su MA, Giang K, Zumer K, et al. Mechanisms of an autoimmunity syndrome in mice caused by a dominant mutation in AIRE. J Clin Invest 2008;118(5):1712–26.
43. Zuklys S, Balciunaite G, Agarwal A, et al. Normal thymic architecture and negative selection are associated with AIRE expression, the gene defective in the autoimmune-polyendocrinopathy-candidiasis-ectodermal dystrophy (APECED). J Immunol 2000;165(4):1976–83.
44. Heino M, Peterson P, Sillanpaa N, et al. RNA and protein expression of the murine autoimmune regulator gene (AIRE) in normal, RelB-deficient and in NOD mouse. Eur J Immunol 2000;30(7):1884–93.
45. Liston A, Gray DH, Lesage S, et al. Gene dosage–limiting role of AIRE in thymic expression, clonal deletion, and organ-specific autoimmunity. J Exp Med 2004; 200(8):1015–26.
46. Hubert FX, Kinkel SA, Webster KE, et al. A specific anti-AIRE antibody reveals AIRE expression is restricted to medullary thymic epithelial cells and not expressed in periphery. J Immunol 2008;180(6):3824–32.
47. Anderson G, Lane PJ, Jenkinson EJ. Generating intrathymic microenvironments to establish T-cell tolerance. Nat Rev Immunol 2007;7(12):954–63.
48. Hamazaki Y, Fujita H, Kobayashi T, et al. Medullary thymic epithelial cells expressing AIRE represent a unique lineage derived from cells expressing claudin. Nat Immunol 2007;8(3):304–11.

49. Gray D, Abramson J, Benoist C, et al. Proliferative arrest and rapid turnover of thymic epithelial cells expressing AIRE. J Exp Med 2007;204(11):2521–8.

50. Pitkanen J, Doucas V, Sternsdorf T, et al. The autoimmune regulator protein has transcriptional transactivating properties and interacts with the common coactivator CREB-binding protein. J Biol Chem 2000;275(22):16802–9.

51. Akiyoshi H, Hatakeyama S, Pitkanen J, et al. Subcellular expression of autoimmune regulator is organized in a spatiotemporal manner. J Biol Chem 2004; 279(32):33984–91.

52. Tao Y, Kupfer R, Stewart BJ, et al. AIRE recruits multiple transcriptional components to specific genomic regions through tethering to nuclear matrix. Mol Immunol 2006;43(4):335–45.

53. Derbinski J, Kyewski B. Linking signalling pathways, thymic stroma integrity and autoimmunity. Trends Immunol 2005;26(10):503–6.

54. Gillard GO, Farr AG. Contrasting models of promiscuous gene expression by thymic epithelium. J Exp Med 2005;202(1):15–9.

55. Gill J, Malin M, Sutherland J, et al. Thymic generation and regeneration. Immunol Rev 2003;195:28–50.

56. Gotter J, Brors B, Hergenhahn M, et al. Medullary epithelial cells of the human thymus express a highly diverse selection of tissue-specific genes colocalized in chromosomal clusters. J Exp Med 2004;199(2):155–66.

57. Johnnidis JB, Venanzi ES, Taxman DJ, et al. Chromosomal clustering of genes controlled by the AIRE transcription factor. Proc Natl Acad Sci U S A 2005; 102(20):7233–8.

58. Derbinski J, Gabler J, Brors B, et al. Promiscuous gene expression in thymic epithelial cells is regulated at multiple levels. J Exp Med 2005;202(1):33–45.

59. Derbinski J, Pinto S, Rosch S, et al. Promiscuous gene expression patterns in single medullary thymic epithelial cells argue for a stochastic mechanism. Proc Natl Acad Sci U S A 2008;105(2):657–62.

60. Anderson MS, Venanzi ES, Klein L, et al. Projection of an immunological self shadow within the thymus by the AIRE protein. Science 2002;298(5597): 1395–401.

61. Ramsey C, Winqvist O, Puhakka L, et al. AIRE deficient mice develop multiple features of APECED phenotype and show altered immune response. Hum Mol Genet 2002;11(4):397–409.

62. Kuroda N, Mitani T, Takeda N, et al. Development of autoimmunity against transcriptionally unrepressed target antigen in the thymus of AIRE-deficient mice. J Immunol 2005;174(4):1862–70.

63. Kont V, Laan M, Kisand K, et al. Modulation of AIRE regulates the expression of tissue-restricted antigens. Mol Immunol 2008;45(1):25–33.

64. Ruthenburg AJ, Li H, Patel DJ, et al. Multivalent engagement of chromatin modifications by linked binding modules. Nat Rev Mol Cell Biol 2007;8(12):983–94.

65. Mikkelsen TS, Ku M, Jaffe DB, et al. Genome-wide maps of chromatin state in pluripotent and lineage-committed cells. Nature 2007;448(7153):553–60.

66. Lan F, Collins RE, De Cegli R, et al. Recognition of unmethylated histone H3 lysine 4 links BHC80 to LSD1-mediated gene repression. Nature 2007;448(7154):718–22.

67. Liston A, Lesage S, Wilson J, et al. AIRE regulates negative selection of organ-specific T cells. Nat Immunol 2003;4(4):350–4.

68. DeVoss J, Hou Y, Johannes K, et al. Spontaneous autoimmunity prevented by thymic expression of a single self-antigen. J Exp Med 2006;203(12):2727–35.

69. Anderson MS, Venanzi ES, Chen Z, et al. The cellular mechanism of AIRE control of T cell tolerance. Immunity 2005;23(2):227–39.

70. Ruan QG, Tung K, Eisenman D, et al. The autoimmune regulator directly controls the expression of genes critical for thymic epithelial function. J Immunol 2007; 178(11):7173–80.
71. Gillard GO, Dooley J, Erickson M, et al. AIRE-dependent alterations in medullary thymic epithelium indicate a role for AIRE in thymic epithelial differentiation. J Immunol 2007;178(5):3007–15.
72. Sakaguchi S, Ono M, Setoguchi R, et al. Foxp3 + CD25 + CD4+ natural regulatory T cells in dominant self-tolerance and autoimmune disease. Immunol Rev 2006;212:8–27.
73. Ribot J, Romagnoli P, van Meerwijk JP. Agonist ligands expressed by thymic epithelium enhance positive selection of regulatory T lymphocytes from precursors with a normally diverse TCR repertoire. J Immunol 2006;177(2):1101–7.
74. Aschenbrenner K, D'Cruz LM, Vollmann EH, et al. Selection of Foxp3+ regulatory T cells specific for self antigen expressed and presented by AIRE+ medullary thymic epithelial cells. Nat Immunol 2007;8(4):351–8.
75. Watanabe N, Wang YH, Lee HK, et al. Hassall's corpuscles instruct dendritic cells to induce CD4 + CD25+ regulatory T cells in human thymus. Nature 2005; 436(7054):1181–5.
76. Bensinger SJ, Bandeira A, Jordan MS, et al. Major histocompatibility complex class II-positive cortical epithelium mediates the selection of CD4(+)25(+) immunoregulatory T cells. J Exp Med 2001;194(4):427–38.
77. Spence PJ, Green EA. Foxp3+ regulatory T cells promiscuously accept thymic signals critical for their development. Proc Natl Acad Sci U S A 2008;105(3):973–8.
78. Chen Z, Benoist C, Mathis D. How defects in central tolerance impinge on a deficiency in regulatory T cells. Proc Natl Acad Sci U S A 2005;102(41):14735–40.
79. Suzuki E, Kobayashi Y, Kawano O, et al. Expression of AIRE in thymocytes and peripheral lymphocytes. Autoimmunity 2008;41(2):133–9.
80. Ramsey C, Hassler S, Marits P, et al. Increased antigen presenting cell-mediated T cell activation in mice and patients without the autoimmune regulator. Eur J Immunol 2006;36(2):305–17.
81. Lee JW, Epardaud M, Sun J, et al. Peripheral antigen display by lymph node stroma promotes T cell tolerance to intestinal self. Nat Immunol 2007;8(2):181–90.
82. Schaller CE, Wang CL, Beck-Engeser G, et al. Expression of AIRE and the early wave of apoptosis in spermatogenesis. J Immunol 2008;180(3):1338–43.
83. Taubert R, Schwendemann J, Kyewski B. Highly variable expression of tissue-restricted self-antigens in human thymus: implications for self-tolerance and autoimmunity. Eur J Immunol 2007;37(3):838–48.
84. Winqvist O, Gustafsson J, Rorsman F, et al. Two different cytochrome P450 enzymes are the adrenal antigens in autoimmune polyendocrine syndrome type I and Addison's disease. J Clin Invest 1993;92(5):2377–85.
85. Krohn K, Uibo R, Aavik E, et al. Identification by molecular cloning of an autoantigen associated with Addison's disease as steroid 17 alpha-hydroxylase. Lancet 1992;339(8796):770–3.
86. Winqvist O, Karlsson FA, Kampe O. 21-Hydroxylase, a major autoantigen in idiopathic Addison's disease. Lancet 1992;339(8809):1559–62.
87. Hedstrand H, Ekwall O, Olsson MJ, et al. The transcription factors SOX9 and SOX10 are vitiligo autoantigens in autoimmune polyendocrine syndrome type I. J Biol Chem 2001;276(38):35390–5.
88. Hedstrand H, Ekwall O, Haavik J, et al. Identification of tyrosine hydroxylase as an autoantigen in autoimmune polyendocrine syndrome type I. Biochem Biophys Res Commun 2000;267(1):456–61.

89. Skoldberg F, Portela-Gomes GM, Grimelius L, et al. Histidine decarboxylase, a pyridoxal phosphate-dependent enzyme, is an autoantigen of gastric entero-chromaffin-like cells. J Clin Endocrinol Metab 2003;88(4):1445–52.

90. Ekwall O, Hedstrand H, Grimelius L, et al. Identification of tryptophan hydroxylase as an intestinal autoantigen. Lancet 1998;352(9124):279–83.

91. Clemente MG, Obermayer-Straub P, Meloni A, et al. Cytochrome P450 1A2 is a hepatic autoantigen in autoimmune polyglandular syndrome type 1. J Clin Endocrinol Metab 1997;82(5):1353–61.

92. Clemente MG, Meloni A, Obermayer-Straub P, et al. Two cytochromes P450 are major hepatocellular autoantigens in autoimmune polyglandular syndrome type 1. Gastroenterology 1998;114(2):324–8.

93. Husebye ES, Gebre-Medhin G, Tuomi T, et al. Autoantibodies against aromatic L-amino acid decarboxylase in autoimmune polyendocrine syndrome type I. J Clin Endocrinol Metab 1997;82(1):147–50.

94. Giraud M, Taubert R, Vandiedonck C, et al. An IRF8-binding promoter variant and AIRE control CHRNA1 promiscuous expression in thymus. Nature 2007; 448(7156):934–7.

# Genetics of Type 1 Diabetes and Autoimmune Thyroid Disease

Simon H.S. Pearce, MD[a],*, Tony R. Merriman, PhD[b]

**KEYWORDS**

- Autoimmunity • Genomics • Grave's disease
- Type 1 diabetes • Genome-wide association

The autoimmune thyroid diseases [AITD] (eg, Graves' disease [GD] and autoimmune hypothyroidism) along with type 1 diabetes (T1D) are common autoimmune endocrine disorders that collectively affect approximately 3% of the population over a lifetime.[1,2] Each has a complex genetic basis, which means that susceptibility alleles at several different loci, along with nongenetic factors, are thought to contribute to disease pathogenesis in varying degrees in each affected individual.[3] These alleles and loci differ among individuals such that in the collective population, a large number (likely to be dozens) of alleles at different loci contribute to disease. Although alleles of the major histocompatibility complex have been known to contribute to the susceptibility to several forms of autoimmunity for more than 35 years,[4,5] the advances in genomics over past 5 years have enabled an acceleration in the identification of novel loci, and hence biochemical pathways, implicated in the development of these conditions. Some of the variants identified seem to modulate T-lymphocyte signaling during and after engagement of the T-cell antigen receptor and have been found to be susceptibility alleles for many different forms of human autoimmunity (**Fig. 1**). Other loci seem to have restricted putative roles, with susceptibility apparently confined to one autoimmune condition or to a specific ancestral group.

Replication has become a prerequisite for the validation of complex disease alleles. For autoimmunity, however, it is expected that different populations with the same disorder may carry different susceptibility alleles,[6] because immune-response gene polymorphism is naturally selected by survival from infectious diseases and exposure to different infective agents has varied markedly with differing population histories. This means that failure to replicate a disease association in a different population

[a] Institute of Human Genetics, University of Newcastle, International Centre for Life, Central Parkway, Newcastle upon Tyne, NE1 3BZ, UK
[b] Department of Biochemistry, University of Otago, Dunedin, New Zealand
* Corresponding author.
*E-mail address:* s.h.s.pearce@ncl.ac.uk (S.H.S. Pearce).

Endocrinol Metab Clin N Am 38 (2009) 289–301
doi:10.1016/j.ecl.2009.01.012
0889-8529/09/$ – see front matter © 2009 Elsevier Inc. All rights reserved.

endo.theclinics.com

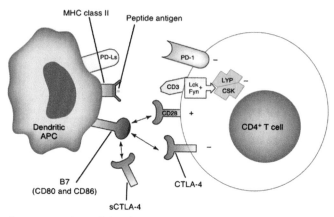

**Fig. 1.** An antigen-presenting cell (APC) interacting with a T cell shows the role of key variant autoimmunity molecules. The dendritic APC presents a cleaved peptide-antigen bound to the groove of the tetrameric class II MHC molecule. This is recognized by a T cell with an antigen receptor (CD3 complex) of appropriate affinity for the peptide–MHC complex. For the T cell to become activated, a second signal must be delivered by the interaction of a co-stimulatory molecule with B7 molecules expressed on the APC. CD28 is a positive costimula-tor that enables T-cell proliferation and activation, but CTLA-4 is an inhibitory costimulator that provides a negative second signal, which causes the T cell to become quiescent or to apoptose. Soluble CTLA-4 (sCTLA-4) might play a role as a natural inhibitor of CD28 engage-ment by binding to APC B7 molecules with a higher affinity than to CD28 and stopping the costimulatory activation of the T cell via CD28–B7 interaction. Lymphoid tyrosine phospha-tase (LYP) is encoded by the *PTPN22* gene and the autoimmunity-associated SNP codes for an arginine (wild-type) to tryptophan change, which produces greater phosphatase activity in the LYP molecule.[22]

may reflect the different selection pressures of the two ancestral groups studied rather than that the association is necessarily false positive; the lack of replication ascribed to heterogeneity in study design or poor statistical power to replicate. In this article, we review recent findings in the field of genetics of AITD and T1D that have started to reveal some of the molecular pathways that are important in the pathogenesis of these autoimmune endocrinopathies. We first examine loci common to AITD and T1D and then loci specific to each disease. Large-scale genomic analyses, including genome-wide association analyses, have just started to furnish useful information and are central to the recent discoveries, particularly in T1D.

## GENETIC EPIDEMIOLOGY

Between a quarter and one third of patients who have GD have a first-degree relative with either GD or autoimmune hypothyroidism, with approximately one eighth of patients who have T1D having a first-degree relative with T1D,[7,8] which suggests a significant contribution of genetic factors to AITD and T1D. Detailed twin studies have suggested that inherited factors make the dominant contribution to disease susceptibility, contributing as much as 70% and 80% of the etiologic risk for T1D and GD, respectively.[9,10] An index of the heritability of a disorder can be gained by as-sessing the risk to a sibling of an affected individual compared with that of the back-ground unrelated population. For GD and T1D, this relative risk estimate, termed $\lambda_s$, has been estimated to be approximately 10 and 15, respectively,[11] which is consistent with the heritability of several other common autoimmune conditions. People with these disorders are often concerned about their children being affected. The risk to someone whose mother is affected by GD of developing either GD or autoimmune hypothyroidism can be calculated to be approximately 15%.[8] Similarly, the risk of T1D if one's father has T1D is approximately 6% but is only 3% if one's mother is affected.[7,12]

## LOCI SHARED BETWEEN AUTOIMMUNE THYROID DISEASE AND TYPE 1 DIABETES

T1D and AITD both occur as a result of organ-specific T-cell–mediated autoimmune attack of endocrine tissues. Given the co-occurrence of AITD and T1D within individuals and families,[13–15] the existence of the same inherited alleles contributing to both diseases has long been predicted. The current genetic data indicate that this is true, although it is becoming increasingly apparent that allelic diversity at a single locus can mediate disease specificity.

### Major Histocompatibility Complex

It has been known for more than 30 years that certain human leukocyte antigen (HLA) alleles, encoded within the major histocompatibility complex (MHC) on chromosome 6p21, are overrepresented in patients who have AITD and T1D.[4,5] In T1D the class II antigen-presenting *HLA-DRB1* gene confers the major risk within the HLA region,[16,17] with the situation less clear in AITD. The exact allele or haplotype combinations that are associated with AITD depend on the nature of the thyroid disease (ie, GD or autoimmune hypothyroidism) and the ancestral origin of the patient group. In white populations of European descent, the *'DR3'* haplotype (*HLA DRB1*0301-DQB1*0201-DQA1*0501*) is typically found in approximately 50% of individuals with GD compared with approximately 25% to 30% of the background population, for an odds ratio (OR) for DR3 of approximately 2 (**Table 1**).[18] In patients with Hashimoto's

**Table 1**
**Confirmed susceptibility loci in autoimmune thyroid disease and type 1 diabetes**

| Gene | Chromosome | Odds Ratio[a] TID | Odds Ratio AITD |
|------|-----------|-------------------|-----------------|
| *MHC locus* | 6p21 | 3–4 | 2 |
| *CTLA4* | 2q33 | 1.2 | 1.5 |
| *PTPN22* | 1p13 | 2.0 | 1.7 |
| *IFIH1* | 2q24 | 1.2 | 1.1 |
| *CD25* | 10p15 | 2.0 | 1.2 |
| *C12orf30* | 12q24 | 1.3 | NA |
| *ERBB3* | 12q13 | 1.3 | NA |
| *PTPN2* | 18p11 | 1.3 | 1.1 |
| *KIAA0350* | 16p13 | 1.2 | NA |
| *CD226* | 18q22 | 1.2 | 1.1 |
| *INS* | 11p15 | 1.3 | NA |
| *FCRL3* | 1q23 | NA | 1.2 |
| *TSHR* | 14q31 | – | 1.3 |

*Abbreviation:* NA, no association.
[a] The increased risk conferred by the susceptibility allele. If the etiologic susceptibility allele is not known, the odds ratio from the most associated allele at a locus is presented.

thyroiditis, HLA associations also have been found with the *HLA 'DR4'* haplotype; however, the effects are less consistent than those found in GD.[19] In T1D, the same *DR3* haplotype is consistently associated with disease, albeit with a larger strength of effect (OR = 3–4) than seen in GD. However, it is the considerably stronger association with the *HLA DRB1\*04-DQB1\*0301-DQA1\*0302* haplotypes in the white population that distinguishes T1D from AITD.[16,17] This *'DR4'* haplotype is observed in 70% to 80% of patients who have T1D, compared with approximately 25% of the background population and confers a risk of OR > 4. This haplotype confers especially strong risk when present in combination with the *DR3* haplotype (increasing risk approximately 20-fold). In non-white populations, the class II haplotypes are a major risk factor for T1D and AITD, although different alleles are often involved.

A recent large-scale analysis of several hundred single nucleotide polymorphism (SNP) markers spread across the *MHC* shows that several different alleles, including not only those classically associated at *HLA-DRB1*, but also within the Class I region, *HLA-A/B*, contribute toward the *MHC* association with T1D.[16] A similar analysis in GD shows that the *HLA-C* region also makes a significant contribution to the *MHC* association.[20] These and numerous other studies have provided firm hints that other genes within the MHC region contribute to T1D and AITD. Because of the tight linkage disequilibrium (close association) of neighboring markers within the MHC, however, higher numbers of affected subjects need to be studied before the contributions of individual disease alleles with weaker effects than HLA-DRB1 and the class I loci are able to be fully resolved. Ultimately, it is likely that variants in some of the many non-HLA genes within the MHC region (eg, complement or notch genes) also may be implicated in disease susceptibility.

We make two observations from these HLA data. First, with an OR for association of the *DR3* haplotype with GD of approximately 2 in many studies, compared with T1D (global OR for association at HLA between 3 and 4), there seems to be a lesser contribution of *HLA* to disease etiology in AITD. Second, the *HLA* molecules serve to process and present peptide fragments as antigens to the T-cell receptor, which determines the antigenic specificity of the adaptive immune response. In AITD, because the *HLA* associations are relatively heterogeneous (different in distinct populations and only present in 50% of patients), this may mean that there is not a single T-cell epitope (for instance, on the thyroid stimulating hormone receptor) that can be identified as being critical for disease onset or progression of AITDs. In T1D, more than two dozen pancreatic β-islet-specific autoantigens have been implicated in disease onset or pathogenesis.[21]

### Lymphoid Tyrosine Phosphatase

An additional locus that contributes to AITD and T1D susceptibility is *PTPN22*, which encodes the lymphoid tyrosine phosphatase (LYP). LYP is a negative regulator of T-cell antigen receptor (CD3) signaling. A coding polymorphism, arginine to tryptophan at codon 620, activates the LYP molecule, paradoxically causing more potent inhibition of the T-cell antigen receptor (CD3) signaling kinases, following engagement with MHC-antigen.[22] The tryptophan allele is carried by approximately 10% of healthy subjects in northern European white populations but is overrepresented in patients who have GD, with a prevalence of approximately 13% and more than 17% in patients who have T1D.[23–26] The OR for the effect of this allele in GD and T1D is 1.5 to 2.0 depending on the population, but because of its comparative rarity,[23,24] it contributes slightly less to overall population disease susceptibility than other genes (eg, *CTLA4* in GD, *INS* in T1D; see later discussion). The effects of the variant tryptophan 620 allele are population specific, because the allele is only present at substantial frequency in white populations, being essentially absent in individuals of Asian and African descent.[27] The mechanism by which the tryptophan 620 LYP variant predisposes to autoimmunity is unknown, but it is possible that it may mediate less efficient "weeding out" of T cells bearing potentially autoreactive T-cell receptors in thymic development,[22,27] leading to an autoimmune proclivity in later life.

## Cytotoxic T-Lymphocyte Antigen-4

Alleles in the cytotoxic T-lymphocyte antigen-4 (CTLA4) gene on chromosome 2q33 have been associated extensively with GD and—in fewer studies—with autoimmune hypothyroidism.[28] CTLA4 is a cell surface immunoglobulin-like receptor involved in the regulation of the costimulatory ("second") signal that regulates T-lymphocyte activation following HLA-peptide antigen encounter and so was a good candidate gene for autoimmunity.[28] Initial associations of CTLA4 alleles with GD by Yanagawa and colleagues[29] were confirmed with a gamut of replication studies in many different GD populations.[30] Based on the association in GD, CTLA4 was also tested for association with T1D, with several studies confirming an effect,[31] although not as strong as that observed in GD. The true disease susceptibility allele at CTLA4 remains to be defined but probably lies within a 6-kb region, including the 3′ untranslated region of the gene.[32] The susceptibility haplotype at CTLA4 is carried by approximately 50% of the healthy white population, and its prevalence increases to 60% in patients who have GD, with an OR for the most associated allele of approximately 1.5.[30,32] The involvement of CTLA4 in genetic susceptibility to autoimmunity crosses species. A CTLA4 variant in the nonobese diabetic mouse model (a model of human T1D) has been implicated in murine autoimmune diabetes.[32]

The mechanism by which a noncoding 3′ untranslated region CTLA4 polymorphisms might modulate the immune response is still far from clear. One theory is that there is a circulating, soluble isoform of the CTLA4 protein that may be able to engage and occupy the CD28/CTLA4 receptors on antigen-presenting cells (known as B7 molecules) and thereby modulate costimulatory signaling (see **Fig. 1**).[32] Despite significant work in this area, this theory still lacks direct experimental evidence to support it.[33] Another recent study suggested a role for CTLA4 polymorphisms at an early stage of T-cell differentiation and lineage commitment, with CTLA4 genotypes being shown to correlate with the number of circulating CD4+, CD25+ T regulatory lymphocytes.[34] It is notable that the allele associations at CTLA4 and at the adjacent inducible costimulator locus seem to be subtly different in other autoimmune diseases (eg, systemic lupus erythematosus) than with AITD.[35] These recent findings call into question the assumption that the detailed pattern of association at CTLA4 would be identical in T1D as that found AITD.[32] There may be an unsuspected level of complexity underlying the mechanistic effect of CTLA4 variants, with a possibility that different variants and etiological mechanisms contribute to different autoimmune conditions.

## CD25 and IFIH1

The CD25 gene encodes the α-chain of the interleukin-2 receptor, a key player in the regulation of lymphocytes through the activity of regulatory T cells, and markers within this gene were found to be associated with T1D, with an OR of approximately 1.3.[36] A replication case-control study using GD probands has confirmed a modest effect, with an OR of 1.24 at the most associated marker.[37] Although association at CD25 needs to be confirmed in a second AITD patient cohort before it is robust, it seems likely to be a further susceptibility locus making a small contribution toward GD pathogenesis. The initial T1D study did not map the specific disease-causative DNA variant within the CD25 gene;[36] however, these findings have been replicated in a second independent T1D patient cohort,[38] and a fine-mapping study has placed the most associated SNP within its 5′ regulatory regions.[39] The most associated allele has been found to correlate with low levels of circulating soluble interleukin-2 receptor, which suggests a mechanism for the functional effect of the variant.[39]

Interferon-induced helicase-1 (IFIH1) was identified as contributing susceptibility to T1D in an intensive study of 6500 nonsynonymous SNP markers.[40] The maximally associated allele encodes an alanine to threonine change; this association has been replicated in probands with GD[41] and in other autoimmune disorders. The effect is weak, with an OR less than 1.2 for T1D in whites.[40,42] The IFIH1 gene is in a region of extended linkage disequilibrium on Chr 2 (analogous to, but not as extensive as, the situation within the MHC), meaning that it is not yet certain whether IFIH1 is the susceptibility gene within the Chr 2 genomic region. Based on its functionality, however, it is the strongest candidate within the region. The functional consequences of the IFIH1 variant are currently unknown, but IFIH1 is believed to have a role in regulating cellular antiviral and apoptotic responses.

## DISEASE-SPECIFIC GENES
### Autoimmune Thyroid Disease

#### Thyroid antigens
Disease-specific loci for GD have started to be identified in recent years. Alleles of SNP markers within the thyroid-stimulating hormone receptor gene have been shown to have unequivocal association with GD in three distinct patient cohorts, including in a genome-wide analysis of functionally significant (nonsynonymous) SNPs.[43–45] The associated variants lie within the regulatory regions and those encoding the extracellular domain of the receptor. Fine mapping studies are in progress to more fully define the disease-associated allele and the mechanism for the disease effect.[43,44] In contrast, several studies have shown weaker evidence for association of GD with polymorphisms in the thyroglobulin (Tg) gene.[46,47] On aggregate, these studies of the Tg gene have not shown convincing evidence for association with GD (although the effect may be different in autoimmune hypothyroidism).[48] Tg is a huge gene of 48 exons, and further work to define and test the enormous diversity of haplotypes is currently awaited.

#### FC-receptor like
A series of molecules with homology to cell surface immunoglobulin (Fc-) receptors lie in a cluster in chromosome 1q21-q23, a region that was implicated in susceptibility to several autoimmune diseases in whole-genome linkage studies.[49] The initial study identified a four-SNP promoter haplotype of FCRL3 as being associated with rheumatoid arthritis and systemic lupus erythematosus in Japanese patient cohorts.[50] This association has been replicated in two studies of GD, and the most associated markers seem to lie in a haplotype block adjacent to FCRL3, encompassing alleles of the FCRL5 gene in whites.[45,51] There is still a substantial amount of fine mapping to be done before we can predict the mechanism by which variants within the FC-receptor like (FCRLs) contribute to AITD pathogenesis. Notably, this association is not replicated in all cohorts of whites with GD, and there is no evidence for association of FCRL3 with T1D.[52–54]

#### CD40
An SNP marker, encoding a change in the context of the initiation of translation codon of the B lymphocyte surface immunoreceptor, CD40 has shown a weak association

with GD in some studies[55,56] but not in others.[57,58] Overall, a meta-analysis of the various studies confirms that *CD40* polymorphism does not have a major influence of GD susceptibility, but an effect with an OR of 1.2 or less cannot entirely be excluded.[59] *CD40* alleles are not associated with T1D.[53]

## Type 1 Diabetes

### The insulin gene

Similar to the discovery of thyroid-stimulating hormone receptor in AITD, genes that encode proteins specific to the insulin-producing cells of the endocrine pancreas are candidate etiologic determinants for T1D. Consequently, variation at a tandem repeat polymorphism in the regulatory region of the insulin gene (*INS*) has been long established as a susceptibility determinant of moderate effect in T1D.[60] The disease-protective allele (class III; longer repeat length) results in higher expression in the thymus and lower expression in the pancreas.[61] It is possible that infants with this allele are better able to delete autoreactive T cells in the thymus (ie, more thymic expression of insulin increases the chance for recognition by autoreactive T cells in the thymus and their consequent deletion).[62] In the pancreas, people with the susceptibility *INS* allele (class I; shorter repeat length) produce higher levels of insulin,[63] which increases the amount of self-antigen available for autoimmune recognition.

## GENOME-WIDE ASSOCIATION ANALYSIS

Two full genome-wide association analyses using a dense set of hundreds of thousands of SNP markers have been published in T1D.[64,65] Combined with follow-up replication studies,[66] this has allowed confirmation of five novel genetic associations centering on *ERBB3*, *C12orf30*, *KIAA3050*, *PTPN2*, and *CD226*. The latter two loci also showed association with GD.[67] Alleles at some of these five novel genes are closely associated with those at neighboring genes; mapping of the precise genetic variants underlying these new associations, which undoubtedly will be achieved in the near future, will confirm the new genes involved in disease pathogenesis. *CD226* is a T-cell costimulatory receptor, and *PTPN2* is a T-cell protein tyrosine phosphatase.[67] These genes further underscore the importance of T-cell activity in T1D and GD. Further work on the other three genes may reveal novel "diabetogenic" pathways.

A full genome-wide association analysis using a dense set of markers has not been published as yet in AITDs. A low-resolution scan using a modest set of 14,500 SNP markers that encoded nonsynonymous protein changes in 1000 GD and controls recently was performed, however.[45] Some of the previously demonstrated associations were not identified, including those at *CTLA4* and *PTPN22*, most likely because of a lack of representation on the gene chip of markers within the most associated haplotype blocks. Association at *MHC* and the *TSHR* was confirmed in an expanded cohort of 2500 GD patients, and the association within the FCRL region was refined to markers within *FCRL3*.[45]

## LESSONS FROM THE PAST AND FUTURE DEVELOPMENTS

Even with the discovery and confirmation of 10 susceptibility loci in T1D, approximately one third of the familial clustering evident in T1D remains unexplained.[67] It is estimated that the HLA region accounts for 41%, the other confirmed nine loci for a further 7%, and the environmental contribution as 20%. Although these estimates are based on analysis of families with two or more affected first-degree relatives, it is clear that numerous loci that are likely to have weak effects are yet to be discovered in T1D. A similar situation exists for AITD.

Although candidate gene studies have had modest success, it remains disappointing that no novel disease-specific AITD susceptibility gene has yet been robustly identified by reverse genetic approaches, despite a substantial amount of effort from several research groups over the last 10 years. The major strategy used previously has been genome-wide scanning for linkage in families with two or more affected individuals. The use of this strategy to reproducibly detect AITD susceptibility genes was, in retrospect, doomed to failure, however, because linkage analysis lends itself to detecting rare susceptibility alleles of strong effect. It is clear that aside from the HLA region, AITD results from the inheritance of common susceptibility alleles of modest effect. The notable success in linkage scanning in complex disease was the discovery of the *CARD15* (NOD2) gene in Crohn's disease,[68,69] in which several rare and penetrant mutant alleles contribute only a small portion of the population attributable risk. In comparison, the genomic region containing the established AITD/T1D susceptibility gene *PTPN22*, with a relatively common susceptibility allele, is not reproducibly linked to either disease.

Previously for AITD and T1D, linkage scanning was the strategy used because of the available genotyping technologies and the existing knowledge of variation in the human genome (requiring only 300–400 microsatellite marker to be typed). Notably, linkage scanning did not result in any novel discoveries in T1D or AITD genetics.[70,71] The advent of SNP genotyping chips has made rapid high-fidelity genotyping of numerous markers, identified as a result of the Human Genome/HapMap Project, in thousands of individuals a reality. Genome-wide association studies have been successful in T1D, and genome-wide association studies are currently underway using dense marker maps of 300,000 or more SNPs in substantial AITD cohorts. They will undoubtedly provide new information that may be helpful in understanding pathogenesis. These genome-wide association analyses have even greater issues with multiple testing than the equivalent linkage studies and have practical limitations in being insensitive to rare etiological variants or variants in recombination "hotspots" with little surrounding linkage disequilibrium.[72] In the coming decades, the development of technologies that enable the affordable sequencing of individual genomes will begin to address these issues. In the meantime, recently released sequencing technologies are enabling the comprehensive testing of individual genes for an influence of rare variants on disease risk, although extremely large cohorts will be required for association testing.

Delineating interactions between genetic variants in pathogenic pathways is necessary to identify genetic effects and understand biochemical mechanisms. For example, genetic interaction has been reported between variants in the genes that encode the CCR5 chemokine receptor and its CCL3L1 chemokine ligand in susceptibility to HIV infection and rheumatoid arthritis.[73] There is a strong argument in favor of testing for genetic interaction even in the absence of a dominant single-locus effect, particularly when a biologic interaction is established. In the presence of interaction, one polymorphism must be considered in the context of a potential second unlinked but interacting polymorphism. Undetected epistasis, the multiplicative effect of two gene products on the same biologic pathway, may be a significant reason why single-locus tests of association fail to replicate across separate cohorts. Testing for genetic interaction on a genome-wide basis in the absence of biologic hypotheses is recommended[74] but is a statistical challenge.[75]

Copy number variations (CNV), which are chromosomal duplications or deletions that encompass more than 1 kb of DNA, are firmly established and mapped across the human genome.[76] Many common CNVs are known to involve coding genes. Many of the genes that exhibit CNV are important in adaptation of humans to their environment (eg, for immunologic or metabolic function). Variations in the copy number of such genes are predicted to have major effects on gene function, and the importance of CNV in disease susceptibility is just starting to become apparent. It is already clear that CNV plays a role in other autoimmune and infectious disorders,[73,77–79] and it could be important in AITD and T1D. These CNVs constitute an underexplored source of genetic variation, and genome-wide assessment of their relevance in AITD and T1D is likely to be published within the next 2 years.

With the recent availability of a superficial understanding of the genetic variation contributing to T1D susceptibility at the genome-wide level in whites, it is possible to begin to assess whether the initial promise of genetic analysis ultimately will be worthwhile in terms of disease prediction or insights into pathogenesis that ultimately could lead to novel therapy. Thus far, with the identification of at least 10 allelic variants that contribute to T1D susceptibility, most of which have weak effect, it seems likely that there will be little clinically relevant gain for disease prediction over and above information long established for *MHC* alleles. The hope, however, remains that novel compounds that target the proteins implicated in autoimmune disease pathogenesis (eg, LYP inhibitors)[80] may translate to the clinic over the next few years or that insights into inherited susceptibility may allow a greater understanding of avoidable environmental precipitants of disease.

## REFERENCES

1. Leese GP, Flynn RV, Jung RT, et al. Increasing prevalence and incidence of thyroid disease in Tayside, Scotland: the Thyroid Epidemiology Audit Research Study. Clin Endocrinol (Oxf) 2008;68(2):311–6.
2. Eurodiab Ace Study Group. Variation and trends in incidence of childhood diabetes in Europe. Lancet 2000;355(9207):873–6.
3. Lander ES, Schork NJ. Genetic dissection of complex traits. Science 1994; 265(5184):2037–48.
4. Grumet FC, Payne RO, Konishi J, et al. HLA antigens as markers for disease susceptibility and autoimmunity in Graves' disease. J Clin Endocrinol Metab 1974;39(6):1115–9.
5. Schernthaner G, Ludwig H, Mayr WR. Juvenile diabetes mellitus: HLA-antigen frequencies dependent on the age of onset of the disease. J Immunogenet 1976;3(2):117–21.
6. Pearce SH, Merriman TR. Genetic progress towards the molecular basis of autoimmunity. Trends Mol Med 2006;12(2):90–8.
7. Tillil H, Köbberling J. Age-corrected empirical genetic risk estimates for first-degree relatives of IDDM patients. Diabetes 1987;36(1):93–9.
8. Vaidya B, Kendall-Taylor P, Pearce SH. The genetics of autoimmune thyroid disease. J Clin Endocrinol Metab 2002;87(12):5385–97.
9. Brix TH, Kyvik KO, Christensen K, et al. Evidence for a major role of heredity in Graves' disease: a population-based study of two Danish twin cohorts. J Clin Endocrinol Metab 2001;86(2):930–4.
10. Kyvik KO, Green A, Beck-Nielsen H. Concordance rates of insulin dependent diabetes mellitus: a population based study of young Danish twins. BMJ 1995; 311(7010):913–7.
11. Vyse TJ, Todd JA. Genetic analysis of autoimmune disease. Cell 1996;85(3): 311–8.
12. el-Hashimy M, Angelico MC, Martin BC, et al. Factors modifying the risk of IDDM in offspring of an IDDM parent. Diabetes 1995;44(3):295–9.

13. Torfs CP, King MC, Huey B, et al. Genetic interrelationship between insulin-dependent diabetes mellitus, the autoimmune thyroid diseases, and rheumatoid arthritis. Am J Hum Genet 1986;38(2):170–87.

14. Payami H, Joe S, Thomson G. Autoimmune thyroid disease in type 1 diabetic families. Genet Epidemiol 1989;6(1):137–41.

15. Somers EC, Thomas SL, Smeeth L, et al. Autoimmune diseases co-occurring within individuals and within families: a systematic review. Epidemiology 2006; 17(2):202–17.

16. Nejentsev S, Howson JM, Walker NM, et al. Localization of type 1 diabetes susceptibility to the MHC class I genes HLA-B and HLA-A. Nature 2007; 450(7171):887–92.

17. Erlich H, Valdes AM, Noble J, et al. HLA DR-DQ haplotypes and genotypes and type 1 diabetes risk: analysis of the type 1 diabetes genetics consortium families. Diabetes 2008;57(4):1084–92.

18. Farid NR, Sampson L, Noel EP, et al. A study of human leukocyte D locus related antigens in Graves' disease. J Clin Invest 1979;63(1):108–13.

19. Tandon N, Zhang L, Weetman AP. HLA associations with Hashimoto's thyroiditis. Clin Endocrinol 1991;34(5):383–6.

20. Simmonds MJ, Howson JM, Heward JM, et al. A novel and major association of HLA-C in Graves' disease that eclipses the classical HLA-DRB1 effect. Hum Mol Genet 2007;16(18):2149–53.

21. Lieberman SM, DiLorenzo TP. A comprehensive guide to antibody and T-cell responses in type 1 diabetes. Tissue Antigens 2003;62(5):359–77.

22. Vang T, Congia M, Macis MD, et al. Autoimmune-associated lymphoid tyrosine phosphatase is a gain of function variant. Nat Genet 2005;37(12): 1317–9.

23. Bottini N, Musumeci L, Alonso A, et al. A functional variant of lymphoid tyrosine phosphatase is associated with type I diabetes. Nat Genet 2004;36(4): 337–8.

24. Velaga MR, Wilson V, Jennings CE, et al. The codon 620 tryptophan allele of the lymphoid tyrosine phosphatase (LYP) gene is a major determinant of Graves' disease. J Clin Endocrinol Metab 2004;89(11):5862–5.

25. Smyth D, Cooper JD, Collins JE, et al. Replication of an association between the lymphoid tyrosine phosphatase locus (LYP/PTPN22) with type 1 diabetes, and evidence for its role as a general autoimmunity locus. Diabetes 2004;53(11): 3020–3.

26. Smyth DJ, Cooper JD, Howson JM, et al. PTPN22 Trp620 explains the association of chromosome 1p13 with type 1 diabetes and shows a statistical interaction with HLA class II genotypes. Diabetes 2008;57(6):1730–7.

27. Gregersen PK, Lee HS, Batliwalla F, et al. PTPN22: setting thresholds for autoimmunity. Semin Immunol 2006;18(4):214–23.

28. Gough SC, Walker LS, Sansom DM. CTLA4 gene polymorphism and autoimmunity. Immunol Rev 2005;204(4):102–15.

29. Yanagawa T, Hidaka Y, Guimaraes V, et al. CTLA-4 gene polymorphism associated with Graves' disease in a Caucasian population. J Clin Endocrinol Metab 1995;80(1):41–5.

30. Vaidya B, Pearce SHS. The emerging role of the CTLA4 gene in autoimmune endocrinopathies. Eur J Endocrinol 2004;150(5):619–26.

31. Nisticò L, Buzzetti R, Pritchard LE, et al. The CTLA-4 gene region of chromosome 2q33 is linked to, and associated with, type 1 diabetes. Hum Mol Genet 1996; 5(7):1075–80.

32. Ueda H, Howson JM, Esposito L, et al. Association of the T-cell regulatory gene CTLA4 with susceptibility to autoimmune disease. Nature 2003;423(6939): 506–11.

33. Anjos SM, Shao W, Marchand L, et al. Allelic effects on gene regulation at the autoimmunity-predisposing CTLA4 locus: a re-evaluation of the 3'+6230G > A polymorphism. Genes Immun 2005;6(4):305–11.

34. Atabani SF, Thio CL, Divanovic S, et al. Association of CTLA4 polymorphism with regulatory T cell frequency. Eur J Immunol 2005;35(7):2157–62.

35. Cunninghame-Graham DS, Wong AK, McHugh NJ, et al. Evidence for unique association signals in SLE at the CD28-CTLA4-ICOS locus in a family-based study. Hum Mol Genet 2006;15(21):3195–205.

36. Vella A, Cooper JD, Lowe CE, et al. Localization of a type 1 diabetes locus in the IL2RA/CD25 region by use of tag single-nucleotide polymorphisms. Am J Hum Genet 2005;76(5):773–9.

37. Brand OJ, Lowe CE, Heward JM, et al. Association of the interleukin-2 receptor alpha (IL-2Ralpha)/CD25 gene region with Graves' disease using a multilocus test and tag SNPs. Clin Endocrinol (Oxf) 2007;66(4):508–12.

38. Qu HQ, Montpetit A, Ge B, et al. Toward further mapping of the association between the IL2RA locus and type 1 diabetes. Diabetes 2007;56(4):1174–6.

39. Lowe CE, Cooper JD, Brusko T, et al. Large-scale genetic fine mapping and genotype-phenotype associations implicate polymorphism in the IL2RA region in type 1 diabetes. Nat Genet 2007;39(9):1074–82.

40. Smyth DJ, Cooper JD, Bailey R, et al. A genome-wide association study of non-synonymous SNPs identifies a type 1 diabetes locus in the interferon-induced helicase (IFIH1) region. Nat Genet 2006;38(6):617–9.

41. Sutherland A, Davies J, Owen CJ, et al. Genomic polymorphism at the interferon-induced helicase (IFIH1) locus contributes to Graves' disease susceptibility. J Clin Endocrinol Metab 2007;92(8):3338–41.

42. Qu HQ, Marchand L, Grabs R, et al. The association between the IFIH1 locus and type 1 diabetes. Diabetologia 2008;51(3):473–5.

43. Hiratani H, Bowden DW, Ikegami S, et al. Multiple SNPs in intron 7 of thyrotropin receptor are associated with Graves' disease. J Clin Endocrinol Metab 2005; 90(5):2898–903.

44. Dechairo BM, Zabaneh D, Collins J, et al. Association of the TSHR gene with Graves' disease: the first disease-specific locus. Eur J Hum Genet 2005; 13(11):1223–30.

45. Wellcome Trust Case Control Consortium, Australo-Anglo-American Spondylitis Consortium, Burton PR, et al. Association scan of 14,500 nonsynonymous SNPs in four diseases identifies autoimmunity variants. Nat Genet 2007;39(11):1329–37.

46. Ban Y, Greenberg DA, Concepcion E, et al. Amino acid substitutions in the thyroglobulin gene are associated with susceptibility to human and murine autoimmune thyroid disease. Proc Natl Acad Sci U S A 2003;100(25):15119–24.

47. Collins JE, Heward JM, Carr-Smith J, et al. Association of rare thyroglobulin gene microsatellite variants with autoimmune thyroid disease. J Clin Endocrinol Metab 2003;88(10):5039–42.

48. Collins JE, Heward JM, Howson JM, et al. Common allelic variants of exons 10, 12, and 33 of the thyroglobulin gene are not associated with autoimmune thyroid disease in the United Kingdom. J Clin Endocrinol Metab 2004;89(12):6336–9.

49. Capon F, Semprini S, Chimenti S, et al. Fine mapping of the PSORS4 psoriasis susceptibility region on chromosome 1q21. J Invest Dermatol 2001;116(5): 728–30.

50. Kochi Y, Yamada R, Suzuki A, et al. A functional variant in FCRL3, encoding Fc receptor-like 3, is associated with rheumatoid arthritis and several autoimmunities. Nat Genet 2005;37(5):478–85.

51. Simmonds MJ, Heward JM, Carr-Smith J, et al. Contribution of single nucleotide polymorphisms within FCRL3 and MAP3K7IP2 to the pathogenesis of Graves' disease. J Clin Endocrinol Metab 2006;91(3):1056–61.

52. Owen CJ, Kelly H, Eden JA, et al. Analysis of the Fc receptor-like-3 (FCRL3) locus in Caucasians with autoimmune disorders suggests a complex pattern of disease association. J Clin Endocrinol Metab 2007;92(3):1106–11.

53. Smyth DJ, Howson JM, Payne F, et al. Analysis of polymorphisms in 16 genes in type 1 diabetes that have been associated with other immune-mediated diseases. BMC Med Genet 2006;7(3):20.

54. Duchatelet S, Caillat-Zucman S, Dubois-Laforgue D, et al. FCRL3 -169CT functional polymorphism in type 1 diabetes and autoimmunity traits. Biomed Pharmacother 2008;62(3):153–7.

55. Tomer Y, Concepcion E, Greenberg DA. A C/T single-nucleotide polymorphism in the region of the CD40 gene is associated with Graves' disease. Thyroid 2002; 12(12):1129–35.

56. Ban Y, Tozaki T, Taniyama M, et al. Association of a C/T single-nucleotide polymorphism in the 5' untranslated region of the CD40 gene with Graves' disease in Japanese. Thyroid 2006;16(5):443–6.

57. Heward JM, Simmonds MJ, Carr-Smith J, et al. A single nucleotide polymorphism in the CD40 gene on chromosome 20q (GD-2) provides no evidence for susceptibility to Graves' disease in UK Caucasians. Clin Endocrinol (Oxf) 2004;61(2): 269–72.

58. Houston FA, Wilson V, Jennings CE, et al. Role of the CD40 locus in Graves' disease. Thyroid 2004;14(7):506–9.

59. Simmonds MJ, Heward JM, Franklyn JA, et al. The CD40 Kozak SNP: a new susceptibility loci for Graves' disease? Clin Endocrinol 2005;63(2):232–3.

60. Barratt BJ, Payne F, Lowe CE, et al. Remapping the insulin gene/IDDM2 locus in type 1 diabetes. Diabetes 2004;53(7):1884–9.

61. Vafiadis P, Bennett ST, Todd JA, et al. Insulin expression in human thymus is modulated by INS VNTR alleles at the IDDM2 locus. Nat Genet 1997;15(3): 289–92.

62. Chentoufi AA, Polychronakos C. Insulin expression levels in the thymus modulate insulin-specific autoreactive T-cell tolerance: the mechanism by which the IDDM2 locus may predispose to diabetes. Diabetes 2002;51(5):1383–90.

63. Vafiadis P, Bennett ST, Colle E, et al. Imprinted and genotype-specific expression of genes at the IDDM2 locus in pancreas and leucocytes. J Autoimmun 1996; 9(3):397–403.

64. Wellcome Trust Case Control Consortium. Genome-wide association study of 14,000 cases of seven common diseases and 3,000 shared control. Nature 2007;447(7145):661–78.

65. Hakonarson H, Grant SF, Bradfield JP, et al. A genome-wide association study identifies KIAA0350 as a type 1 diabetes gene. Nature 2007;448(7153):591–4.

66. Hakonarson H, Qu HQ, Bradfield JP, et al. A novel susceptibility locus for type 1 diabetes on Chr12q13 identified by a genome-wide association study. Diabetes 2008; doi: 10.2337/db07–1305.

67. Todd JA, Walker NM, Cooper JD, et al. Robust associations of four new chromosome regions from genome-wide analyses of type 1 diabetes. Nat Genet 2007; 39(7):857–64.

68. Hugot JP, Chamaillard M, Zouali H, et al. Association of NOD2 leucine-rich repeat variants with susceptibility to Crohn's disease. Nature 2001;411(6837):599–603.
69. Ogura Y, Bonen DK, Inohara N, et al. A frameshift mutation in NOD2 associated with susceptibility to Crohn's disease. Nature 2001;411(6837):603–6.
70. Mein CA, Esposito L, Dunn MG, et al. A search for type 1 diabetes susceptibility genes in families from the United Kingdom. Nat Genet 1998;19(3):297–300.
71. Taylor JC, Gough SC, Hunt PJ, et al. A Genome-wide screen in 1119 relative pairs with autoimmune thyroid disease. J Clin Endocrinol Metab 2006;91(2):646–53.
72. Terwilliger JD, Hiekkalinna T. An utter refutation of the "Fundamental theorem of the HapMap". Eur J Hum Genet 2006;14(4):426–37.
73. McKinney C, Merriman ME, Chapman PT, et al. Evidence for an influence of chemokine ligand 3-like 1 (CCL3L1) gene copy number on susceptibility to rheumatoid arthritis. Ann Rheum Dis 2008;67(3):409–13.
74. Daly MJ, Altshuler D. Partners in crime. Nat Genet 2005;37(4):337–8.
75. Zhang Y, Liu JS. Bayesian inference of epistatic interactions in case-control studies. Nat Genet 2007;39(9):1167–73.
76. Redon R, Ishikawa S, Fitch KR, et al. Global variation in copy number in the human genome. Nature 2006;444(7118):444–54.
77. Gonzalez E, Kulkarni H, Bolivar H, et al. The influence of CCL3L1 gene-containing segmental duplications on HIV-1/AIDS susceptibility. Science 2005;307(5714):1434–40.
78. Aitman TJ, Dong R, Vyse TJ, et al. Copy number polymorphism in Fcgr3 predisposes to glomerulonephritis in rats and humans. Nature 2006;439(7078):851–5.
79. Fanciulli M, Norsworthy PJ, Petretto E, et al. FCGR3B copy number variation is associated with susceptibility to systemic but not organ-specific autoimmunity. Nat Genet 2007;39(6):721–3.
80. Xiao Yu X, Sun J-P, He Y, et al. Structure, inhibitor, and regulatory mechanism of a lymphoid-specific tyrosine phosphatase implicated in autoimmune diseases. Proc Natl Acad Sci U S A 2007;104(50):19767–72.

# Advances in Type 1 Diabetes Therapeutics: Immunomodulation and β-Cell Salvage

Frank Waldron-Lynch, MD, PhD[a,b], Kevan C. Herold, MD[a,b,*]

**KEYWORDS**

• Type 1 diabetes • Immune therapy • Autoimmunity • β-cell

Type 1 diabetes is the commonest severe chronic autoimmune endocrine disease accounting for 90% of childhood-onset diabetes and 5% to 10% of adult diabetes. In the United States there are 30,000 new cases annually with 1 in 300 children and 1 in 100 adults affected.[1] Worldwide the incidence of type 1 diabetes is increasing at approximately 2% to 5% per year,[2] with the median age of diagnosis decreasing.[3,4] Overall there are between 10 and 20 million people affected worldwide with significant health care and societal costs.[5]

## IMMUNOPATHOGENESIS OF TYPE 1 DIABETES

The etiology of insulin deficiency is a loss of immune tolerance to pancreatic β cells leading to β-cell dysfunction and, with disease progression, destruction.[6,7] Much clinical and experimental evidence supports that Type 1 diabetes is an autoimmune-mediated disease, which develops in genetically susceptible individuals and reflects the loss of immune tolerance; possibly caused by a normal immune response to altered-self or a loss of the normal mechanisms that prevent responses to self. Murine models of type 1 diabetes have been bred to investigate the immunopathogenesis of the disease and to test therapeutic strategies; the most widely studied model is the non-obese diabetic (NOD) mouse.[8–10] Evidence from this and other models has supported the pivotal role of T cells as the key mediators in the degeneration of pancreatic β cells with contributions from other immune cells such as B cells that may play a role in the initiation and amplification of autoimmune responses.[11,12]

Supported by grants: DK068678, DK063608, DK61035, the Juvenile Diabetes Research Foundation, and the William Brehm Foundation.

[a] Department of Immunobiology, Yale University, 10 Amistad Street, 131D, New Haven, CT 06520, USA
[b] Department of Internal Medicine, 333 Cedar Street, New Haven, CT 06520, USA
* Corresponding author. Department of Immunobiology, Yale University, 10 Amistad St, 131D, New Haven, CT 06520.
E-mail address: Kevan.herold@yale.edu (K.C. Herold).

Endocrinol Metab Clin N Am 38 (2009) 303–317
doi:10.1016/j.ecl.2009.01.005
0889-8529/09/$ – see front matter © 2009 Elsevier Inc. All rights reserved.

endo.theclinics.com

At the clinical onset of type 1 diabetes a mononuclear infiltrate of macrophages, B lymphocytes, and T lymphocytes has been observed in biopsies of pancreatic islets in NOD mice and in patients.[13,14] There are, however, clear differences between the lesions that are seen in humans and mice that suggest differences in the pathogenic mechanisms that lead to the common end point of hyperglycemia and β-cell destruction in both cases. In the islets of NOD mice, a very cellular infiltrate is observed that ranges from an infiltrative, destructive insulitis to periinsulitis, which is generally considered to be nondestructive. CD4+ T cells predominate in the lesions. About 50% of the infiltrating cells are B lymphocytes, but there is very little known about the role of these cells in the pathogenesis of insulitis apart from the clear demonstration that they are required. In contrast, the extent of the cellular infiltration in humans is much more modest. CD8+ T cells are more numerous than CD4+ T cells, which are rarely seen, and there is increased Class I major histocompatibility complex (MHC) expression by islet cells. Moreover, innate immune cells can be found. In a recent report of a group of newly diagnosed type 1 diabetes patients, natural killer (NK) cell and viral inclusions were found in three of the six patients, whereas the others had a predominately T-cell infiltrate suggesting that at diagnosis there may be interindividual variability in the pathogenic process.[15]

The strongest genetic association for type 1 diabetes is within the *MHC* region on chromosome 6p21, most strongly within the MHC Class II locus. Other genetic loci linked to the disease include the insulin gene promoter, *CTLA4*, *PTPN22*, the interleukin-2 receptor α chain, and *IFIH1*,[16] but the strength of the genetic effects at these loci are considerably less (see article by authors elsewhere in this issue). Nonetheless, the significance of the logarithm of odds or association score itself does not establish the biologic relevance of the genetic locus, because it may be difficult to identify differences in the frequencies of alleles that are vital for the disease pathogenesis but prevalent in a population. A recent study from the Wellcome Trust Case Control Consortium has identified four additional regions of genetic association.[17]

There is strong experimental evidence from the NOD mouse model that insulin may be the primary autoantigen that the adaptive immune response is directed against in type 1 diabetes, and human data also support the importance of insulin as an antigen.[18,19] In a recent study, Nakayama and colleagues[20,21] found that NOD mice that expressed only an immunologically different form of insulin were protected from development of diabetes and insulitis. A number of autoantigens have been identified. Glutamic acid decarboxylase-65 (GAD65), the original "64K" antigen recognized by islet cell surface antibodies from patients, has been suggested to be a primary antigen by some, but not all, investigators. Others, such as pancreatic islet-specific glucose-6-phosphatase catalytic subunit related protein (IGRP), are recognized by pathogenic T cells but appear to be secondary in the timing of their appearance and role in the disease. For example, NOD mice that are tolerant to proinsulin do not develop IGRP reactive T cells or diabetes. However, mice tolerant to IGRP develop insulitis and progress to diabetes. Even transgenic mice that express IGRP-reactive T cells do not progress to diabetes when tolerant to proinsulin. The tolerance can be broken and diabetes can be induced when islet inflammation, induced with streptozotocin, is provided.[22]

Pancreatic β-cell destruction is a chronic process. Observational studies, beginning with discordant twins and triplets that were followed until the onset of diabetes, and more recent studies in relatives of subjects with diabetes have described the progression of disease. The risk of diabetes appears to be related to the number of autoantibodies that are recognized, suggesting that progression of disease is associated with spreading of the autoantigenic repertoire. In the Diabetes Prevention Trial-1 (DPT-1), individuals with four positive autoantibodies were found to have a risk of disease that exceeded 60% after 5 years. Likewise, metabolic impairment, although not detectable at the earliest stages of disease, also is a good marker of progression. Relatives of patients with type 1 diabetes who are younger than 18 years and are autoantibody positive with impaired glucose tolerance have a greater than 90% risk for the diagnosis of disease within 6 years.

## CURRENT THERAPY AND OUTCOMES

Standard therapy at diagnosis of type 1 diabetes involves the replacement of insulin to prevent life-threatening ketoacidosis. This replacement therapy has been incrementally optimized over more than 80 years with the development of insulin analogs, education programs, glucose monitoring, and cardiovascular risk factor modification to improve clinical outcomes.[23] The Diabetes Control and Complications Trial (DCCT) in 1993 demonstrated that intensive glycemic control reduced the microvascular complications of retinopathy by 34% to 76%, microalbuminuria by 35%, and neuropathy by 65%.[24] The primary data from the DCCT failed to identify a threshold for HbA1c below which complications did not occur, suggesting that at least for microvascular complications, the goal of therapy should be to approximate normal glucose control, although subsequent analyses have questioned this inference. Further advances in medical therapy have led to reduced macrovascular complications, with intensive pharmacologic therapy to control blood pressure and lipids.[25] Despite these advances, most patients are still unable to achieve glycemic targets, with fewer that 5% of patients in the intensively treated group achieving glycemic targets despite considerable clinical support.[24] Intensive insulin therapy is also associated with the significant side effects of increased serious hypoglycaemia,[26] weight gain,[27] and excessive diurnal glucose fluctuations.[28] Unfortunately, type 1 diabetic patients continue to have a reduced life expectancy of 10 to 15 years because of macrovascular and microvascular complications.[29] This has led to significant efforts to develop immunotherapy and islet transplant therapies to prevent the onset or cure type 1 diabetes.

## MODEL OF CURATIVE TREATMENT

A successful treatment strategy to reverse the pathogenesis of type 1 diabetes needs three components: a remission-induction therapy to arrest immune-mediated destruction of the β cells combined with maintenance therapy to prevent reemergence of autoimmunity, followed by tropic or augmentation therapy to expand β-cell mass, thereby ensuring insulin independence.[30] In this article we discuss the use of immunomodulation to induce remission from autoimmunity and ideally to restore tolerance to pancreatic β cells. Finally, we describe mechanisms to expand endogenous pancreatic islets. A key consideration with these potential treatments is that they need to be acceptable to patients with type 1 diabetes and produce similar if not better outcomes than current insulin replacement therapy.

## ANTIGEN-SPECIFIC IMMUNE MODULATION
### Mechanism

Antigen-specific approaches attempt to direct the immune system away from polyclonal diabetogenic T-cell responses by modulating responses to specific key antigens (**Fig. 1**).[31] Initially, it was though that restoration of self-tolerance may occur through anergy or deletion of self-reactive T cells at high doses of antigen. More recently, data from animal models have shown that antigen-specific regulatory T cells

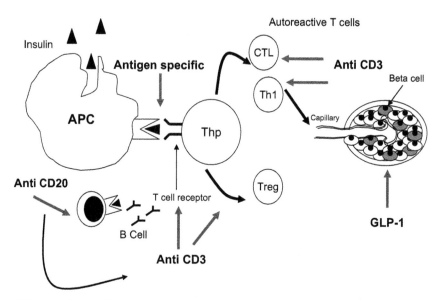

**Fig.1.** Therapeutic targets in type 1 diabetes. An autoantigen is presented to an antigen presenting cell (APC). The antigen is processed to epitopes which are bound and displayed on Class II MHC molecule. Recognition of the antigen/MHC complex by autoantigen reactive, but undifferentiated T cells (Thp) causes their activation and differentiation into effector T cells and activation of other effector T cells that are capable of directly destroying beta cells. In addition to presenting antigen, APCs produce proinflammatory cytokines such as interleukin (IL-1) and tumor necrosis factor (TNF) that lead to the recruitment and activation of autoreactive T-cells. B lymphocytes can serve as antigen presenting cells and are required for disease development. Antigen specific therapies with insulin, Diapep277 or Glutamic acid decarboxylase (GAD65) have been proposed to down-regulate T cell activation and/or induce regulatory T cells (Treg). Anti-CD3 monoclonal antibodies (mAb) bind to the T cell receptor complex and are thought to induce a transient depletion of pathogenic T cells followed by induction of a Tregs. Anti-CD20mAb causes depletion of auto reactive B cells. Glucagon-like peptide 1 (GLP-1) improves recovery of residual β-cell function.

(Tregs) can inhibit even a polyclonal autoreactive T-cell response following direct contact, by bystander or linked suppression in which other cells in the environment of the Tregs are inhibited, and themselves can then regulate immune responses (infectious tolerance).[32,33] The specificity of the response means that the tolerogenic actions avoid the complications of systemic immunosuppression. An important issue for the therapeutic application of this mechanism is an understanding of the activation requirements that induce regulatory versus effector T cells. In the NOD mouse, intranasal administration of insulin can exacerbate diabetes when the peptide used for immunization includes a Class I MHC cytotoxic T lymphocyte (CTL) epitope, but causes protection from diabetes when the CTL epitope is eliminated and the mice are administered the Class II binding peptide. In human trials to date, there has not been evidence for exacerbation of disease following vaccination with antigens.[34]

### Human Trials—Insulin, Diapep277, GAD65

#### Insulin

Therapeutic trials have been undertaken in humans to test whether antigen therapy could be successful in the prevention of diabetes in individuals with a high risk for development of disease, based on their familial relationship to patients with diabetes and autoantibody status (secondary prevention), or in patients with recent-onset type 1 diabetes (intervention study).[35] The choice of antigens was largely determined from previous success in ameliorating type 1 diabetes in rodent models[36] and very small human trials.[37,38] The largest trial, DPT-1, involved the screening of 100,000 first- and second-degree relatives for type 1 diabetes–associated autoantibodies. High-risk individuals were then invited to participate and randomized to three groups: treatment with oral insulin, treatment with low-dose subcutaneous insulin twice a day, or observation alone. At completion of DPT-1, no difference was observed in progression to diabetes between the treatment and control subjects. Subsequently, a subgroup analysis demonstrated that oral insulin had a treatment effect in subjects with high titers of insulin antibodies (IAA), suggesting the possible importance of matching treatment to the dominant autoimmune epitope.[39] A new trial has been commenced in relatives expressing IAA to determine the utility of the treatment.[40] Similarly studies with intranasal insulin have shown immunomodulatory effects in humans[41] and results from phase II trials are awaited to determine efficacy.[42]

### Diapep277

The peptide Diapep277 corresponds to positions 437 to 460 of the human heat shock protein 60 (HSP 60). In children and in murine models of type 1 diabetes, this peptide has been found to be an immunodominant epitope.[43] HSP 60 is found located on the membranes of the β-cell secretary granules and shares significant homology to bacterial HSP65.[44,45] In rodent models of type 1 diabetes, Diapep277 had been demonstrated to significantly reduce the development of diabetes when combined with dietary modifications.[46] Initially Diapep277 was thought to change the phenotype of T-cell responses from a Th1 (cellular) to a Th2 (humoral) response. More recent studies have suggested that HSP60 can interact with T cells directly through TLR2.[47,48] Initially a phase II randomized controlled double-blind trial in newly diagnosed type 1 patients demonstrated preserved endogenous insulin production and less requirement for exogenous insulin at 10 months.[49] However, recent trials over a 2-year duration demonstrated that whereas there was some preservation of C-peptide secretion, there was no effect on daily insulin requirement or HbA1c levels in the treated groups.[50–53]

### GAD65

Glutamic acid decarboxylase 65 (GAD65) is a protein that has been identified as a major islet autoantigen in type 1 diabetes.[54] Autoreactive T-cell responses to GAD65 are found in type 1 patients and individuals at high risk of development of type 1 diabetes.[55] In the NOD mice, administration of GAD65 by oral, nasal, and intravenous routes was able to prevent diabetes.[56,57] A primary safety trial of GAD65 as an antigen-specific therapy in a small number of patents with latent autoimmune diabetes of adulthood (LADA) showed increasing C-peptide levels and the induction of Treg.[58] A similar study has been performed in children by Diamyd and publication of the complete results is awaited.[59]

### NON–ANTIGEN SPECIFIC
#### Diabetes Prevention—Nicotinamide

Several diabetes prevention trials have been undertaken to determine if the administration of the B vitamin nicotinamide would avoid the development of type 1 diabetes in susceptible children. Nicotinamide had previously been demonstrated to prevent diabetes in rodent models.[60,61] In addition, limited studies in humans had suggested that nicotinamide could provide β-cell protection after the diagnosis of type 1 diabetes. These observations led to the European-Canadian Nicotinamide Diabetes Intervention Trial (ENDIT) to determine the effect of nicotinamide on the development of type 1 diabetes. In total 30,000 relatives were screened at 324 centers in 20 countries for entry with 522 eligible children identified. No difference was observed between the treated and untreated group in the rate of development of diabetes.[62] Similarly, pilot studies with nicotinamide plus cyclosporin, vitamin E, and intensive insulin therapy have also failed to demonstrate efficacy in treatment of new-onset type 1 diabetes.[63–65]

### Non–Antigen-Specific Immunomodulation

The first intervention trials of immunosuppressive agents in recent-onset type 1 diabetes involved testing agents that had been previously used successfully in solid organ transplantation protocols to deplete or inactivate T cells. Cyclosporin A and azathioprine with prednisolone reduced the need for administration of subcutaneous insulin and reduced the rate of C-peptide loss.[66–69] This therapeutic approach did not restore self-tolerance, as the beneficial effects were limited to the duration of the therapy and patients relapsed after withdrawal of therapy.[70] The significant chronic side effects of these drugs combined with the need for constant administration precluded widespread clinical use.[71] Recently, a new combination strategy of two doses of daclizumab (anti-CD25 antibody) with daily administration of mycophenolate mofetil has commenced clinical trials. Enrollment was completed in January 2007 with the study planned for a 2-year duration (see **Fig. 1**).[40]

### Anti-CD3 Monoclonal Antibodies

Anti-CD3 monoclonal antibodies (mAb) were initially developed and used successfully to treat solid organ allograft rejection in humans.[72,73] Anti-CD3 mAb binds to the T-cell receptor-CD3 complex down-regulating T-cell–mediated antigen responses (antigenic modulation) and inducing anergy in activated T cells.[74,75] Preclinical trials on the NOD mouse demonstrated that a single short course of anti-CD3 mAb produced and maintained remission from diabetes without the need for continuous administration.[76] In addition, the immunomodulation was selective, with the murine responses to exogenous antigens being normal several weeks after treatment.[77] Modification of the Fc region of the antibody to prevent Fc-receptor (FcR) binding eliminated the cytokine release syndrome and prevented major T-cell depletion.[78] In the NOD model, the mechanism of action of the bivalent modified FcR-nonbinding anti-human CD3 mAb (hOKT3γ1 [Ala-Ala]) appears to be in two consecutive phases. The first phase involves a transient depletion of pathogenic T cells. The second induces a subset of Tregs that suppress the activity of pathogenic T cells establishing immune tolerance and accounting for the duration of treatment effect.[79–81]

The first human trials of patients with recent-onset type 1 diabetes using the hOKT3γ1(Ala-Ala) antibody demonstrated that a single course of treatment led to a maintenance of C-peptide responses at 1 year post diagnosis. At 2 years post diagnosis, treated patients had lower HbA1c and reduced insulin usage. C-peptide responses had declined but remained significantly higher than in the untreated group, indicating preservation of β-cell mass.[82,83] Similar clinical findings were reported by Keymeulen and colleagues[84] who used the ChAglyCD3 mAb (glycosylated anti-CD3 FcR non-binding) at higher doses. Patients in the treated group at 18 months had maintained baseline insulin production and had lower exogenous insulin requirement. The best outcomes were observed in patients with the greatest insulin secretary capacity at enrollment. In both treatments a mild cytokine release syndrome was reported, likely related to a degree to T-cell activation. In the trial of the ChAglyCD3, a transient self-limiting reactivation of Epstein-Barr virus with clinical symptoms was also reported.

The improvements in C-peptide responses and metabolic parameters in humans following anti-CD3 mAb are not maintained indefinitely, despite evidence from the NOD mouse that remission was permanent.[85] The etiology of the temporary remission in humans is unclear but may relate to the reemergence or development of autoreactive T cells after an initial clearance, owing to the chronic autoimmune process underlying type 1 diabetes.[86] The transient reestablishment of immune homeostasis with anti-CD3 mAb may provide a therapeutic window to intervene and consolidate self-tolerance to the pancreatic islets with other immunomodulatory agents.[87] Among the combination approaches that have shown efficacy in rodent models is the administration of antigen at the time of the anti-CD3 mAb. In the NOD mouse, this was shown to induce antigen-specific regulatory T cells that could modulate disease.[88]

## Rituximab (anti-CD20)

Early studies, using anti-IgM to deplete B lymphocytes had shown that these cells were required for the initiation of insulitis and diabetes in the NOD mouse. It was widely believed that any role for B cells must be at the initiation of the disease, possibly as antigen-presenting cells, because at the time of onset, T lymphocytes and even T-cell clones were capable of adoptively transferring disease to naïve animals. Moreover, there was little evidence that immunoglobulins played a significant pathologic role, although a prior study had shown that the offspring of B-cell deficient NOD mothers did not develop diabetes, indicating that transplacental passage of a factor was required. The lack of a suitable anti-CD20 antibody for use in rodents limited studies of the B-cell mechanisms that might be involved in diabetes. Therefore, it was not until the availability of a transgenic mouse in which human CD20 was expressed on B lymphocytes that the effects of anti-CD20 mAb could be tested. Surprisingly, not only did the anti-CD20 mAb prevent the onset of diabetes in these NOD mice when administered at 4 or 9 weeks of age, but it also induced reversal of diabetes and produced lasting tolerance when administered at the time of hyperglycemia onset. Studies by these investigators suggest that treatment with anti-CD20 mAb induced a population of B cells with regulatory properties. The effects of anti-CD20 in human type 1 diabetes will be known with the completion of a Rituximab trial, scheduled in fall 2008.[89]

### PANCREATIC β-CELL THERAPY

Human islet cells have the capacity to expand and contract according to metabolic demands. During normal growth and pregnancy β-cell mass expands to meet metabolic demands.[90] In type 1 diabetes, children or adolescents do not appear to achieve full adult β-cell mass before the development of clinically overt diabetes.[91] Although the residual β-cells are present at the diagnosis of type 1 diabetes, they are functionally impaired in their responses to glycemia.[92] Further loss of β-cell mass may be temporarily delayed by the restoration of euglycemia via the administration of subcutaneous insulin as clinically evident by the temporary reduction in insulin requirements during a honeymoon phase of disease.[93] However following the honeymoon period there is persistent decline in endogenous insulin production.[94]

Studies in hyperglycemic NOD mice demonstrate that β-cells are present before treatment but are dysfunctional in insulin secretion. Following anti-CD3 mAb therapy there is a recovery in β-cell function. The apparent increase in β-cell mass observed is accounted for by recovery in β-cell function with a lesser contribution from regeneration of new β cells.[95] The incretin, glucagon-like peptide 1 (GLP-1) receptor, has been demonstrated to stimulate β-cell replication in rodents.[96] A constant infusion of GLP-1 in prediabetic NOD mice reduces the rate of β-cell apoptosis and increases β-cell mass, delaying the onset of diabetes.[97] In humans, high levels of GLP-1 found after gastric bypass have been postulated to contribute to the overgrowth of pancreatic β cells (nesidioblastosis) that rarely occurs postoperatively.[98,99] Both GLP-1 and the inhibitor of dipeptidyl transferase IV (DPPIV), an enzyme (Sitagliptin) that metabolizes GLP-1, are widely used in the treatment of type 2 diabetes.[100] A sequential treatment of immunomodulation with antilymphocyte serum followed by exendin-4 (GLP-1 receptor agonist) induced complete remission in 90% of diabetic NOD mice treated.[101] A recent study of diabetic NOD mice treated with anti-CD3 mAb and exendin-4 improved the rate of remission of diabetes compared with anti-CD3 mAb alone. However, the effect of exendin-4 was to improve the recovery of residual β-cell function after treatment with anti-CD3 mAb. Not surprisingly, the effects of treatment were greatest in mice with the largest residual β-cell mass.[102] These results provide evidence that a combination of immunomodulation followed by metabolic treatment may have additive effects in individuals with a degree of preserved β-cell islet function.

## FUTURE THERAPY
### Earlier Intervention with Effective Therapies

As the results from ongoing intervention trials of non–antigen-specific therapies become available, the balance between the certainty of prediction of diabetes and the safety and efficacy of these agents will need to be reconsidered. Newer analyses from DPT-1 suggest that serologic markers and metabolic studies can identify relatives of patients at extraordinary risk for the future development of diabetes. For example, among unaffected first-degree relatives younger than 18, those with glucose intolerance have a greater than 90% risk of meeting the diagnostic criteria for diabetes within a 6-year period.[103] Furthermore, individuals with four autoantibodies (IAA, anti-ICA512, anti-GAD65, and ICA) have a greater than 50% risk of fulfilling the diagnosis within 5 years.[104] Agents that would have been considered appropriate only for patients with established disease might in the future be considered for use in these high-risk individuals, even before frank hyperglycemia is present, with the goal of preserving functional β-cell mass.

### Combination Therapy

From human studies of antigen-specific and non–antigen-specific therapies and islet transplantation, it has become apparent that it is unlikely that a single therapeutic approach will be successful in ensuring adequate β-cell mass in all type 1 diabetes patients. The difficulties in the development of treatment protocols largely relate to our lack of a complete understanding of the immune mechanisms that precipitate and drive the disease process, and the etiology of β-cell failure late in the course of the disease.[30] However, given that these processes may be different, it would appear appropriate to combine and sequence treatments to determine if outcomes can be improved.[105] Care should be taken in the immunosuppressive combinations, because establishment of dominant tolerance requires the generation, de novo, of Tregs and may be inhibited by specific immunosuppressive drugs that block T-cell activation signals.[106] Similarly, the administration of Sirolimus and Tacrolimus, the systemic immunosuppressants used in the Edmonton transplantation protocol, have been found to inhibit β-cell regeneration in a murine model of diabetes.[107]

Preclinical studies combining nasal proinsulin (antigen specific) with anti-CD3 mAb (antigen nonspecific) in NOD mice demonstrated greater efficacy than either monotherapy. This outcome was mediated in vivo by induction of insulin-specific Tregs that could transfer dominant tolerance to recent-onset diabetic recipients suppressing autoaggressive CD8 responses.[88] This finding has raised the possibility of cell-based tolerogenic therapy.[108]

## The Need for Biomarkers

One of the most vexing problems in the field has been the absence of validated biomarkers for the autoimmune response that can be used to judge the activity of the disease and the responses to therapies. Measurement of autoantibody titers does not appear to be a good marker of the process because they have not been shown to change with interventions in which the natural history of the disease has been altered, such as following anti-CD3 mAb. Without a biomarker, trials frequently need to be performed for 1 year or longer, until there is evidence of a change in metabolic function. This measurement is not optimal because it reflects the end point of the process that one hopes to block, rather than a measure of the process itself. Some biomarker assays have shown discriminant ability in comparing responses in subjects with type 1 diabetes with healthy controls in blinded studies. Others provide mechanistic insights but have not been widely tested. Most evaluated approaches have used classic cellular immunologic methods. Newer technologies including MHC tetramers and gene expression signatures are now being developed and tested, and have been used in other autoimmune diseases.[109,110]

## SUMMARY

New immunotherapeutics have shown efficacy in altering the natural course of type 1 diabetes. They have not completely reversed the metabolic dysfunction, and the potential contribution of spontaneous β-cell regeneration to recovery, when the autoimmune process has been arrested, is not clear in humans. A number of new immunomodulatory approaches, both antigen specific and non–antigen specific, will be evaluated in the next few years. However, even with successful immunotherapy, full restoration of metabolic control is likely to require the addition of therapy to augment β-cell function or mass. An approach that would obviate this would be to prevent progression of the disease from the prediagnosis stage. New information on the risks of disease in autoantibody relatives with metabolic dysfunction indicates that successful intervention in this group would be appropriate.

## REFERENCES

1. La Porte RE, Matsushima M, Chang YF. Prevalence and incidence of insulin-dependant diabetes. 2nd Edition. Bethesda: National Institutes of Health, NIH publ; 1995. No. 95-1468.
2. Onkamo P, Vaananen S, Karvonen M, et al. World wide increase in the incidence of Type 1 diabetes—analysis of the data on published incidence trends. Diabetologia 1999;42:1395–403.
3. Dahlquist G, Mustonen L. Analysis of 20 years of prospective registration of childhood onset diabetes time trends and birth cohort effects. Swedish Childhood Study Group. Acta Paediatr 2000;89:1231–7.
4. Weet I, De Leeuw IH, Du Caju MV, et al. The incidence of type 1 diabetes in the age group 0-39 years has not increased in Antwerp (Belgium) between 1989 and 2000. Diabetes Care 2002;25:840–6.

5. World Health Organization. Available at: http://www.who.int/en. Accessed December 1, 2008.
6. Atkinson MA. ADA Outstanding Scientific Achievement Lecture 2004. Thirty years of investigating the autoimmune basis for type 1 diabetes: why can't we prevent or reverse this disease? Diabetes 2005;54:1253–63.
7. Steele C, Hagopian WA, Gitelman S, et al. Insulin secretion in type 1 diabetes. Diabetes 2004;53(2):426–33.
8. Delovitch TL, Singh B. The nonobese diabetic mouse as a model of autoimmune diabetes: immune dysregulation gets the NOD. Immunity 1997;7(6):727–38.
9. Wen L, Chen NY, Tang J, et al. The regulatory role of DR4 in a spontaneous diabetes DQ8 transgenic model. J Clin Invest 2001;107(7):871–80.
10. Roy CJ, Warfield KL, Welcher BC, et al. Human leukocyte antigen-DQ8 transgenic mice: a model to examine the toxicity of aerosolized staphylococcal enterotoxin B. Infect Immun 2005;73(4):2452–60.
11. Wicker LS, Leiter EH, Todd JA, et al. Beta 2-microglobulin-deficient NOD mice do not develop insulitis or diabetes. Diabetes 1994;43(3):500–4.
12. Serreze DV, Silveira PA. The role of B lymphocytes as key antigen-presenting cells in the development of T cell-mediated autoimmune type 1 diabetes. Curr Dir Autoimmun 2003;6:212–27.
13. Foulis AK, McGill M, Farquharson MA. Insulitis in type 1 (insulin-dependent) diabetes mellitus in man–macrophages, lymphocytes, and interferon-gamma containing cells. J Pathol 1991;165(2):97–103.
14. Itoh N, Hanafusa T, Miyazaki A, et al. Mononuclear cell infiltration and its relation to the expression of major histocompatibility complex antigens and adhesion molecules in pancreas biopsy specimens from newly diagnosed insulin-dependent diabetes mellitus patients. J Clin Invest 1993;92:2313–22.
15. Dotta F, Censini S, van Halteren AG, et al. Coxsackie B4 virus infection of beta cells and natural killer cell insulitis in recent-onset type 1 diabetic patients. Proc Natl Acad Sci U S A 2007;104(12):5115–20.
16. Wang WY, Barratt BJ, Clayton DG, et al. Genome-wide association studies: theoretical and practical concerns. Nat Rev Genet 2005;6(2):109–18.
17. Todd JA, Walker NM, Cooper JD, et al. Robust associations of four new chromosome regions from genome-wide analyses of type 1 diabetes. Nat Genet 2007;39(7):857–64.
18. Kent SC, Chen Y, Bregoli L, et al. Expanded T cells from pancreatic lymph nodes of type 1 diabetic subjects recognize the insulin epitope. Nature 2005;435:224–8.
19. Mannering SI, Harrison LC, Williamson NA, et al. The insulin A-chain epitope recognized by human T cells is post translationally modified. J Exp Med 2005;202:1191–7.
20. Nakayama M, Abiru N, Moriyama H, et al. Prime role for an insulin epitope in the development of type 1 diabetes in NOD mice. Nature 2005;435(7039):220–3.
21. Jahromi MM, Eisenbarth GS. Cellular and molecular pathogenesis of type 1A diabetes. Cell Mol Life Sci 2007;64:865–72.
22. Krishnamurthy B, Mariana L, Gellert SA, et al. Autoimmunity to both proinsulin and IGRP is required for diabetes in nonobese diabetic 8.3 TCR transgenic mice. J Immunol 2008;180(7):4458–64.
23. American Diabetes Association. Standards of medical care in diabetes—2008. Diabetes Care 2008;31:S12–54.
24. Diabetes Control and Complications Trial Research Group. The effect of intensive treatment of diabetes on the development and progression of long-term complications in insulin-dependent diabetes mellitus. N Engl J Med 1993;329:977–86.

25. Perkin BA, Ficocrello LH, Silva KH, et al. Regression of microalbuminuria in type 1 diabetes. N Engl J Med 2003;348:2085–93.
26. Diabetes Control and Complications Trial Research Group. Hypoglycemia in the Diabetes Control and Complications Trial. Diabetes 1997;46(2):271–86.
27. Purnell JQ, Hokanson JE, Marcovina SM, et al. Effect of excessive weight gain with insulin therapy of type 1 diabetes on lipid levels and blood pressure: results from the DCCT. The Diabetes Control and Complications Trial. JAMA 1998;280: 140–6.
28. Boland E, Monsod T, Delucia M, et al. Limitations of conventional methods of self monitoring of blood glucose: lessons learned from three days of continuous glucose sensing in paediatric patients with type 1 diabetes. Diabetes Care 2001;24(11):1858–62.
29. Liu E, Eisenbarth GS. Type IA diabetes mellitus-associated autoimmunity. Endocrinol Metab Clin North Am 2002;31:391–410, vii–viii.
30. Waldron-Lynch F, von Herrath M, Herold KC. Towards a curative therapy in type 1 diabetes: remission of autoimmunity, maintenance and augmentation of β cell mass. 2007 Defining Optimal Immunotherapies for Type 1 Diabetes. Novartis Found Symp 2009;292:146–55.
31. Fousteri G, Bresson, von Herrath M. Rational development of antigen-specific therapies for type 1 diabetes. Adv Exp Med Biol 2007;601:313–9.
32. Cobbold SP, Nolan KF, Graca L, et al. Regulatory T cells and dendritic cells in transplantation tolerance: molecular markers and mechanisms. Immunol Rev 2003;196:109–24.
33. St. Clair EM, Turka LA, Saxon A, et al. New reagents on the horizon for immune tolerance. Annu Rev Med 2007;58:329–46.
34. Graca L, Chen TC, Le Moine A, et al. Dominant tolerance: activation thresholds for peripheral generation of regulatory T cells. Trends Immunol 2005;26:131–5.
35. Haller MJ, Gottieb PA, Schatz DA. Type 1 diabetes intervention trials 2007: where are we and where are we going? Curr Opin Endocrinol Diabetes Obes 2007;14:283–7.
36. Roep BO. Are insights gained from NOD mice sufficient to guide clinical translation? Ann N Y Acad Sci 2007;1103:1–10.
37. Keller RJ, Eisenbarth GS, Jackson RA. Insulin prophylaxis in individuals at high risk of type 1 diabetes. Lancet 1993;341:927–8.
38. Fuchtenbusch M, Rabl W, Grassi B, et al. Delay of type 1 diabetes in high risk, first degree relatives by parental antigen administration: the Schwabling Insulin Prophylaxis Pilot Trial. Diabetologia 1998;41:536–41.
39. Skyler JS, Krischer JP, Wolfsorf J, et al. Effects of oral insulin in relatives of patients with type 1 diabetes. Diabetes Prevention Trial-Type 1. Diabetes Care 2005;28:1068–76.
40. Available at: http://www.diabetestrialnet.org. Accessed December 1, 2008.
41. Harrison LC, Honeyman MC, Steele CE, et al. Pancreatic beta-cell function and immune responses to insulin after administration of intranasal insulin to humans at risk for type 1 diabetes. Diabetes Care 2004;27(10):2348–55.
42. Available at: http://www.thegeorgeinstitute.org. Accessed December 1, 2008.
43. Horvath L, Cervenak L, Orosazlan M, et al. Antibiodies against different epitopes of heat shock protein 60 in children with type 1 diabetes mellitus. Immunol Lett 2002;80(3):155–62.
44. Brudzynski K, Martinez V, Gupta RS. Secretory granule autoantigen in insulin-dependent diabetes mellitus is related to 62 kDa heat-shock protein (hsp60). J Autoimmun 1992;5(4):453–63.

45. Cohen IR. Peptide therapy for type 1 diabetes: the immunological homunculus and the rational for vaccination. Diabetologia 2002;45:1468–74.
46. Brugman S, Klatter FA, Visser J, et al. Neonatal administration of DiaPep277 combined with hydrolysed casein diet, protects against Type 1 diabetes in BB-DP rat. An experimental study. Diabetologia 2004;47(7):1331–3.
47. Zanin-Zhorov A, Bruck R, Tal G, et al. Heat shock protein 60 inhibits Th1-mediated hepatitis model via innate regulation of Th1/Th2 transcription factors and cytokines. J Immunol 2005;174(6):3227–36.
48. Nussbaum G, Zanin-Zhorov A, Quintana F, et al. Peptide p277 of HSP60 signals T cells: inhibition of inflammatory chemotaxis. Int Immunol 2006;18: 1413–9.
49. Raz I, Elias D, Avron A, et al. Beta cell function in new-onset type 1 diabetes and immunomodulation with heat-shock protein peptide (DiaPep277): a randomised, double-blind, phase II trial. Lancet 2001;358:1749–53.
50. Elias D, Raz I, Avron A, et al. Treatment of new-onset type 1 diabetes with peptide DiaPep277 is safe and associated with preserved beta-cell function: extension of a randomised, double-blind, phase II trial. Diabetes Metab Res Rev 2007;23:292–8.
51. Roep B, Huurman V, Decochez K, et al. Therapy with the hsp60 peptide Dia-Pep277 in C-peptide positive type 1 diabetes patients. Diabetes Metab Res Rev 2007;23:269–75.
52. Schloot N, Meierhoff G, Lengyel C, et al. Effect of heat shock protein peptide Di-aPep277 on β-cell function in paediatric and adult patients with recent-onset diabetes mellitus type 1: two prospective, randomised, double blind phase II trials. Diabetes Metab Res Rev 2007;23:276–85.
53. Lazar L, Ofan R, Weintrob N, et al. Heat-shock protein peptide DiaPep277 treatment in children with newly diagnosed type 1 diabetes: a randomised, double-blind phase II study. Diabetes Metab Res Rev 2007;23:286–91.
54. Baekkeskov S, Aanstoot HJ, Christgau S, et al. Identification of the 64K autoantigen in insulin-dependent diabetes as the GABA-synthesizing enzyme glutamic acid decarboxylase. Nature 1990;347:151–6.
55. Oling V, Marttila J, Ilonen J, et al. GAD65 and proinsulin-specific CD4 + T cells detected by MHC class II tetramers in peripheral blood of type 1 diabetes patients and at-risk subjects. J Autoimmun 2005;25:235–43.
56. Tian J, Atkinson MA, Clare-Salzler M, et al. Nasal administration of glutamate decarboxylase (GAD65) peptides induces Th2 responses and prevents murine insulin-dependent diabetes. J Exp Med 1996;183:1561–7.
57. Tian J, Clare-Salzler M, Herschenfeld A, et al. Modulating autoimmune responses to GAD inhibits disease progression and prolongs islet graft survival in diabetes-prone mice. Nat Med 1996;2(12):1348–53.
58. Agardh CD, Cilio CM, Lethagen A, et al. Clinical evidence for the safety of GAD65 immunomodulation in adult-onset autoimmune diabetes. J Diabet Complications 2005;19:238–46.
59. Available at: http://www.diamyd.com. Accessed December 1, 2008.
60. Yamada K, Nonaka K, Hanafusa T, et al. Preventive and therapeutic effects of large-dose nicotinamide injections on diabetes associated with insulitis. An observation in nonobese diabetic (NOD) mice. Diabetes 1982;31(9): 749–53.
61. Reddy S, Bibby NJ, Elliott RB. Early nicotinamide treatment in the NOD mouse: effects on diabetes and insulitis suppression and autoantibody levels. Diabetes Res 1990;15:95–102.

62. European Nicotinamide Diabetes Intervention Trial (ENDIT) group. European Nicotinamide Diabetes Intervention Trial (ENDIT): a randomised controlled trial if intervention before the onset of type 1 diabetes. Lancet 2004;363:925–31.
63. Crino A, Schiaffinin R, Manfrini S, et al. A randomized trial of nicotinamide and vitamin E in children with recent onset type 1 diabetes (IMDIAB IX). Eur J Endocrinol 2004;150:719–24.
64. Crino A, Schiaffini R, Ciampalini P, et al. A two year observational study of nicotinamide and intensive insulin therapy in patients with recent onset type 1 diabetes mellitus. J Pediatr Endocrinol Metab 2005;18:749–54.
65. Pozzilli P, Visalli N, Boccuni ML, et al. Randomized trial comparing nicotinamide and nicotinamide plus cyclosporin in recent onset insulin-dependent diabetes (IMDIAB 1). The IMDIAB Study Group. Diabet Med 1994;11:98–104.
66. Stiller CR, Dupre J, Gent M, et al. Effects of cyclosporine immunosuppression in insulin-dependent diabetes mellitus of recent onset. Science 1984;223(4643): 1362–7.
67. Stiller CR, Dupre J, Gent M, et al. Effects of cyclosporine in recent-onset juvenile type 1 diabetes: impact of age and duration of disease. J Pediatr 1987;111(6 Pt 2): 1069–72.
68. Silverstein J, Maclaren N, Riley W, et al. Immunosuppression with azathioprine and prednisone in recent-onset insulin-dependent diabetes mellitus. N Engl J Med 1988;319(10):599–604.
69. Bougneres PF, Carel JC, Castano L, et al. Factors associated with early remission of type I diabetes in children treated with cyclosporine. N Engl J Med 1988;318(11):663–70.
70. Bougnères PF, Landais P, Boisson C, et al. Limited duration of remission of insulin dependency in children with recent overt type I diabetes treated with low-dose cyclosporin. Diabetes 1990;39(10):1264–72.
71. Parving HH, Tarnow L, Nielsen FS, et al. Cyclosporine nephrotoxicity in type 1 diabetic patients. A 7-year follow-up study. Diabetes Care 1999;22(3):478–83.
72. Cosimi AB, Burton RC, Colvin RB, et al. Treatment of acute renal allograft rejection with OKT3 monoclonal antibody. Transplantation 1981;32:535–9.
73. Friend PJ, Hale G, Chatenoud L, et al. Phase I study of an engineered aglycosylated humanized CD3 antibody in renal transplant rejection. Transplantation 1981;32:535–9.
74. Smith JA, Tso JY, Clark MR, et al. Nonmitogenic anti-CD3 monoclonal antibodies deliver a partial T cell receptor signal and induce clonal anergy. J Exp Med 1997; 185:1413–22.
75. Chatenoud L, Baudrihaye MF, Kreis H, et al. Human in vivo antigenic modulation induced by the anti-T cell OKT3 monoclonal antibody. Eur J Immunol 1982; 12(11):979–82.
76. Chatenoud L, Thervet E, Primo J, et al. Anti-CD3 antibody induces long-term remission of overt autoimmunity in nonobese diabetic mice. Proc Natl Acad Sci U S A 1994;91:123–7.
77. Chatenoud L, Primo J, Bach JF. CD3 antibody-induced dominant self tolerance in overtly diabetic NOD mice. J Immunol 1997;158:2947–54.
78. Herold KC, Burton JB, Francois, et al. Activation of human T cells by FcR nonbinding anti-CD3 mAb, hOKT3gamma1 (Ala-Ala). J Clin Invest 2003;111: 409–18.
79. Belghith M, Bluestone JA, Barriot S, et al. TGF-beta-dependent mechanisms mediate restoration of self-tolerance induced by antibodies to CD3 in overt autoimmune diabetes. Nat Med 2003;9(9):1202–8.

80. Bisikirska B, Colgan J, Luban J. TCR stimulation with modified anti-CD3 mAb expands CD8 T cell population and induces CD8CD25 Tregs. J Clin Invest 2005;115(10):2904–13.
81. You S, Leforban B, Garcia C, et al. Adaptive TCG-β-dependent regulatory T cells control autoimmune diabetes and are a privileged target of anti-CD3 antibody treatment. Proc Natl Acad Sci U S A 2007;104:6335–40.
82. Herold KC, Hagopian W, Auger JA, et al. Anti-CD3 monoclonal antibody in new-onset type 1 diabetes mellitus. N Engl J Med 2002;346(22):1692–8.
83. Herold KC, Gitelman SE, Masharani U, et al. A single course of anti-CD3 mono-clonal antibody hOKT3{gamma}1(Ala-Ala) results in improvement in C-peptide responses and clinical parameters for at least 2 years after onset of type 1 dia-betes. Diabetes 2005;54(6):1763–9.
84. Keymeulen B, Vandemeulebroucke E, Ziegler AG, et al. Insulin needs after CD3-antibody therapy in new-onset type 1 diabetes. N Engl J Med 2005;352(25):2598–608.
85. Ablamunits V, Sherry NA, Kushner JA, et al. Autoimmunity and Beta cell regen-eration in mouse and human type 1 diabetes: the peace is not enough. Ann N Y Acad Sci 2007;1103:19–32.
86. Von Herrath M, Sanda S, Herold K. Type 1 diabetes as a relapsing-remitting disease? Nat Rev Immunol 2007;7:988–94.
87. Chatenoud L, Bluestone JA. CD3-specfic antibodies: a portal to the treatment of autoimmunity. Nat Rev Immunol 2007;7:622–32.
88. Bresson D, Togher L, Rodrigo E, et al. Anti-CD3 and nasal proinsulin combina-tion therapy enhances remission from recent-onset autoimmune diabetes by inducing Tregs. J Clin Invest 2006;116:1371–81.
89. Bour-Jordan H, Bluestone JA. B cell depletion: a novel therapy for autoimmune diabetes? J Clin Invest 2007;117(12):3642–5.
90. Bonner-Weir S. Perspective: postnatal pancreatic β cell growth. Endocrinology 2000;141:1926–9.
91. Tsai EB, Sherry NA, Palmer JP, et al. The rise and fall of insulin secretion in type 1 diabetes mellitus. Diabetologia 2006;49:261–70.
92. Sherry NA, Kushner JA, Glandt M, et al. Effects of autoimmunity and immune therapy on beta-cell turnover in type 1 diabetes. Diabetes 2006;55:3238–45.
93. Chase HP, MacKenzie TA, Burdick J, et al. Redefining the clinical remission period in children with type 1 diabetes. Pediatr Diabetes 2004;5(1):16–9.
94. Palmer JP, Fleming GA, Greenbaum CJ, et al. C-peptide is the appropriate outcome measure for type 1 diabetes clinical trials to preserve beta-cell func-tion: report of an ADA workshop, 21–22 October 2001. Diabetes 2004;53(1):250–64.
95. Sherry NA, Tsai EB, Herold KC. Natural history of β-cell function in type 1 dia-betes. Diabetes 2005;54:S32–9.
96. Xu G, Stoffers DA, Habener JF. Exendin-4 stimulates both beta-cell replication and neogenesis, resulting in increased beta-cell mass and improved glucose tolerance in diabetic rats. Diabetes 1999;48(12):2270–6.
97. Zhang J, Tokui Y, Yamagata K, et al. Continuous stimulation of human glucagon-like peptide-1 (7-36) amide in a mouse model (NOD) delays the onset of auto-immune type 1 diabetes. Diabetologia 2007;50:1900–9.
98. Service GJ, Thompson GB, Service FJ, et al. Hyperinsulinemic hypoglycaemia with nesidoblastosis after gastric-bypass surgery. N Engl J Med 2005;353:249–54.

99. Cummings DE, Overduin J, Foster-Schubert KE, et al. Gastric bypass for obesity: mechanisms of weight loss and diabetes resolution. J Clin Endocrinol Metab 2004;89:2608–15.
100. Amori RE, Lau J, Pittas AG. Efficacy and safety of incretin therapy in type 2 diabetes: systematic review and meta-analysis. JAMA 2007;298(2):194–206.
101. Ogawa N, List JF, Habener JF, et al. Cure of overt diabetes in NOD mice by transient treatment with anti-lymphocyte serum and exendin-4. Diabetes 2004;53(7): 1700–5.
102. Sherry NA, Chen W, Kushner JA, et al. Exendin-4 improves reversal of diabetes in NOD mice treated with anti-CD3 monoclonal antibody by enhancing recovery of β-cells. Endocrionology 2007;148:5138–44.
103. Sherr J, Sosenko J, Skyler JS, et al. Prevention of type 1 diabetes: the time has come. Nat Clin Pract Endocrinol Metab 2008;4:334–43.
104. Skyler JS. Prediction and prevention of type 1 diabetes: progress, problems, and prospects. Clin Pharmacol Ther 2007;81:768–71.
105. Bresson D, Von Herrath M. Moving to efficient therapies in type 1 diabetes: to combine or not to combine. Autoimmun Rev 2007;6:315–22.
106. Cobbold SP, Adams E, Graca L, et al. Immune privilege induced by regulatory T cells in transplantation tolerance. Immun 2006;213:239–55.
107. Nir T, Melton DA, Dor Y. Recovery from diabetes in mice β cell regeneration. J Clin Invest 2007;117:2553–61.
108. Bluestone JA, Thomson AW, Shevach EM, et al. What does the future hold for cell-based tolergenic therapy? Nat Rev Immunol 2007;7:650–4.
109. Seyfert-Margolis V, Gisler TD, Asare AL, et al. Analysis of T-cell assays to measure autoimmune responses in subjects with type 1 diabetes. Diabetes 2006;55:2588–94.
110. Bennett L, Palucka AK, Arce E, et al. Interferon and granulopoiesis signatures in systemic lupus erythematosus blood. J Exp Med 2003;197(6):711–23.

# The Thyroid-Stimulating Hormone Receptor: Impact of Thyroid-Stimulating Hormone and Thyroid-Stimulating Hormone Receptor Antibodies on Multimerization, Cleavage, and Signaling

Rauf Latif, PhD[a],*, Syed A. Morshed, PhD[a],
Mone Zaidi, MD[b], Terry F. Davies, MD[a]

**KEYWORDS**

- TSH receptor • Multimerization • Oligomerization
- Signaling • TSHR antibodies • Autoimmune thyroid disease

The thyroid-stimulating hormone receptor (TSHR) (**Fig. 1**) is a G-protein coupled receptor anchored to the surface of thyroid epithelial cells (or thyrocytes). The hormone TSH, synthesized by anterior pituitary thyrotrope cells, binds to the TSHR and regulates thyroid growth and development, as well as thyroid hormone synthesis and release.[1] The TSHR is also the major autoantigen in Graves' disease and is the target of antigen-specific T cells and autoantibodies that either stimulate the gland, leading to hyperthyroidism, or block endogenous TSH leading to hypothyroidism.[1] The transmission of these extracellular signals following the binding of TSH or

Supported in part by DK069713 and DK052464 from National Institute of Diabetes and Digestive and Kidney Diseases, the VA Merit Award Program, and the David Owen Segal Endowment.
[a] Thyroid Research Unit, Mount Sinai School of Medicine and the James J. Peters VA Medical Center, New York, NY 10468, USA
[b] Thyroid Research Unit and the Mount Sinai Bone Program, Mount Sinai School of Medicine, New York, NY 10029, USA
* Corresponding author. 130 West Kingsbridge Road, Bronx, NY 10468.
*E-mail address:* rauf.latif@mssm.edu (R. Latif).

Endocrinol Metab Clin N Am 38 (2009) 319–341
doi:10.1016/j.ecl.2009.01.006
0889-8529/09/$ – see front matter. Published by Elsevier Inc.
endo.theclinics.com

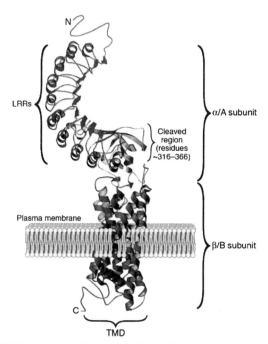

**Fig. 1.** Structure of TSH receptor. This model of the TSHR shows the seven transmembrane domains (TMDs) as spirals embedded within the lipid bilayer of the plasma membrane. The short cytoplasmic tail and the TMDs together make up the β/B subunit of the receptor. The unique 50aa long cleaved region (residues 316–366 aa) is as indicated. The nine leucine rich repeats (LRRs) each consisting of 20–24 aa, are depicted as spirals (α and β pleated sheets) on the ectodomain of the receptor and make up the major portion of the α/A subunit. The LRRs have a characteristic horseshoe shape with a concave inner surface. C, C- terminus; N, N-terminus. (*Adapted from* Davies TF, Ando T, Lin RY, Tomer Y, Latif R. Thyrotropin receptor-associated diseases: from adenomata to Graves disease. J Clin Invest 2005;115:1972–83; with permission.)

autoantibodies to the large extracellular domain of the TSHR is orchestrated via G proteins coupled to transmembrane loops of the TSHR in the inner leaflet of the plasma membrane resulting in activation of a myriad of signaling pathways. This, in turn, leads to proliferation and survival of the thyrocyte. Our understanding of this complex signaling and regulation has broadened in the past decade following better insights into TSHR structure-function and the dynamic changes of the TSHR on the cell surface. This article provides an update on the posttranslational changes in the TSHR, their impact on structure-function, and emphasizes the role of TSHR antibodies (TSHR-Abs) and the insights they have provided.

## THE THYROID-STIMULATING HORMONE RECEPTOR IN DEVELOPMENT, HEALTH, AND DISEASE
### The Thyroid-Stimulating Hormone Receptor in Thyroid Maturation

Since the cloning of the TSHR in 1989[2–4] the gross structure of the TSHR and its function in regulating thyroid cell signaling and proliferation have been exhaustively studied in both primary thyroid cells and TSHR transfected cell culture models. There are several comprehensive reviews on this topic.[5] Further, studies of the role of the TSHR in thyroid development and differentiation have revealed that TSH and the TSHR have pivotal roles in regulating the size and function of the thyroid gland but are not required for early thyroid development. Studies have established that the TSHR plays an important role in the growth of the gland and activation of the TSH/TSHR signaling pathway concurrent with the expression of genes needed for thyroid hormone synthesis and secretion.[5] Such important insights have come from studying abnormal thyroid morphogenesis using various TSHR-defective mice. Several mutant mouse lines derived to possess a nonfunctional TSHR (eg, Tshr[hyt]/Tshr[hyt])[6] showed that the thyroid gland developed to a much smaller size than normal at 2 months of age in the absence of a functional TSHR. Furthermore, the expression levels of thyroid peroxidase (TPO; the enzyme responsible for Tg iodination) and the sodium iodine symporter (NIS; which transports iodine into the thyroid cell) were greatly reduced. Conversely, no significant changes were detected in the amounts of thyroglobulin (Tg), and transcription factors such as paired box gene 8 (PAX8), and thyroid transcription factors (TTF) 1 and 2. Similarly, in our TSHR knockout (TSHR-KO) mouse model, formed by homologous recombination,[7] we found that the thyroid glands were smaller than those of control littermates. Histology of these thyroid glands showed that the TSHR-KO thyroid had fewer follicles and more non–follicle-associated interstitial cells within the gland when compared with wild-type thyroid. Hence, comparing TSHR gene expression with thyroid morphology and other thyroid-specific gene expression in fetal and neonatal thyroid has suggested that the TSHR is essential for terminal thyroid maturation and growth but not essential for the early thyroid organogenesis or migration to its normal anatomical position.[8] The role of the TSHR in humans has been studied by examining fetal thyroid gland formation, which occurs during 7 to 9 weeks of gestation and thyroid embryogenesis is largely complete by 12 weeks. At 12 weeks, the fetal thyroid is capable of concentrating iodide and synthesizing thyroid hormones, which lessens the dependence on maternal thyroid hormone in the second trimester. Fetal TSH is first detectable at 10 weeks of gestation by bioassay and radioimmunoassay.[9] Consistent with the rodent studies, loss of functional maturation of the TSHR in babies, as well as in babies born to mothers with potent TSHR-blocking antibodies, causes hypothyroidism and hypoplastic glands but the thyroid gland in these individuals is located normally.[8] The data, therefore, agree that TSH/TSHR signaling is essential for full thyroid maturation and function. However, the exact role that the TSHR plays in glandular maturation remains unclear, but may be revealed by future embryonic thyroid cell–derived systems able to recapitulate the entire developmental program.[8,10,11]

### Extra-Thyroidal Expression of Thyroid-Stimulating Hormone Receptor

TSHR expression at the mRNA level and, in some cases, at the protein level, has been well documented in extrathyroidal tissues.[12,13] The TSH receptor is highly expressed in adipocytes and bone cells and we discuss in the following sections these two important tissues where the role of the TSHR is well established.

### The role of the thyroid-stimulating hormone receptor in adipocytes

TSH has been shown to induce lipolysis[14] and TSHR-specific immunoreactivity has been demonstrated in fibroblasts and adipose tissue obtained from healthy individuals and patients with Graves' ophthalmopathy and pretibial myxedema.[15] A recent study has shown that TSH stimulates adipogenesis in cultured embryonic stem cells independent of adipogenic factors.[16] In human orbital fibroblasts, TSHR activation renders preadipocytes refractory to PPARgamma-induced adipogenesis, although TSHR activation stimulates early differentiation.[17] Hence, TSHR signal transduction appears to modulate a variety of cellular processes in fibroblasts and adipocytes although it is unclear precisely how TSHR signals interdigitate with the complex network of signaling leading to adipogenesis.[18]

### The role of the thyroid-stimulating hormone receptor in bone

TSHR expression in osteoclasts has been clearly demonstrated and the TSHR has been implicated in the modulation of bone cell function.[19,20] Indeed, our studies provided the first evidence that exogenous administration of low doses of TSH positively influenced bone remodeling by inhibiting osteoclast differentiation and activating osteoblast differentiation, thus eliciting both antiresorptive and anabolic bone effects in aged and ovariectomized rats.[21] The antiresorptive actions of exogenous TSH administration were shown by its ability to prevent the progressive bone loss typically induced immediately after gonadectomy of sexually mature female rats. The anabolic effect of TSH administration was shown by its ability to enhance both trabecular and cortical bone formation 7 months later in aged animals that had established osteopenia, characterized by low bone turnover rates and reduced bone volume. Claims that TSH has no role in bone biology[22] have, therefore, proven premature.

### The Thyroid-Stimulating Hormone Receptor in Disease

Congenital abnormalties in the TSHR and somatic mutations in thyroid adenomata have provided rich insights into structure-function of this complex receptor glycoprotein.[10] In addition, the receptor is the target of the immune response in patients with Graves' disease where both T and B cells are found that recognize TSHR epitopes. TSHR-stimulating antibodies bind to the receptor leading to overstimulation of the gland, thereby increasing levels of the circulating T3 and T4 hormones. The role of TSHR as an antigen in Hashimoto's thyroiditis (HT) is less well established. Whereas TSHR autoantibodies of the blocking variety may be seen in approximately 15% of patients with HT, whether the TSHR serves as a primary T-cell antigen and contributes to the cause of glandular destruction by cytotoxic T cells in HT is unlikely.[23] However, the generation of high-affinity TSHR monoclonal antibodies with stimulating, blocking, or no functional activity from several laboratories, including our own[24–26] has further advanced the understanding of TSHR signaling both in vitro and in vivo and has given us the tools to study posttranslational changes in the TSHR.[27,28]

### THYROID-STIMULATING HORMONE RECEPTOR STRUCTURE AND FUNCTION

The *TSHR* gene on chromosome 14q31[29] codes for a 764 amino acid protein, which is divided into a signal peptide of 21 amino acids, a large glycosylated ectodomain of 394 residues encoded by 9 exons and the remaining 349 residues, encoded by the 10th and largest exon, which constitutes the 7 transmembrane domains and cytoplasmic tail. The sequence also revealed two nonhomologous segments within the TSHR ectodomain (residues 38–45 and 316–366) not found in the closely related glycoprotein hormone receptors (ie, the luteinizing hormone [LH] and follicle-stimulating hormone [FSH] receptors).[1] Initial TSH cross-linking studies indicated that the mature TSHR contained two subunits[30] and its subsequent molecular cloning indicated that both subunits were coded by a single gene so that intramolecular cleavage must have occurred[30,31]—a phenomenon not observed with the LH and FSH receptors (**Fig. 2**). The cysteine clusters in the N-terminus have been shown to be important for the proper folding and intracellular trafficking of the receptor,[1] whereas clusters at the C-terminus of the ectodomain serve in disulfide bond formation after intramolecular cleavage, which forms the large extracellular (or ecto) domain (mostly the α or A subunit) and the short membrane-anchored and intracellular portion of the receptor (the β or B subunit) (see **Fig. 1**). The TSHR ectodomain comprises mainly nine leucine-rich repeats (LRRs) and an N-terminal tail, encoded by exons 2 to 8, which forms the binding domain for TSH and almost all types of TSHR autoantibodies that arise in autoimmune thyroid

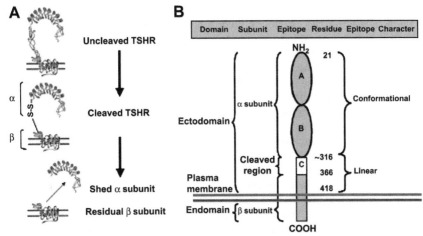

| Domain | Subunit | Epitope Residue | Epitope Character |

Fig. 2. TSHR structure, posttranslational processing, and epitope geography. (A) Three forms of the TSHR: the TSH holoreceptor undergoes cleavage and loses residues approximately 316 to 366. This results in the formation of a two-subunit structure (α/A and ß/B) connected by disulfide bonds and is referred to as the cleaved TSHR. Upon reduction, the α/A subunit (making up much of the ectodomain) is shed from the cell surface and leaves the ß/B subunits on the membrane. (B) Schematic representation of the structure of the TSHR and the epitopes recognized by TSHR-mAbs. An approximately 50-AA region removed by TSHR cleavage (cleaved region) is shown in white. The capital letters (A–C) indicate the three major epitopes recognized in a hamster model of GD.[120] Epitopes shown as oval indicate conformational recognition, and squares indicate linear recognition regions. Note that the ectodomain consists of more than just the TSHR α/A subunit. (Adapted from Ando T, Latif R, Davies TF. Antibody-induced modulation of TSH receptor post-translational processing. J Endocrinol 2007;195:179–86; with permission.)

diseases (AITD). The LRRs are 20 to 25 residue protein motifs consisting of a β strand and α helix turns. When assembled, the LRRs determine a horseshoelike structure with the β strands making a concave inner surface, which is the major TSH binding region. The seven transmembrane domains are joined intracellularly by connecting loops that interact with G proteins when the receptor is activated, whereas the exoplasmic loops, outside the cell, appear to have ancillary roles in receptor structure and activation.[32,33] Another important region in the structure of the TSHR is the "hinge" region. The hinge region extends from residues 277 to 418 and is approximately 141 amino acids, one of the largest hinge regions among the glycoprotein hormone receptors. Earlier it was believed that the hinge region was only an inert structural bridge between the ligand-binding luceine-rich domain (LRD) and signal-transducing transmembrane unit. However, based on several modeling studies of glycoprotein hormone receptors,[34–37] the hinge region may not be a simple structural linker but may contribute to signal transduction[38] by undergoing structural change in response to ligand binding as evidenced by progressive deletions of the hinge region, which reduced the sensitivity to TSH-stimulated cyclic adenosine monophosphate (cAMP).[38]

It has been shown that the TSHR is capable of binding to Gα and Gq and this interaction takes place via critical regions of the transmembrane domain.[39] However, the intracellular ICL2-ICL3 interaction is critical for selective Gq activation.[40] Investigation of the two nonhomologous segments within the ectodomain showed that deletion of residues 38 to 45 abrogated TSH binding,[41] whereas deletion of residues 316 to 366 did not[42] and the TSHR-transfected cells were still capable of TSH-mediated signaling. A detailed mutational analysis of residues 38 to 45 showed that Cys 41 was the critical residue required for TSH binding[43] and data also indicated that Cys41 interaction with other neighboring Cys residues in the TSHR ectodomain, via disulfide bonds, was essential for high-affinity TSH binding.[1,41,44] Hence, cysteine bonding helped restrain the structure critical for TSH ligand binding.[41]

Studies using mutagenesis and synthetic peptides originally showed the existence of multiple TSH-binding sites in the region of the LRRs of the ectodomain compatible with the existence of a conformational binding site.[45,46] Another approach has used a panel of epitope-mapped TSHR antibodies to block labeled TSH binding to the native TSHR. This approach defined TSH binding based on TSHR sequences recognized by the antibodies and suggested three distinct TSH binding regions in the TSHR (amino acids 246–260, 277–296, and 381–385).[47,48] These regions may fold together to form a complex TSH binding pocket. Comparative modeling and docking studies of the TSHR have further advanced our understanding of this discontinuous TSH binding pocket. In the comparative modeling studies the LRD of the TSHR was modeled on the template of porcine ribonuclease inhibitor and the transmembrane domain (TMD) was based on the classical group A rhodopsin receptor TM domains. The structure of the TSHR LRD and TMD were joined together through the TSHR cleavage domain modeled using the structure of human tissue inhibitor of matrix metalloproteinase-2 (TIMP-2).[37] These studies revealed the electrostatic potential interaction sites of TSH and also revealed the basic differences in the binding specificity and affinity of various ligands to the receptor. This clarified the weak interaction of FSH and human chorionic gonadotropin to the TSHR.[49]

By producing a truncated extracellular region of the TSHR encompassing the LRR region, it has been finally possible to crystallize the human TSHR extracellular domain (amino acids 1–260) complexed to the Fab fragment of a human TSHR-stimulating antibody.[50] In this complex, the antibody binds perpendicular to the concave horseshoe-shaped LRD encompassing a large region using an extensive network of polar, ionic, and hydrophobic bonding.[50] It is also remarkable that TSH showed almost identical binding features to that of the Fab fragment of the stimulating monoclonal antibody although with much fewer contact points. Unlike the FSH-FSHR complex that contained two FSH-FSHR complexes suggesting dimer formation, this study of the TSHR revealed no evidence of ectodomain dimers in the presence of the Fab or TSH suggesting that the TSHR, unlike the LHR or FSHR, does not dimerize on ligand binding.[49,50] Thus, dimerization/multimerization is certainly not ligand induced and TSH binding may be capable of dissociating most constitutively oligomeric receptors.[51]

## POSTTRANSLATIONAL CHANGES IN THE THYROID-STIMULATING HORMONE RECEPTOR

The TSHR, like other G-protein coupled receptors (GPCR), undergoes several different types of posttranslational modification, some of which take place in the endoplasmic reticulum (ER)–Golgi apparatus while others take place on the cell surface. In addition to the ER-Golgi carbohydrate modifications of the ectodomain, the TSHR also undergoes proteolysis, unique to this receptor among the family of glycoprotein receptors, as evidenced by the presence of a cleaved region. Studies from our laboratory have shown that TSHR dimerization/multimerization is another important modification that occurs constitutively within the thyroid cell. These posttranslational modifications lead to a heterogeneous pool of receptors on the cell surface. The TSHR is, therefore, subject to changes in its half-life[52] and its affinity for TSH binding, resulting in altered activation and signaling.[53]

## Glycosylation and Sulfation

The TSHR has six potential glycosylation sites on the large extracellular domain, which constitutes about 30% to 40% of its molecular weight. Thus, in native thyrocytes and transfected cells the full-length TSHR appears as a 100- and 120-KDa protein. The former is the mannose-rich precursor not expressed on the membrane.[54,55] The latter is the fully matured glycosylated receptor that is expressed on the plasma membrane.[54] Glycosylation seems to play a quantitative role in folding and surface expression of the TSHR and is not involved in TSH binding.[56] In contrast, sulfation of the hinge region has been shown to be critical for the binding of TSH to the receptor[57] and it is sulfation of the second tyrosine residue in the motif YDY distal to the hinge region that is functionally important for high-affinity binding.[58] Thus, it seems that sulfation of this critical residue is needed to maintain the receptor in its correct conformation.

## Palmitoylation and Disulfide-Bond Formation

Cysteine 699 in the cytoplasmic domain of the receptor is palmitoylated. Mutation of this site leads to delay in the trafficking of functionally normal receptors to the cell surface.[59] It is well known that in addition to acylation of the protein, palmitoylation is another modification that is important in targeting some receptors into lipid rafts.[53] The extracellular domain (residues aa 1–412) of the TSHR has 11 cysteine residues, 10 of which are distributed into 2 cysteine clusters.[1] Cysteines 24, 29, 31, and 41 of the N-terminus cluster have been shown to undergo a combination of disulfide bonding of which cysteine 41, which is unique to the TSHR, has been shown to be the most critical residue. Mutation of this cysteine leads to loss of TSH binding, indicating that cysteine 41 is responsible for forming the correct tertiary structure required for the binding of TSH.[41] The cysteine clusters at 283 to 301 and 390 to 408 at the C terminus of the LRD, demarking the 50 amino acid cleaved region (residues aa 317–366), are disulfide bonded and link the $\alpha$ subunit of the ectodomain to the latter half of the cleaved $\beta$ subunit in cleaved receptors. How the response to the ligand is transmitted to the transmembrane domain in these cleaved receptors is still unclear. However, it has been observed that the ectodomain by itself is capable of forming dimers and tetramers when expressed in bacterial or mammalian systems. The entire ectodomain (aa 1–412) when expressed as a glycan phosphatidylinositol (GPI)-linked protein in Chinese hamster ovary (CHO) cells also shows the propensity to form multimers,[60] indicating the role these cysteines might or might not have in multimerization.

## Thyroid-Stimulating Hormone Receptor Multimerization

Until 10 years ago it was believed that only tyrosine kinase receptors were capable of forming dimers and oligomers;[61] however, the advent of newer biophysical techniques such as FRET/BRET (Foster resonance energy transfer/bioluminescence energy transfer) has allowed the identification of GPCR dimers/oligomers. We found that the TSHR also forms oligomers in both TSHR-transfected cells and native thyrocytes.[28,62] Whereas unstimulated TSHRs were found in multimeric forms,[28] this multimeric state was reversed by TSH, consistent with the crystallization data discussed above.[51] The phenomenon of TSHR dimerization or formation of higher-order complexes of the TSHR is not recent. It was reported earlier that recombinant TSHR ectodomain generated in bacteria and insect cells could form multimers,[63] as could full-length receptor and β-subunits expressed in mammalian cells.[44,64] The existence of these higher molecular weight complexes was confirmed in native porcine and human thyroid tissue.[65,66] However, these early observations were dismissed as "caramelization" of TSHR glycans owing to the heating of samples above 50°C[1] resulting in artifactual aggregates. Further studies from our laboratory established the presence of constitutive homo interactions between TSH receptors by FRET in living cells, which was confirmed using BRET.[28,67] Using acceptor photobleaching, FRET, and co-immunoprecipitation experiments, we confirmed that oligomeric complexes of the TSHR decreased in a dose-dependent manner when treated with TSH,[51] although, interestingly, this was not seen in transiently transfected cells.[67] However, studies of TSHR movement on the surface of cells using fluorescent recovery after photobleaching have also shown that ligand treatment increased their mobility by decreasing their size, further confirming the dynamic behavior of the constitutively oligomeric TSHRs on the cell surface after exposure to ligand.

### The Function of Thyroid-Stimulating Hormone Receptor Multimerization

As described previously, it has been established that glycoprotein receptors such as FSHR, LHR, and TSHR have the propensity to homo-oligomerize in both native and transfected cells.[68] However, the functional significance of oligomerization in even the most well characterized GPCRs, such as the rhodopsin receptor, is not fully clear. Recent studies using atomic force microscopy have established that rhodopsin receptors in native tissue exist as oligomeric arrays and it has been conceptualized that cooperative interactions within these oligomeric arrays are critical for the propagation of an external signal across the cell membrane.[69] Hence, multimeric GPCRs are increasingly being recognized as scaffolds for the formation and localization of signaling complexes in the cell. Indeed, the magnitude and manner of the receptor response is most likely determined by the complex relationship among the ligand, receptor, G protein, and other associated proteins, as these forms may have functional roles in protein trafficking, internalization, and receptor stability, as well as signaling.[69] Using receptor binding and desorption experiments Urizar and colleagues[67] have shown that homodimerization of the TSHR is associated with strong negative cooperativity, an allosteric mechanism where ligand binding at one site reduces the binding affinity at another site on the molecule or dimer. In addition, the role of oligomerization in trafficking of the wild-type receptor has been elegantly studied to explain the cause of TSH resistance in rare cases of congenital hypothyroidism. Using FRET and co-immunoprecipitation, it has been shown that the defective mutant receptor is capable of entrapping the wild-type receptor in the endoplasmic reticulum owing to dimerization.[70] Hence, a growing body of evidence vividly indicates that GPCRs exist as dimeric/oligomeric complexes in heterologous and native systems with varied physiological roles such as signaling, trafficking, and internalization.

### Lipid Rafts and Multimerization

Lipid rafts are sphingolipid- and cholesterol-rich membrane microdomains on the plasma membrane. The association of sphingolipids with cholesterol condenses the packing of the sphinogolipids, leading to an enhanced mobility within the membrane. Lipid rafts have been associated with signal transduction within cells by their sequestering of signaling proteins. Using cholera toxin labeled with Alexa 594 and BodipyFL, which binds to lipid rafts enriched in $G_{M1}$ gangliosides, we showed that TSHRs were localized to these $GM_1$-enriched lipid rafts, and moved out of the rafts on TSH activation,[71] a phenomenon we were able to confirm biochemically. Indeed, the multimeric forms of the receptor were preferentially partitioned into these lipid microdomains and the multimers were dynamically regulated by receptor-specific and post–receptor-specific modulators.[72] These data suggested that TSHR multimers, following the binding of TSH, dissociated and moved out of the rafts rather than our initial hypothesis that receptors would move into lipid rafts to facilitate signaling.[13] The composition of the minimal functional signaling units within these lipid rafts remains to be understood.

### Thyroid-Stimulating Hormone Receptor Cleavage

A posttranslational proteolytic event clips the TSHR into two subunits.[73,74] This intramolecular cleavage results in removal of the unique intervening approximately 50 amino acid polypeptide segment in the ectodomain (aa 316–366) (see **Fig. 2**).[31,73] This cleavage step may involve a matrix metalloprotease-like enzyme acting at the cell surface,[75,76] such as ADAM 10.[77] Following cleavage, the α/A and β/B subunits are disulfide bonded by cysteine residues flanking the now absent cleaved 50 amino acid region; a structure also compatible with molecular modeling of the TSHR.[37] Subsequently, these α-β disulfide links are broken by protein disulfide isomerase (PDI)[78] and also by progression of β subunit degradation toward the membrane.[55] This unbonding leads to loss of the α subunit from the membrane-bound receptor, most likely by surface shedding.[79] This helps explain the large excess of TSHR β versus TSHR α/A subunits (up to 3:1) found in normal thyroid membrane preparations.[31,54] However, TSHR signal transduction may not be dependent on ectodomain cleavage as demonstrated by a noncleavable construct, although subtle aspects of this phenomenon have not been explored.[13,42] In primary thyrocytes, many of the TSHRs are fully glycosylated and cleaved,[31] although β/B subunits predominate.[31,80] However, in transfected cells the holoreceptor is the dominant form because of inefficient receptor processing.[54,55] It should also be noted that the phenomenon of subunit shedding has been demonstrated only in vitro in primary thyrocytes and transfected cells.[75,78,81] There has been no convincing report demonstrating the shedding of TSHRs in vivo although it has been hypothesized that shed receptors might act as an antigenic reservoir for initiating autoimmune responses in Graves' disease.[82]

### Role of Thyroid-Stimulating Hormone Receptor Cleavage

The pathophysiological relevance of cleavage has largely remained enigmatic. TSH itself probably has a role in posttranslational modifications[74,75,78] and we found that TSH stimulation modestly enhanced cleavage in a time- and dose-dependent manner.[24,81] This observation was compatible with the hypothesis that TSHR cleavage is important in receptor signaling. In fact, we had earlier observed that the cleaved form of the TSHR was better able to bind Gsα, also suggesting cleavage of the TSH receptor may be associated with receptor activation in transfected CHO cells.[83] However, an uncleavable TSHR construct could still signal via cAMP, although other pathways may still be impaired.[42] The role of cleavage in receptor trafficking and internalization has also been studied using truncated receptors, which are physiologically equivalent to cleaved and shed receptors. It was found that they had faster internalization and a shorter half-life indicating that cleavage may also have a major influence on receptor trafficking.[84]

## THYROID-STIMULATING HORMONE RECEPTOR SIGNALING PATHWAYS
### Receptor Activation

The transmembrane domain of the TSHR mainly activates the classical G-protein-coupled effectors such as Gs, Gq, different subtypes of Gi, and Go, as well as G12 and G13.[85] Stimulation of the receptor leads to dissociation of trimeric G proteins into Gα and Gβγ subunits, which in turn trigger a complex signaling network

(**Fig. 3**).[86] Unlike other glycoprotein receptors, the TSHR is constitutively active and susceptible to enhanced constitutive activation by mutation, deletions, and even mild trypsin digestion.[87,88] Studies using mutational analyses have suggested that the putative electrostatic interactions between the ectodomain and the extracellular loops of the transmembrane domains (TMD) in the TSHR may be critical for the maintenance of a relatively inactive "closed" state.[32] When these constraints are absent or removed, for example by a mutation or ligand binding, an "open" conformation ensues. This two-state "model" predicts that the "open" format of the receptor, when stabilized, would lead to full activation. Further support for this model came from the development of enhanced constitutive activation when the TSHR ectodomain was truncated, suggesting that the presence of the ectodomain dampened a constitutively active β subunit.[32,89,90] Additionally, recent TSHR computer modeling and docking studies[37] have shown that several mutations in the TMD that are associated with increased TSHR basal activity are caused by the formation of new interactions that may stabilize the "open" activated form of the receptor.

### Classical Pathway

Most of the activities of the TSHR are mediated by Gs protein, which activates the adenylate cyclase (AC)/cAMP cascade leading to the activation of either the protein kinase-dependent *Rap1-b-Raf-ERK-Elk1* cascade or the PKA-independent EPAC1-*Rap1b-Raf-ERK-Elk1* signaling pathway in order to regulate thyroid function (see **Fig. 3**). Both these pathways include the extracellular regulated kinase (ERK), which is a downstream component of a well-conserved signaling module. Raf activates MEK1/2, which are dual-specificity protein kinases, which then activate ERK1/2.[91]

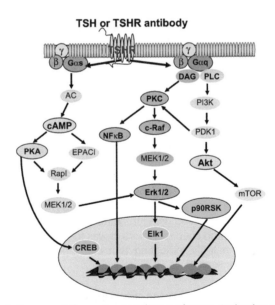

**Fig. 3.** A simplified diagram of the major signaling pathways. Activation of TSH receptor on the cell surface by TSH or TSHR antibodies results in the activation of two major classes of G proteins. This activation is relayed to second messengers via the major signaling pathways such as cAMP/PKA/ERK, PI3/Akt, PKC/NFκB, and PKC/c-raf/ERK/P90RSK and mTOR being a major player of proliferation. These pathways interact with each resulting in a multitude of cross-talks but for simplicity sake these have been omitted.

This *Raf-MEK-ERK* pathway is also a key downstream effector of the Ras small GTPase, which requires receptor tyrosine kinase (RTK) activation by various growth factors.[92] Both Elk-1 and p90RSK are important downstream transcription factors in these ERK1/2 activation pathways.[93]

An alternate TSHR effector pathway, via Gq, mediates the activation of the PLC-β and the Gγ subunit.[94] Once activated, PLC hydrolyzes phosphatidylinositol bisphosphate (PIP$_2$) to inositol 3,4,5-trisphosphate (IP$_3$) and diacylglycerol (DAG).[95] Akt is activated as a result of PI3-kinase activity, because Akt requires the formation of the "PIP3" molecule in order to be translocated to the cell membrane. With PIP3, Akt is then phosphorylated by another kinase called PDK1, and is thereby activated.[96] The Akt signaling pathway has been shown to be required most notably for cellular proliferation and survival.[97]

PI3 and DAG are also involved in the activation of Ca+ and PKC isoenzymes, respectively, whereas PDK1 kinase is involved in the activation of atypical PKC isoenzymes.[96] Hence PDK1 plays a central role in many signal transduction pathways involving Akt, PKC isoenzymes, p70 S6 kinase, and RS kinase.[98–100] In a recent study using PCC13 rat thyroid cells it was observed that the release of Gβγ in response to TSH activated phosphoinositide-3 kinase and regulated gene expression in thyroid cells. Gβγ overexpression lead to an inhibition of NIS expression by causing a decrease in Pax8 binding to the NIS promoter.[101]

### Nonclassical Pathways

TSH has also been shown to activate a variety of additional pathways with important functions adding to the complexity of the TSHR signaling system (see **Fig. 3**).

### Nuclear factor kappa B

Activation of transcription factors of the nuclear factor kappa B (NFκB) by TSH has been reported.[102] NFκB-activating agents can induce the phosphorylation of IκB's, targeting them for rapid degradation through a ubiquitin-proteosome pathway, releasing NFκB to enter the nucleus, where it regulates gene expression.[103] A recent study has shown that TSH-mediated NFκB activation releases interleukin (IL)-6 in human abdominal subcutaneous adipocytes and cultured CHO cells expressing the TSHR.

### Mitogen-activated protein kinase

In addition to the downstream TSHR signaling responses, each arm of the effectors is under the influence of a wide variety of growth factors. These factors work via mitogen-activated protein kinase (MAPK) cascades, which are key signaling systems involved in the regulation of normal cell proliferation, survival, and differentiation.[104] TSH increases intracellular cAMP, which rapidly stimulates the MAP kinase cascade independent of PKA (see **Fig. 3**). The molecular mechanism of ERK1/2 activation by TSH is cAMP–dependent but PKA independent and involves the activation of Rap1 and B-raf.[104]

### Janus kinases/signal transducer and activator of transcription

It has also been shown that TSH activates the Janus kinases (JAK)/signal transducer and activator of transcription (STAT) pathway via the TSHR.[105]

### Murine target of rapamycin

Central to the pathway that induces cell growth in mammals is the murine target of rapamycin (mTOR), an evolutionarily conserved ser/thr kinase that is inhibited by the drug rapamycin.[106] Recent studies have shown that the proliferative response to chronic TSHR stimulation by TSH relies heavily on the activation of the mTOR pathway. This action of TSH via mTOR observed in rat thyrocytes in culture has been shown to be independent of AKT activation in vivo.[107]

## THE THYROID-STIMULATING HORMONE RECEPTOR AS ANTIGEN

The TSHR is a major immune target in AITD. The reasons for the failure of tolerance to this widely expressed antigen are uncertain but include a complex mixture of genetic susceptibility and environmental influences (as reviewed).[108]

### The Different Types of Thyroid-Stimulating Hormone Receptor Autoantibodies

Autoantibodies to the TSHR (TSHR-Abs) may influence thyroid function by stimulating the TSHR and promoting excessive thyroid growth, hormone production, and hormone secretion causing Graves' disease (GD).[1,27,109] TSHR-Abs may also block the action of TSH and induce hypothyroidism as seen in some patients with the atrophic form of Hashimoto's thyroiditis.[110] In addition, GD patients may have both these types of TSHR-Abs resulting in the blocking TSHR-Abs blunting activation induced by stimulating TSHR-Abs (Fig. 4).[111] The stimulating and blocking TSHR-Abs are clinically detectable, but indistinguishable, by competition assays using labeled TSH binding to the normally conformed TSHR (the TSH-binding inhibition assays). A third type of antibody, which does not interfere with TSH binding, has been termed "neutral" and cannot, therefore, be measured by receptor competition assays but rather require immunoprecipitation or immunoblot analysis. These types of antibody were considered unimportant or artifactual when first reported,[1] but their frequency in animal models of Graves' disease has aroused interest in them once again (see later in this article). Nevertheless, the major characteristic of TSHR-Abs is their influence on thyroid function via the TSHR by either stimulating or blocking the receptor from activation. This occurs despite the low serum concentrations of TSHR-Abs (10 μg/mL).[112] The estimated serum concentration of TSHR-Ab is significantly less than that of thyroid antibodies to TPO and Tg, indicating their necessarily high affinity. In addition, TSHR-Abs are commonly oligoclonal and of the IgG1 subclass as shown by isotyping of heavy and light chains,[113,114] although other isotypes have been reported.[115]

### Thyroid-Stimulating Hormone Receptor Autoantibody Conformational Epitopes

It has been recently shown, by using mouse monoclonal TSHR-Abs, that there are multiple antibody-binding sites on the TSHR that compete for TSH binding in the TSH-binding pocket.[47] Most stimulating antibodies and some blocking TSHR-Abs bind to conformational epitope(s) on the α subunit[25,26,116,117] and binding to the LRD region of the ectodomain has been shown for stimulating mAbs to the TSHR.[118]

### Thyroid-Stimulating Hormone Receptor Autoantibody Linear Epitopes

In addition to these conformationally dependent TSHR-Abs, it has been repeatedly shown that sera from patients with autoimmune thyroid disease may contain additional TSHR-Abs recognizing linear epitopes of the TSHR ectodomain and the β domain.[1,119] For example, the presence of blocking antibodies that recognize linear epitopes in the β subunit was shown by binding inhibition of mouse-blocking TSHR-mAbs using Graves' sera.[119] Recent studies of animal models of GD have also demonstrated the presence of TSHR-Abs that recognize linear epitopes.[47,52] These TSHR-Abs were isolated as monoclonal antibodies that did not stimulate the TSHR nor block the action of TSH and, therefore, were of the "neutral" variety (see Fig. 4).

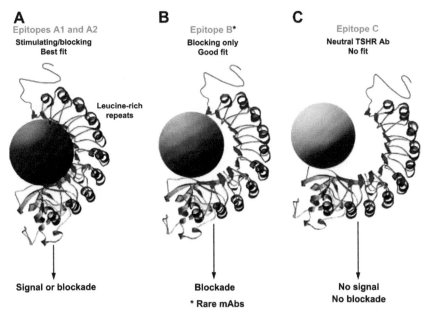

**Fig. 4.** Model of TSHR antibody binding to the ectodomain. The TSH binding-pocket, represented by the LRRs, is shown by spirals representing the α helix and the β pleated sheets represented by the wide arrows. The region represents the unique cleaved region (316–366 aa) of the receptor as indicated in **Fig. 1**. (*A*) Epitope A1 represents the site where thyroid-stimulating antibodies bind in part to the LRRs, bringing about a structural change in the receptor that leads to signal transduction; Epitope A2 represents a similar competing site, where TSH blocking antibodies bind (both illustrated as a best fit). (*B*) Epitope B is the least common site, where TSHR-blocking antibodies may bind but do not compete with antibodies binding to Epitope A. They bind in part to the LRR region but do not bring about the required structural change for signal transduction yet are still able to hinder TSH binding to this site (illustrated as good fit). (*C*) Epitope C is where neutral antibodies bind to the cleaved region and/or the N terminus of the TSHR ectodomain, bringing no appropriate structural alteration to the TSHR and thus leaving the LRR region free for TSH, and other TSHR antibodies, to bind. Thus, neutral antibodies result in no signal transduction and do not block TSH binding therefore illustrated as no fit. (*Adapted from* Davies TF, Ando T, Lin RY, Tomer Y, Latif R. Thyrotropin receptor-associated diseases: from adenomata to Graves disease. J Clin Invest 2005;115:1972–83; with permission.)

### Thyroid-Stimulating Hormone Receptor Autoantibodies in Animal Models

As alluded to earlier, in TSHR-immunized animals, both stimulating and blocking antibodies have been isolated.[120,121] In addition, the cleaved region itself has been shown to be one of the major linear epitopes for "neutral" TSHR-Abs[52,121] explaining the lack of TSH competition because this region is out of the TSH-binding pocket.[47] In our hamster model of GD[120,121] induced by immunizing with the Nagayama adenovirus vector expressing full-length human TSHR,[122] we found anti-TSHR sera recognizing three distinct epitopes termed A, B, and C.[121] Two of the three epitopes were conformational within the α subunit: Epitope A for both stimulating and blocking Abs, which should be closely related to the sites that stimulating and blocking TSHR-Abs bind, as seen in GD, and Epitope B exclusively for blocking Abs. The third epitope was a group of cleaved region linear epitopes recognized by monoclonal neutral TSHR-Abs (Epitope C). Epitope C was distinct from, and thus did not overlap with, other conformational epitopes,[121] which is compatible with the fact that the sole presence of such "neutral antibodies" could not induce hyperthyroidism by themselves.[121]

## INFLUENCE OF THYROID-STIMULATING HORMONE RECEPTOR AUTOANTIBODIES ON THYROID-STIMULATING HORMONE RECEPTOR POSTTRANSLATIONAL PROCESSING
### Cleavage

We have recently shown that many TSHR-Abs, including the neutral TSHR-mAbs, inhibit TSHR posttranslational cleavage and increase the surface expression of the TSHR (see **Fig. 2**). This regulated posttranslational processing of TSHR by TSHR-Abs has been observed in thyroid cells and not just TSHR-transfected cells, implying a functional significance. How this may be relevant to Graves' disease has yet to be fully understood. Our thyroid stimulating monoclonal antibody (MS-1) inhibited TSHR cleavage, and also induced a slowing of TSHR mobility suggesting the induction of heavier forms of the TSHR as dimers/multimers.[51] This may not be surprising, as antibodies are divalent. Therefore, we proposed that cleavage-inhibiting TSHR-Abs stabilized the TSHR ectodomain by maintaining dimeric or multimeric TSHR forms owing to the IgG bivalency. The mechanism by which this multimerization may inhibit intra-molecular cleavage of the TSHR is unknown. However, our data suggested that a structural inhibition of the cleavage enzyme(s) is the most likely. Evidence for this conclusion comes from the fact that the TSHR-Ab–induced inhibition of cleavage was epitope dependent. We showed that two neutral antibodies that bound to residues 335 to 354 showed differing regulation of cleavage even with overlapping epitopes. Because neither of these mAbs bound to the proximal (residues 322–341) or distal (352–371) TSHR peptides,[52,121] it appeared that any TSHR-Ab that bound proximal to residue 341 inhibited cleavage and TSHR-Abs that bound distal to 352 failed to inhibit cleavage. This conclusion proved true for all the monoclonal TSHR-Abs we examined. The detailed molecular explanation for such activities will need to await the identification and structure of the cleavage enzyme(s) involved in this phenomenon. These data were also the first to show potential biological activity of neutral TSHR-Abs on the TSHR. However, neutral Abs may be detected in individuals without GD and, as discussed earlier, TSHR-Abs to the cleaved region have been detected in animals immunized with TSHR antigen that failed to develop hyperthyroidism.[120,121,123]

### Dimerization

As discussed earlier, monoclonal TSHR-stimulating antibody (MS-1), which like all antibodies is divalent, did not act like TSH in that it failed to enhance constitutive cleavage in TSHR-transfected cells. This strongly suggested that monomerization of the receptors may be an important preliminary process to the cleavage event as evidenced by the fact that the MS-1-Fab fragment did indeed act like TSH.[81] On the other hand, such an observation is less compatible with the hypothesis that cleavage is important for signal transduction unless the quality of the signal initiated by an antibody is different from that initiated by TSH. Clearly, there is a complex relationship between dimerization and cleavage of the TSHR, which continues to require clarification.

### Lipid Rafts

By studying the effect of TSHR-stimulating antibody on TSHR movement in live cells, we observed that TSHR-Abs, like TSH, were able to move multimeric receptors out of lipid rafts.[72] However, unlike TSH, some of the receptors outside the rafts remained in a dimeric state because of the bivalent nature of the TSHR-Abs. Hence, TSHR-Abs are capable of stabilizing these dimeric structures. The effects of blocking and neutral TSHR-Abs have not yet been studied.

## Summary

Taken together, these recent data introduce a new concept by which TSHR antibodies regulate posttranslational processing of the TSHR. It now seems plausible that the potential antibody-mediated persistence of excess uncleaved TSHRs could result in an increased thyroid antigenic load at the thyroid cell surface.

## THYROID-STIMULATING HORMONE RECEPTOR AUTOANTIBODY–INDUCED SIGNAL TRANSDUCTION

### Stimulating Thyroid-Stimulating Hormone Receptor Autoantibodies

The recent development of monoclonal antibodies to the TSHR has enabled us to investigate TSHR signaling events in vitro and in vivo. We have hypothesized that different TSHR-Abs may have unique signaling imprints at the TSHR, thus altering cellular functions. Although our stimulating antibodies used primarily TSH signaling pathways, there were some differences in signaling activities and signal strengths. Most importantly, the human M22 antibody,[116] which had the highest affinity for the TSHR, demonstrated significantly greater PKA activation than TSH in a rat thyroid cell model,[124] and there were subtle differences in PKA activity induced by other stimulating antibodies. This suggested that antibody binding to amino acids not contacted by TSH on the TSHR may be responsible for such high PKA activity. Furthermore, the high affinity of this antibody may have driven the higher cAMP levels that contributed to a high degree of cell proliferation. M22 also increased p90RSK, a downstream molecule of ERK regulation suggesting activation of additional signaling modules downstream. Two other potent stimulating antibodies (KSAb1 and KSAb2) provoked phosphorylation of the intracellular ERK1/2 pathway in primary thyrocytes indicating that multiple signaling pathways may be involved in the pathogenesis of GD.[125]

### Blocking Thyroid-Stimulating Hormone Receptor Autoantibodies

Epitopes for TSHR blocking antibodies appear to be widely distributed[47,126] on the $\alpha$ subunit and there is also at least one linear epitope on the $\beta$ subunit.[119,123] To help determine their functional consequences we characterized signaling molecules in exposed rat thyroid cells and found that some blocking antibodies resulted not only in signal molecule activation but they showed different pathway dominance as weak agonists. For example, some activated the c-Raf-ERK pathway but not p90RSK, whereas others did not activate c-Raf-ERK but activated p90RSK. Although these findings may arise from differences in their binding domains, the differences may be because of interference with the constitutive activity of signaling molecules in these cells. More study is necessary to correlate the effector mechanisms used by blocking TSHR-Abs with their different epitopes.

### Neutral Thyroid-Stimulating Hormone Receptor Autoantibodies

It has been generally thought that neutral TSHR antibodies should have no influence on TSH action. As discussed earlier, however, we first found that such neutral antibodies were able to inhibit TSH cleavage, which raised the question of their importance in pathophysiology.[52] We have characterized the influence of some such neutral mAbs on TSH signaling cascades and downstream effectors and found in some cases suppression of multiple signaling modules, including cell proliferation, whereas others caused activation of many of them. A conformational monoclonal

**Table 1**
**Proposed neoclassification of TSHR antibodies**

| Antibody Class | CAMP Signaling[a] | Non-CAMP Signaling[b] | TSH Binding |
|---|---|---|---|
| Stimulators | +++ | ++ | Block |
| True blockers | − | +/− | Block |
| False blockers | +/− | ++ | Block |
| True neutrals | − | − | Do Not Block |
| False neutrals | − | + | Do Not Block |

This classification is derived from studies on nonclassical signaling pathways performed in our laboratory using rat thyrocytes (FRTL5).
[a] Classical signaling pathway.
[b] Nonclassical signaling pathway.

antibody with a possible binding site at the LRD (residues 260–289) has been described as an inverse agonist that suppressed TSHR constitutive activity[127,128] of cAMP generation. These findings, together with ours, raise the possibility that multiple domains in this molecular stretch of the TSHR may exist that suppress or stimulate the TSHR.

*Summary*

Stimulating antibodies use signaling pathways similar to the TSH activation modules contributing to cell activation and growth. Both TSH blocking and neutral TSHR antibodies distinguished different signaling networks and resulted in variable signal responses indicating that some may be weak agonists or inverse agonists. These observations help explain how TSHR-Abs may contribute to different clinical phenotypes in autoimmune thyroid disease. With the information obtained on epitope specificity and signal transduction properties of monoclonal TSHR-Abs, it is apparent that a new nomenclature is needed for TSHR-Abs as proposed in **Table 1**. Hopefully this type of nomenclature will reduce the confusion so apparent in this field.

SUMMARY

The TSHR is central to thyrocyte function and a variety of other cells including adipocytes and osteoclasts. The TSHR may also be affected by genomic and somatic mutations and is also one of the major autoantigens for the autoimmune thyroid diseases. The immensely complex posttranslational processing of the TSHR is slowly being unraveled and a number of the physiologic mechanisms involved have been delineated. Nevertheless, the possible roles of multimerization and cleavage in TSHR signal transduction still require further insight. Similarly, the propensity for multimeric receptors to accumulate in lipid rafts and their functional role needs further clarification. Recent studies, however, have begun to characterize monoclonal antibodies to the TSHR and these have revealed their often unique biologic activities, which vary from full agonists to total antagonists and everything in between. Such a variety of TSHR antibodies may help explain the multiple clinical phenotypes seen in AITD. Discovering the detailed epitopes of these antibodies will provide a much greater understanding of the structure/function relationship of the TSHR.

## REFERENCES

1. Rapoport B, Chazenbalk GD, Jaume JC, et al. The thyrotropin (TSH) receptor: interaction with TSH and autoantibodies. Endocr Rev 1998;19:673–716.
2. Misrahi M, Loosfelt H, Atger M, et al. Cloning, sequencing and expression of human TSH receptor. Biochem Biophys Res Commun 1990;166:394–403.
3. Nagayama Y, Kaufman KD, Seto P, et al. Molecular cloning, sequence and functional expression of the cDNA for the human thyrotropin receptor. Biochem Biophys Res Commun 1989;165:1184–90.
4. Parmentier M, Libert F, Maenhaut C, et al. Molecular cloning of the thyrotropin receptor. Science 1989;246:1620–2.
5. De Felice M, Postiglione MP, Di Lauro R. Minireview: thyrotropin receptor signaling in development and differentiation of the thyroid gland: insights from mouse models and human diseases. Endocrinology 2004;145:4062–7.
6. Postiglione MP, Parlato R, Rodriguez-Mallon A, et al. Role of the thyroid-stimulating hormone receptor signaling in development and differentiation of the thyroid gland. Proc Natl Acad Sci U S A 2002;99:15462–7.
7. Marians RC, Ng L, Blair HC, et al. Defining thyrotropin-dependent and -independent steps of thyroid hormone synthesis by using thyrotropin receptor-null mice. Proc Natl Acad Sci U S A 2002;99:15776–81.
8. Brown RS. Minireview: developmental regulation of thyrotropin receptor gene expression in the fetal and newborn thyroid. Endocrinology 2004;145:4058–61.
9. Burrow GN, Fisher DA, Larsen PR. Maternal and fetal thyroid function. N Engl J Med 1994;331:1072–8.
10. Davies TF, Ando T, Lin RY, et al. Thyrotropin receptor-associated diseases: from adenomata to Graves disease. J Clin Invest 2005;115:1972–83.
11. Thomas D, Friedman S, Lin RY. Thyroid stem cells: lessons from normal development and thyroid cancer. Endocr Relat Cancer 2008;15:51–8.
12. Bahn RS, Dutton CM, Natt N, et al. Thyrotropin receptor expression in Graves' orbital adipose/connective tissues: potential autoantigen in Graves' ophthalmopathy. J Clin Endocrinol Metab 1998;83:998–1002.
13. Davies T, Marians R, Latif R. The TSH receptor reveals itself. J Clin Invest 2002;110:161–4.
14. Vizek K, Razova M, Melichar V. Lipolytic effect of TSH, glucagon and hydrocortisone on the adipose tissue of newborns and adults in vitro. Physiol Bohemoslov 1979;28:325–31.
15. Daumerie C, Ludgate M, Costagliola S, et al. Evidence for thyrotropin receptor immunoreactivity in pretibial connective tissue from patients with thyroid-associated dermopathy. Eur J Endocrinol 2002;146:35–8.
16. Lu M, Lin RY. TSH stimulates adipogenesis in mouse embryonic stem cells. J Endocrinol 2008;196:159–69.
17. Zhang L, Baker G, Janus D, et al. Biological effects of thyrotropin receptor activation on human orbital preadipocytes. Invest Ophthalmol Vis Sci 2006;47:5197–203.
18. Cawthorn WP, Sethi JK. TNF-alpha and adipocyte biology. FEBS Lett 2008;582:117–31.
19. Abe E, Marians RC, Yu W, et al. TSH is a negative regulator of skeletal remodeling. Cell 2003;115:151–62.
20. Abe E, Sun L, Mechanick J, et al. Bone loss in thyroid disease: role of low TSH and high thyroid hormone. Ann N Y Acad Sci 2007;1116:383–91.

21. Sun L, Vukicevic S, Baliram R, et al. Intermittent recombinant TSH injections prevent ovariectomy-induced bone loss. Proc Natl Acad Sci U S A 2008;105:4289–94.

22. Bassett JH, Williams AJ, Murphy E, et al. A lack of thyroid hormones rather than excess thyrotropin causes abnormal skeletal development in hypothyroidism. Mol Endocrinol 2008;22:501–12.

23. Stassi G, De MR. Autoimmune thyroid disease: new models of cell death in autoimmunity. Nat Rev Immunol 2002;2:195–204.

24. Ando T, Latif R, Pritsker A, et al. A monoclonal thyroid-stimulating antibody. J Clin Invest 2002;110:1667–74.

25. Costagliola S, Franssen JD, Bonomi M, et al. Generation of a mouse monoclonal TSH receptor antibody with stimulating activity. Biochem Biophys Res Commun 2002;299:891–6.

26. Sanders J, Jeffreys J, Depraetere H, et al. Thyroid-stimulating monoclonal antibodies. Thyroid 2002;12:1043–50.

27. Ando T, Latif R, Davies TF. Concentration-dependent regulation of thyrotropin receptor function by thyroid-stimulating antibody. J Clin Invest 2004;113:1589–95.

28. Latif R, Graves P, Davies TF. Oligomerization of the human thyrotropin receptor: fluorescent protein-tagged hTSHR reveals post-translational complexes. J Biol Chem 2001;276:45217–24.

29. Libert F, Lefort A, Gerard C, et al. Cloning, sequencing and expression of the human thyrotropin (TSH) receptor: evidence for binding of autoantibodies. Biochem Biophys Res Commun 1989;165:1250–5.

30. Kajita Y, Rickards CR, Buckland PR, et al. Analysis of thyrotropin receptors by photoaffinity labelling. Orientation of receptor subunits in the cell membrane. Biochem J 1985;227:413–20.

31. Loosfelt H, Pichon C, Jolivet A, et al. Two-subunit structure of the human thyrotropin receptor. Proc Natl Acad Sci U S A 1992;89:3765–9.

32. Vlaeminck-Guillem V, Ho SC, Rodien P, et al. Activation of the cAMP pathway by the TSH receptor involves switching of the ectodomain from a tethered inverse agonist to an agonist. Mol Endocrinol 2002;16:736–46.

33. Neumann S, Claus M, Paschke R. Interactions between the extracellular domain and the extracellular loops as well as the 6th transmembrane domain are necessary for TSH receptor activation. Eur J Endocrinol 2005;152:625–34.

34. Claus M, Jaeschke H, Kleinau G, et al. A hydrophobic cluster in the center of the third extracellular loop is important for thyrotropin receptor signaling. Endocrinology 2005;146:5197–203.

35. Fan QR, Hendrickson WA. Structure of human follicle-stimulating hormone in complex with its receptor. Nature 2005;433:269–77.

36. Moyle WR, Xing Y, Lin W, et al. Model of glycoprotein hormone receptor ligand binding and signaling. J Biol Chem 2004;279:44442–59.

37. Nunez MR, Sanders J, Jeffreys J, et al. Analysis of the thyrotropin receptor-thyrotropin interaction by comparative modeling. Thyroid 2004;14:991–1011.

38. Mizutori Y, Chen CR, McLachlan SM, et al. The thyrotropin receptor hinge region is not simply a scaffold for the leucine-rich domain but contributes to ligand binding and signal transduction. Mol Endocrinol 2008;22(5):1171–82.

39. Claus M, Neumann S, Kleinau G, et al. Structural determinants for G-protein activation and specificity in the third intracellular loop of the thyroid-stimulating hormone receptor. J Mol Med 2006;84:943–54.

40. Neumann S, Krause G, Claus M, et al. Structural determinants for G protein activation and selectivity in the second intracellular loop of the thyrotropin receptor. Endocrinology 2005;146:477–85.

41. Wadsworth HL, Chazenbalk GD, Nagayama Y, et al. An insertion in the human thyrotropin receptor critical for high affinity hormone binding. Science 1990; 249:1423–5.
42. Chazenbalk GD, Nagayama Y, Russo D, et al. Functional analysis of the cytoplasmic domains of the human thyrotropin receptor by site-directed mutagenesis. J Biol Chem 1990;265:20970–5.
43. Wadsworth HL, Russo D, Nagayama Y, et al. Studies on the role of amino acids 38–45 in the expression of a functional thyrotropin receptor. Mol Endocrinol 1992;6:394–8.
44. Graves PN, Davies TF. New insights into the thyroid-stimulating hormone receptor. The major antigen of Graves' disease. Endocrinol Metab Clin North Am 2000;29:267–86, vi.
45. Nagayama Y, Russo D, Wadsworth HL, et al. Eleven amino acids (Lys-201 to Lys-211) and 9 amino acids (Gly-222 to Leu-230) in the human thyrotropin receptor are involved in ligand binding. J Biol Chem 1991;266: 14926–30.
46. Smits G, Campillo M, Govaerts C, et al. Glycoprotein hormone receptors: determinants in leucine-rich repeats responsible for ligand specificity. EMBO J 2003; 22:2692–703.
47. Jeffreys J, Depraetere H, Sanders J, et al. Characterization of the thyrotropin binding pocket. Thyroid 2002;12:1051–61.
48. Nagayama Y, Wadsworth HL, Russo D, et al. Binding domains of stimulatory and inhibitory thyrotropin (TSH) receptor autoantibodies determined with chimeric TSH-lutropin/chorionic gonadotropin receptors. J Clin Invest 1991;88:336–40.
49. Sanders J, Miguel RN, Bolton J, et al. Molecular interactions between the TSH receptor and a thyroid-stimulating monoclonal autoantibody. Thyroid 2007;17: 699–706.
50. Sanders J, Chirgadze DY, Sanders P, et al. Crystal structure of the TSH receptor in complex with a thyroid-stimulating autoantibody. Thyroid 2007; 17:395–410.
51. Latif R, Graves P, Davies TF. Ligand-dependent inhibition of oligomerization at the human thyrotropin receptor. J Biol Chem 2002;277:45059–67.
52. Ando T, Latif R, Davies TF. Antibody-induced modulation of TSH receptor post-translational processing. J Endocrinol 2007;195:179–86.
53. Kursawe R, Paschke R. Modulation of TSHR signaling by posttranslational modifications. Trends Endocrinol Metab 2007;18:199–207.
54. Misrahi M, Ghinea N, Sar S, et al. Processing of the precursors of the human thyroid-stimulating hormone receptor in various eukaryotic cells (human thyrocytes, transfected L cells and baculovirus-infected insect cells). Eur J Biochem 1994;222:711–9.
55. Tanaka K, Chazenbalk GD, McLachlan SM, et al. Subunit structure of thyrotropin receptors expressed on the cell surface. J Biol Chem 1999;274:33979–84.
56. Nagayama Y, Nishihara E, Namba H, et al. Identification of the sites of asparagine-linked glycosylation on the human thyrotropin receptor and studies on their role in receptor function and expression. J Pharmacol Exp Ther 2000;295:404–9.
57. Costagliola S, Panneels V, Bonomi M, et al. Tyrosine sulfation is required for agonist recognition by glycoprotein hormone receptors. EMBO J 2002;21: 504–13.
58. Bonomi M, Busnelli M, Persani L, et al. Structural differences in the hinge region of the glycoprotein hormone receptors: evidence from the sulfated tyrosine residues. Mol Endocrinol 2006;20:3351–63.

59. Kosugi S, Mori T. Cysteine-699, a possible palmitoylation site of the thyrotropin receptor, is not crucial for cAMP or phosphoinositide signaling but is necessary for full surface expression. Biochem Biophys Res Commun 1996; 221:636–40.

60. Latif R, Michalek Chris, Morshed Syed, et al. Dimerization of the TSH receptor ectodomain [abstract].

61. Breitwieser GE. G protein-coupled receptor oligomerization: implications for G protein activation and cell signaling. Circ Res 2004;94:17–27.

62. Graves PN, Vlase H, Bobovnikova Y, et al. Multimeric complex formation by the thyrotropin receptor in solubilized thyroid membranes. Endocrinology 1996;137: 3915–20.

63. Vlase H, Graves PN, Magnusson RP, et al. Human autoantibodies to the thyrotropin receptor: recognition of linear, folded, and glycosylated recombinant extracellular domain. J Clin Endocrinol Metab 1995;80:46–53.

64. Ban T, Kosugi S, Kohn LD. Specific antibody to the thyrotropin receptor identifies multiple receptor forms in membranes of cells transfected with wild-type receptor complementary deoxyribonucleic acid: characterization of their relevance to receptor synthesis, processing, structure, and function. Endocrinology 1992;131:815–29.

65. Graves PN, Vlase H, Bobovnikova Y, et al. Multimeric complex formation by the natural TSH receptor. Endocrinology 1996;137:3915–20.

66. Grossman RF, Ban T, Duh QY, et al. Immunoprecipitation isolates multiple TSH receptor forms from human thyroid tissue. Thyroid 1995;5:101–5.

67. Urizar E, Montanelli L, Loy T, et al. Glycoprotein hormone receptors: link between receptor homodimerization and negative cooperativity. EMBO J 2005;24: 1954–64.

68. Persani L, Calebiro D, Bonomi M. Technology insight: modern methods to monitor protein-protein interactions reveal functional TSH receptor oligomerization. Nat Clin Pract Endocrinol Metab 2007;3:180–90.

69. Park PS, Filipek S, Wells JW, et al. Oligomerization of G protein-coupled receptors: past, present, and future. Biochemistry 2004;43:15643–56.

70. Calebiro D, de FT, Lucchi S, et al. Intracellular entrapment of wild-type TSH receptor by oligomerization with mutants linked to dominant TSH resistance. Hum Mol Genet 2005;14:2991–3002.

71. Latif R, Ando T, Daniel S, et al. Localization and regulation of thyrotropin receptors within lipid rafts. Endocrinology 2003;144:4725–8.

72. Latif R, Ando T, Davies TF. Lipid rafts are triage centers for multimeric and monomeric thyrotropin receptor regulation. Endocrinology 2007;148:3164–75.

73. Chazenbalk GD, Tanaka K, Nagayama Y, et al. Evidence that the TSH receptor ectodomain contains not one, but two, cleavage sites. Endocrinology 1997;138: 2893–9.

74. Misrahi M, Milgrom E. Cleavage and shedding of the TSH receptor. Eur J Endocrinol 1997;137:599–602.

75. Couet J, Sar S, Jolivet A, et al. Shedding of human TSH receptor ectodomain: involvement of a matrix metalloprotease. J Biol Chem 1996;271:4545–52.

76. de Bernard S, Misrahi M, Huet JC, et al. Sequential cleavage and excision of a segment of the thyrotropin receptor ectodomain. J Biol Chem 1999;274: 101–7.

77. Kaczur V, Puskas LG, Nagy ZU, et al. Cleavage of the human thyrotropin receptor by ADAM10 is regulated by thyrotropin. J Mol Recognit 2007;20: 392–404.

78. Couet J, de Bernard S, Loosfelt H, et al. Cell surface protein disulfide-isomerase is involved in the shedding of human thyrotropin receptor ectodomain. Biochemistry 1996;35:14800–5.
79. Couet J, Sar S, Jolivet A, et al. Shedding of human thyrotropin receptor ectodomain Involvement of a matrix metalloprotease. J Biol Chem 1996;271(8): 4545–52.
80. Chen CR, Chazenbalk GD, Wawrowsky KA, et al. Evidence that human thyroid cells express uncleaved, single-chain thyrotropin receptors on their surface. Endocrinology 2006;147:3107–13.
81. Latif R, Ando T, Davies TF. Monomerization as a prerequisite for intramolecular cleavage and shedding of the thyrotropin receptor. Endocrinology 2004;145: 5580–8.
82. Vassart G, Costagliola S. A physiological role for the posttranslational cleavage of the thyrotropin receptor? Endocrinology 2004;145:1–3.
83. Ciullo I, Latif R, Graves P, et al. Functional assessment of the thyrotropin receptor-beta subunit. Endocrinology 2003;144:3176–81.
84. Quellari M, Desroches A, Beau I, et al. Role of cleavage and shedding in human thyrotropin receptor function and trafficking. Eur J Biochem 2003;270:3486–97.
85. Allgeier A, Offermanns S, Van Sande J, et al. The human thyrotropin receptor activates G-proteins Gs and Gq/11. J Biol Chem 1994;269:13733–5.
86. Kimura T, Van KA, Golstein J, et al. Regulation of thyroid cell proliferation by TSH and other factors: a critical evaluation of in vitro models. Endocr Rev 2001;22: 631–56.
87. Van SJ, Massart C, Costagliola S, et al. Specific activation of the thyrotropin receptor by trypsin. Mol Cell Endocrinol 1996;119:161–8.
88. Vassart G, Pardo L, Costagliola S. A molecular dissection of the glycoprotein hormone receptors. Trends Biochem Sci 2004;29:119–26.
89. Szkudlinski MW, Fremont V, Ronin C, et al. Thyroid-stimulating hormone and thyroid-stimulating hormone receptor structure-function relationships. Physiol Rev 2002;82:473–502.
90. Zhang M, Tong KP, Fremont V, et al. The extracellular domain suppresses constitutive activity of the transmembrane domain of the human TSH receptor: implications for hormone-receptor interaction and antagonist design. Endocrinology 2000;141:3514–7.
91. Marshall CJ. MAP kinase kinase kinase, MAP kinase kinase and MAP kinase. Curr Opin Genet Dev 1994;4:82–9.
92. Dremier S, Milenkovic M, Blancquaert S, et al. Cyclic AMP-dependent protein kinases, but not Epac, mediate TSH/cyclic AMP-dependent regulation of thyroid cells. Endocrinology 2007;148(10):4612–22.
93. Frodin M, Gammeltoft S. Role and regulation of 90 kDa ribosomal S6 kinase (RSK) in signal transduction. Mol Cell Endocrinol 1999;151:65–77.
94. Stoyanov B, Volinia S, Hanck T, et al. Cloning and characterization of a G protein-activated human phosphoinositide-3 kinase. Science 1995;269:690–3.
95. Kasri NN, Holmes AM, Bultynck G, et al. Regulation of InsP3 receptor activity by neuronal Ca2+-binding proteins. EMBO J 2004;23:312–21.
96. Toker A, Newton AC. Cellular signaling: pivoting around PDK-1. Cell 2000;103: 185–8.
97. Balendran A, Hare GR, Kieloch A, et al. Further evidence that 3-phosphoinositide-dependent protein kinase-1 (PDK1) is required for the stability and phosphorylation of protein kinase C (PKC) isoforms. FEBS Lett 2000;484: 217–23.

98. Downward J. Mechanisms and consequences of activation of protein kinase B/Akt. Curr Opin Cell Biol 1998;10:262–7.

99. Downward J. Signal transduction. New exchange, new target. Nature 1998;396: 416–7.

100. Williams MR, Arthur JS, Balendran A, et al. The role of 3-phosphoinositide-dependent protein kinase 1 in activating AGC kinases defined in embryonic stem cells. Curr Biol 2000;10:439–48.

101. Zaballos MA, Garcia B, Santisteban P. G{beta}{gamma} dimers released in response to TSH activate phosphoinositide 3-kinase and regulate gene expression in thyroid cells. Mol Endocrinol 2008;22(5):1183–99.

102. Cao X, Kambe F, Seo H. Requirement of thyrotropin-dependent complex formation of protein kinase A catalytic subunit with inhibitor of {kappa}B proteins for activation of p65 nuclear factor-{kappa}B by tumor necrosis factor-{alpha}. Endocrinology 2005;146:1999–2005.

103. Baeuerle PA, Henkel T. Function and activation of NF-kappa B in the immune system. Annu Rev Immunol 1994;12:141–79.

104. Iacovelli L, Capobianco L, Salvatore L, et al. Thyrotropin activates mitogen-activated protein kinase pathway in FRTL-5 by a cAMP-dependent protein kinase A-independent mechanism. Mol Pharmacol 2001;60:924–33.

105. Park YJ, Park ES, Kim MS, et al. Involvement of the protein kinase C pathway in thyrotropin-induced STAT3 activation in FRTL-5 thyroid cells. Mol Cell Endocrinol 2002;194:77–84.

106. Schmelzle T, Hall MN. TOR, a central controller of cell growth. Cell 2000;103: 253–62.

107. Brewer C, Yeager N, Di CA. Thyroid-stimulating hormone initiated proliferative signals converge in vivo on the mTOR kinase without activating AKT. Cancer Res 2007;67:8002–6.

108. Tomer Y, Davies TF. Searching for the autoimmune thyroid disease susceptibility genes: from gene mapping to gene function. Endocr Rev 2003;24:694–717.

109. Rees Smith B, McLachlan SM, Furmaniak J. Autoantibodies to the thyrotropin receptor. Endocr Rev 1988;9:106–21.

110. Ando T, Latif R, Davies TF. Thyrotropin receptor antibodies: new insights into their actions and clinical relevance. Best Pract Res Clin Endocrinol Metab 2005;19:33–52.

111. Kim WB, Chung HK, Park YJ, et al. The prevalence and clinical significance of blocking thyrotropin receptor antibodies in untreated hyperthyroid Graves' disease. Thyroid 2000;10:579–86.

112. Atger M, Misrahi M, Young J, et al. Autoantibodies interacting with purified native thyrotropin receptor. Eur J Biochem 1999;265:1022–31.

113. Weetman AP, Yateman ME, Ealey PA, et al. Thyroid-stimulating antibody activity between different immunoglobulin G subclasses. J Clin Invest 1990;86:723–7.

114. Zakarija M. Immunochemical characterization of the thyroid-stimulating antibody (TSAb) of Graves' disease: evidence for restricted heterogeneity. J Clin Lab Immunol 1983;10:77–85.

115. Metcalfe R, Jordan N, Watson P, et al. Demonstration of immunoglobulin G, A, and E autoantibodies to the human thyrotropin receptor using flow cytometry. J Clin Endocrinol Metab 2002;87:1754–61.

116. Sanders J, Evans M, Premawardhana LD, et al. Human monoclonal thyroid stimulating autoantibody. Lancet 2003;362:126–8.

117. Smith BR, Sanders J, Furmaniak J. TSH receptor antibodies. Thyroid 2007;17: 923–38.

118. Costagliola S, Bonomi M, Morgenthaler NG, et al. Delineation of the discontinuous-conformational epitope of a monoclonal antibody displaying full in vitro and in vivo thyrotropin activity. Mol Endocrinol 2004;18:3020–34.
119. Minich WB, Lenzner C, Morgenthaler NG. Antibodies to TSH-receptor in thyroid autoimmune disease interact with monoclonal antibodies whose epitopes are broadly distributed on the receptor. Clin Exp Immunol 2004;136:129–36.
120. Ando T, Imaizumi M, Graves P, et al. Induction of thyroid-stimulating hormone receptor autoimmunity in hamsters. Endocrinology 2003;144:671–80.
121. Ando T, Latif R, Daniel S, et al. Dissecting linear and conformational epitopes on the native thyrotropin receptor. Endocrinology 2004;145:5185–93.
122. Nagayama Y, Kita-Furuyama M, Ando T, et al. A novel murine model of Graves' hyperthyroidism with intramuscular injection of adenovirus expressing the thyrotropin receptor. J Immunol 2002;168:2789–94.
123. Schwarz-Lauer L, Pichurin PN, Chen CR, et al. The cysteine-rich amino terminus of the thyrotropin receptor is the immunodominant linear antibody epitope in mice immunized using naked deoxyribonucleic acid or adenovirus vectors. Endocrinology 2003;144:1718–25.
124. Morshed SA, Latif R, Davies TF. Characterization of thyrotropin receptor antibody-induced signaling cascades. Endocrinology 2009;150(1):519–29.
125. Gilbert JA, Gianoukakis AG, Salehi S, et al. Monoclonal pathogenic antibodies to the thyroid-stimulating hormone receptor in Graves' disease with potent thyroid-stimulating activity but differential blocking activity activate multiple signaling pathways. J Immunol 2006;176:5084–92.
126. Ando T, Davies TF. Monoclonal antibodies to the thyrotropin receptor. Clin Dev Immunol 2005;12:137–43.
127. Costagliola S, Rodien P, Many MC, et al. Genetic immunization against the human thyrotropin receptor causes thyroiditis and allows production of monoclonal antibodies recognizing the native receptor. J Immunol 1998;160:1458–65.
128. Chen CR, McLachlan SM, Rapoport B. Suppression of thyrotropin receptor constitutive activity by a monoclonal antibody with inverse agonist activity. Endocrinology 2007;148:2375–82.

# Toward Better Models of Hyperthyroid Graves' Disease

Selçuk Dağdelen, MD[a,b,*], Yi-chi M. Kong, PhD[c], J. Paul Banga, PhD[a]

**KEYWORDS**

• Graves' disease • Experimental models • Autoimmunity

Hyperthyroid Graves' disease occurs spontaneously only in humans, in whom the clinical manifestations are well recognized to be mediated by autoantibodies to the thyroid-stimulating hormone (TSH) receptor (TSHR). The disease can be induced in experimental animals such as mice by special techniques leading to in vivo expression of the TSHR. These techniques include inoculation with syngeneic cells expressing TSHR or by gene delivery methods such as plasmid cDNA or adenovirus vectors encoding the TSHR or its A-subunit. Depending on the strain, which can include certain inbred, outbred, or transgenic humanized mice, the immunized animals develop thyroid-stimulating antibodies (TSAbs), which closely resemble those present in patients with Graves' disease and may also be accompanied by goiter. More recently, models have been developed whereby chronic stimulation of the thyroid gland is mediated by passive transfer of monoclonal antibodies (mAbs) with strong thyroid-stimulating properties. In addition, other chronic models that use special immunization techniques to induce a prolonged thyroid-stimulating antibody response have also been described. Models that incorporate thyroid inflammation by depleting regulatory T cells before immunization with adenovirus vectors are becoming increasingly close to the clinical condition in patients. Sustained studies over the past decade have led to progressively more realistic models of Graves' disease, providing the basis for further immunologic investigations and facilitating the evaluation of new treatments for the

Dr. Dağdelen is supported by a Research Fellowship at King's College London by the Hacettepe University School of Medicine and Turkish Society of Endocrinology and Metabolism.

[a] Department of Diabetes and Endocrinology, King's College London School of Medicine, Denmark Hill Campus, The Rayne Institute, 123 Coldharbour Lane, London, SE5 9NU, UK
[b] Department of Endocrinology and Metabolism, Hacettepe University, School of Medicine, Ankara, Turkey
[c] Department of Immunology and Microbiology, Wayne State University School of Medicine, 540 E. Canfield Avenue, Detroit MI 48201, USA
* Corresponding author. Department of Diabetes and Endocrinology, King's College London School of Medicine, Denmark Hill Campus, The Rayne Institute, 123 Coldharbour Lane, London, SE5 9NU, UK.
*E-mail address:* selcuk.dagdelen@kcl.ac.uk (S. Dağdelen).

Endocrinol Metab Clin N Am 38 (2009) 343–354
doi:10.1016/j.ecl.2009.01.003
0889-8529/09/$ – see front matter © 2009 Published by Elsevier Inc.

disease. Ultimately, such work should also lead to a complete model of Graves' disease that incorporates extrathyroidal complications such as eye disease.

## EXPERIMENTAL MODELS OF GRAVES' DISEASE
### The First Successful Model

The cloning of TSHR in 1989 was instrumental in the momentum to develop models of Graves' disease.[1–4] In 1996 the first model for Graves' disease was described, generally referred to as the Shimojo model.[5] The model was based on the premise that aberrant expression of major histocompatibility (MHC) class II on thyroid epithelial cells resulted in these cells acting as antigen-presenting cells (APCs) to initiate and propagate the autoimmune insult.[6] Fibroblast L cells, which express accessory costimulatory molecules, were transfected to express human TSHR and MHC class II antigens and were used as nonprofessional APCs.[5] Multiple injections of the transfected fibroblasts into syngeneic AKR/N mice resulted in the induction of anti-TSHR antibodies in all of the animals, measured as TSH-binding inhibiting immunoglobulin activity. Nevertheless, only a small proportion of the animals developed hyperthyroidism (15% to 20%), as defined by elevated serum T4 levels and the production of TSAbs.[1] Furthermore, this model has several other drawbacks. Besides being restricted to one syngeneic strain of inbred mice (H-2 k), there is the drawback of nonspecific activation of the immune system due to the high levels of costimulation by the injected cells. In addition, several months are required to develop the model. Despite these limitations, the model has been successfully established in a number of laboratories, including the authors', and, as the first model of hyperthyroid Graves' disease, it represents a landmark in the field.[7]

### Models That Followed the Shimojo

#### Similar models

Variations on the Shimojo model are also reported. The use of an adjuvant with the transfected fibroblasts expressing MHC class II and TSHR improved the disease incidence in the model. In particular, use of a Th2 adjuvant comprising alum and pertussis toxin increased the incidence of elevated serum T4 to approximately 50% of the animals.[8] In a corollary to this model, outbred hamsters immunized with Chinese hamster ovary cells transfected to express human TSHR allowed the development of another rodent model, although outside the usual realm of a mouse model.[9] Although these Shimojo-like approaches improved on the original model in terms of disease incidence, they all generally behaved in a similar fashion in terms of a complete lack of thyroid inflammation.[9]

A notable exception was the model in BALB/c mice reported by Prabhakar's laboratory in 1999 using syngeneic B-cell lymphoma cells transfected to express TSHR.[10] B cells constitutively express MHC class II with accessory costimulatory molecules and act as professional APCs; therefore, the B-cell immunization model appears to be more suited than the fibroblast model for the induction of disease. This B-cell approach with adjuvant immunization was reported to show hyperthyroidism in 100% of the animals and was accompanied by considerable thyroid inflammation.[10] Despite its high penetrance, for some unknown reason attempts to reproduce this model have been less successful than for the other models described previously, which have been widely replicated. Nevertheless, in the laboratories that have attempted to reproduce the B-cell immunization model, hyperthyroidism has been reported in 50% of the animal groups, although far below the initial reported 100% incidence.[11] In the same report, another variation on the model used injection of BALB/c mice with xenogeneic human embryonic kidney 293 cells transfected to express TSHR ectodomain.[10] Although the rationale for using this xenogeneic system is difficult to perceive, the majority of the animals developed hyperthyroidism. This report also described the use of soluble ectodomain of TSHR protein in adjuvant to induce disease in BALB/c mice.[10]

## DNA Delivery Models

### Plasmid DNA injections in inbred mice
In contrast to the cellular models, other approaches have relied on vaccination with TSHR plasmid DNA in eukaryotic expression vectors. Challenging BALB/c mice by intramuscular injection of naked plasmid coding for human TSHR produced anti-TSHR antibodies, but no hyperthyroidism was evident.[12] Using outbred animals injected in the same manner resulted in hyperthyroidism, although the disease incidence was low at 15%.[13] Low-grade thyroid infiltrates were reported in both the BALB/c and the outbred strains of mice.[12,13] Variation in the injection site to an intradermal placement did not have a significant effect on disease incidence;[14] however, replication of this model has proved notoriously difficult in a number of laboratories, including the authors'.[15–17]

### Plasmid DNA injection in HLA transgenic mice
The MHC allele, HLA-DRB1*0301, associates most strongly with human thyroid autoimmune disease.[18] The authors used humanized mice made transgenic for HLA class II genes to assess the development of hyperthyroidism by the plasmid DNA injection route.[19] These transgenic animals lacked endogenous MHC class II, leading to the expression of the human allele only. To further improve on the model, we used transgenic mice with a background of autoimmunity-prone genes derived from the NOD mouse. In contrast to the transgenic animals lacking NOD background genes, which failed to develop hyperthyroidism, almost one third of the transgenic animals on the NOD background developed hyperthyroidism.[19,20] Interestingly, both of the transgenic strains developed thyroid inflammation, indicating that the genes regulating thyroid infiltration and those responsible for hyperthyroidism are distinct.

### DNA delivery by adenovirus injections
Adenoviral vectors are well recognized to be effective vehicles for delivery of antigen to induce potent T- and B-cell antibody responses.[21] With this improved method of gene delivery, Nagayama and his team showed that injections of recombinant adenovirus coding for TSHR were highly efficient in inducing anti-TSHR antibodies in a variety of inbred strains of mice.[22] Moreover, in BALB/c animals, over 50% of the mice showed hyperthyroidism as assessed by elevated serum T4 levels, whereas other strains such as C57BL/6 were less susceptible, and CBA/J, DBA/1J, and SJL/J animals were completely resistant.[22] There was no thyroid inflammation apparent in any strain with this procedure. The beauty of this model is that a variety of mouse strains can be tested for disease susceptibility.[7] Furthermore, at least in female BALB/c mice, the number of animals susceptible to disease was greater than 50%, allowing immunologic investigations to be initiated, which were not possible with the earlier models due to the low disease incidence.[7] The adenovirus model, like the Shimojo model, did not show any gender bias, and, together with the lack of thyroid gland infiltrate, differs considerably from the human condition.[22–24]

The TSHR is unique among the G-protein coupled receptor families for undergoing cleavage of the N-terminal ectodomain (known as the A-subunit) from the transmembrane and the intracellular regions (known as the B-subunit).[25] In fact, this property of the TSHR has been implicated as one of the prime reasons for its role as an autoantigen[26] and provides an explanation for the preferential binding of TSAbs to the ectodomain when compared with the wild-type, full-length molecule.[27,28] These findings led McLachlan and Rapoport to assess the efficacy of adenovirus expressing the A-subunit of the TSHR (coding for amino acid residues 1 to 289) in inducing hyperthyroidism.[28] As anticipated, the use of AdTSHR289 virus led to a further increase in disease incidence, occurring in as many as 80% of the animals when compared with the wild-type, full-length receptor, making the model even more suited for immunologic studies. To date, this model has proved to be highly reproducible and is the most widely used, including the authors' laboratories.[29–32]

## IMPROVEMENTS IN RECENT MODELS OF GRAVES' DISEASE

Inevitably with time, newer experimental models of Graves' disease have been developed. With the development of mAbs to the TSHR, which act as powerful agonists for the receptor, passive transfer of small quantities of the mAbs into normal animals leads to in vivo stimulation of the thyroid gland, resulting in rapid induction of hyperthyroidism.[29,32–35] Some of the recent models appear to be superior, whereas others provide features not present in the earlier models.[7] All of the newer models are based in the mouse, which is amenable to immunologic manipulations.

### Acute and Chronic Models of Hyperthyroidism by Passive Transfer

Although it is well accepted that the antibodies to the TSHR in Graves' patients are responsible for the hyperthyroidism, it has been difficult to study the mechanism for this in patients. Understanding why the TSHR fails to show refractoriness (desensitization) in Graves' patients despite continuous stimulation in vivo by serum TSAbs is of fundamental importance. The difficulty in studying this mechanism is complicated further because the serum antibodies comprise multiple antibodies to the TSHR, with a range of thyroid stimulating (full and partial agonists) and blocking properties.[36] Moreover, there is a paucity of these antibodies in patient serum, which hampers purification for structure/function analysis.[36]

Both acute and chronic models of antibody-mediated thyroid stimulation by passive transfer of mAbs with powerful agonist activity for the TSHR have been described.[29,33–35] In an acute setting, intravenous injection of a mAb with TSAb activity at low nanogram doses in mice induces rapid elevation of serum T4 levels within 12 to 24 hours that is maintained for a few days before returning to baseline levels.[29,33–35] The more interesting and important chronic exposure studies by passive transfer to replicate the situation in Graves' patients have given contradictory results.[33,35] In a xenogeneic study, chronic stimulation with a TSAb mAb produced by hamster hybridoma grown as ascites in immunodeficient mice resulted in refractoriness of the thyroid gland after 2 weeks, with serum T4 levels in treated mice maintained at similar levels to the untreated control animals.[33] In the authors' chronic exposure study, two different mouse mAbs with strong thyroid-stimulating activity were used but with subtle differences in the characteristics of their stimulation kinetics of the receptor.[29] Weekly intravenous injections of 10 µg of IgG into mice over a period of 9 weeks resulted in the serum levels of T4 continually maintained above baseline, resembling the sustained hyperthyroid status in patients with Graves' disease without receptor desensitization.[35] The different outcomes in the two chronic models described may relate to differences in the stimulatory mAbs, both qualitative and quantitative. It is likely that the xenogeneic hybridoma cells produced more TSAb, thereby saturating the receptors, although the catabolic rate and quantities produced were not reported.[33,35]

## Improved DNA Delivery Model

The earlier plasmid DNA delivery models have proven unreliable in terms of low disease incidence and reproducibility in several laboratories. A much improved plasmid DNA model using in vivo electroporation (electrovaccination) has been recently described for efficient in vivo gene delivery of the TSHR for induction of Graves' disease.[37] Using cDNA coding for the holoreceptor and depending on the plasmid construct, hyperthyroidism was induced in 12% to 32% of the animal population. Disease incidence was elevated significantly to 80% to 95% when the A-subunit (TSHR289) fused with a sequence of histidine residues was used. The novel feature reported for this protocol to induce "murine Graves' disease" was the longevity of the induced antibody to TSHR, which persisted for several months.[37] In other genetic delivery models, such as the adenovirus protocol, the induced antibody declines soon after the final injection. In principle, the electrovaccination model with its high disease incidence and longevity of the induced antibody perfectly replicates the situation in Graves' patients by continuous chronic stimulation of the thyroid gland by the persisting antibody. Despite the lack of thyroid inflammation in this model, it represents a huge leap forward as an ideal model to study the immunology and therapeutic interventions for Graves' disease. The electrovaccination model has not yet been repeated in an independent laboratory, and reports of its use are keenly awaited.

## Models with Thyroid Inflammation

Graves' disease in humans is frequently accompanied by foci of lymphocyte infiltration as well as extrathyroidal complications of thyroid eye disease and pretibial myxedema.[38] Attempts to generate experimental models of thyroid eye disease in animals with TSHR-induced hyperthyroidism have shown little promise.[11,39,40] Currently, no viable models exist for this condition, although the possibility remains that a second autoantigen may be important for this condition.[41] When outbred mice or humanized DR3 transgenic NOD animals are immunized with TSHR cDNA, the induced hyperthyroidism is sometimes accompanied by thyroid inflammation comprising a low-grade lymphocyte infiltrate (**Fig. 1A, B**).[13,19] These findings contrast with the pathologic features of the gland after chronic stimulation, which show hyperplastic thyroid follicles in the absence of inflammatory cells (see **Fig. 1C**).[35] Thyroid inflammation has also been reported in BALB/c animals with the B-cell immunization model of M12 cells expressing TSHR.[10] It is unclear whether the immune response to the TSHR is solely responsible for the lymphocytic infiltrate into the thyroid gland or whether other thyroid antigens such as thyroid peroxidase (TPO) and thyroglobulin (Tg), which are the common autoantigens in destructive (Hashimoto's) thyroiditis, are recruited into the autoimmune insult following intensified TSHR stimulation.[18,42] In the authors' humanized DR3 transgenic NOD model, one animal with a focal infiltrate into the gland was also weakly positive for anti-Tg antibodies;[19] however, it was unclear whether the anti-Tg response was generated as a consequence of TSHR stimulation or the genetic susceptibility of NOD mice to spontaneously develop a low incidence of anti-Tg antibodies and thyroiditis with age.

C57BL/6 mice are normally resistant to disease induction; however, Nagayama and colleagues[43,44] have shown that depletion of $CD4^+CD25^+$ or $CD8^+CD122^+$ regulatory T cells (Tregs) with anti-CD25 or anti-CD122, respectively, followed by immunization of adenovirus coding for TSHR289 protein leads to hyperthyroidism in this strain, accompanied by lymphocytic infiltration and follicular cell destruction. Intriguingly, BALB/c mice that are normally permissive to hyperthyroidism do not show infiltration following depletion of Tregs.[43] On the other hand, BALB/c mice that are normally resistant to the

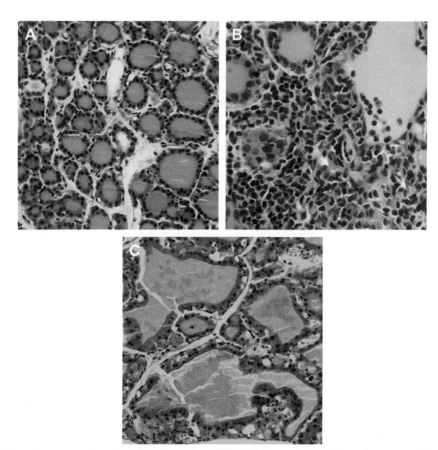

Fig. 1. Representative thyroid sections from TSHR DNA-immunized mice or from mice after chronic stimulation with anti-TSHR mAb injections. Sections from a mouse (A) given vector control and an immunized mouse (B) showing greater than 10% to 20% thyroid infiltration (original magnification, 100× and 200×, respectively). (C) Enlarged thyroid with hyperplastic follicles after chronic stimulation with weekly injections of mAb with powerful thyroid stimulating properties (magnification 200×). (From Flynn JC, Rao PV, Gora M, et al. Graves' hyperthyroidism induced in HLA-DRB1*0301 (DR3) transgenic mice by immunization with thyrotropin receptor DNA. Clin Exp Immunol 2004; 135(1):39 [panels A and B]; and Flynn JC, Gilbert JA, Meroueh C, et al. Chronic exposure in vivo to thyrotropin receptor stimulating monoclonal antibodies sustains high thyroxine levels and thyroid hyperplasia in thyroid autoimmunity-prone HLA-DRB1*0301 transgenic mice. Immunology 2007;122(2):265 [panel C]; with permission.)

induction of thyroiditis with mouse Tg readily develop thyroiditis after depletion of Tregs.[45] Similarly, in a novel transgenic BALB/c model in which the A-subunit of TSHR is targeted to the thyroid, McLachlan and coworkers showed that depletion of Tregs by injection of anti-CD25 followed by adenovirus A-subunit immunizations led to an intense infiltration of the thyroid gland, demonstrating that peripheral T-cell regulation was essential in a model in which central tolerance fails to completely delete TSHR-specific T cells in the thymus.[46] Interestingly, in those animals, there was a strong antibody response to mouse TPO and Tg, giving compelling evidence that antigen spreading from the TSHR to the other thyroid antigens was responsible for the inflammation in the thyroid gland. It is unknown whether the repeated anti-CD25 injections had any effect on TSHR-specific effector T cells.[46]

Although early models of Graves' disease, depending on the strain of animals and the method of TSHR immunization, can result in a mild inflammatory infiltrate into the thyroid gland, some of the studies have not been repeated extensively in independent laboratories to verify the findings. Manipulation of variants of the models, particularly those in which the Treg populations have been depleted, appears to be characterized by inflammatory infiltrates. Nevertheless, it remains uncertain whether TSHR as the sole antigen can provoke inflammation of the thyroid gland or whether spill-over of the immune response to other thyroid antigen targets such as TPO and Tg is responsible for this effect. Studies on the isolated T- and B-cell populations infiltrating the thyroid gland and a characterization of their antigen specificity are clearly necessary to ascertain the role of TSHR stimulation in provoking the inflammatory reaction in thyroid tissue in these models.

## HOW MODELS HAVE BEEN USED TO STUDY THE IMMUNOLOGY OF GRAVES' DISEASE

Spontaneous development of Graves' disease is limited to the human population only. The term *spontaneous* is used because the inductive events are not known. Although it is mediated by T and B cells of the adaptive immune system, detailing the immunology of the disease has proven difficult, particularly because there is a paucity of the "disease-inducing" antibodies in the serum.[36] Furthermore, isolation of the pathogenic T- and B-cell populations has proved difficult[47–49]; hence, the development of animal models of Graves' disease has proved useful for studying the pathogenesis of the disorder. Moreover, intervention therapies can be tested on the models at a preventive and therapeutic level to provide better treatment options for the disease. A brief discussion is provided herein of some of the studies that have taken place on the models of Graves' disease to understand the immunology of the disorder. Greater detail is provided elsewhere in another review.[50]

CD4$^+$ T-helper cells can be divided into two main subsets depending on their cytokine profile as Th1 and Th2 cells.[51] More recently, this simplistic categorization has become more complicated with the definition of the CD4$^+$ subsets into other subpopulations termed *Th17*[52] and *Tregs*. The Tregs have been further divided into natural and induced Treg populations, although, for autoimmune diseases, the induced Tregs are likely an expanded population of natural Tregs with similar antigen specificity (reviewed by T.A. Chatila elsewhere in this issue).[53] Studies aimed at modifying the Th1 and Th2 balance of the immune response to TSHR have shown that, before the onset of disease (preventive setting), polarization of the immune response to the Th1 type can be beneficial, whereas after the onset of disease (as would occur in the human condition), skewing the response to the Th1 or Th2 type has no effect on the course of the disorder.[11,30,54–57]

B-cell targeting has also been used in the Graves' models because it may perturb secretion of the pathogenic TSAbs and also affect antibody independent functions. Targeting of autoreactive B cells has been achieved by interfering with the survival factors essential for B-cell development and maintenance of antibody production. These survival factors belong to the tumor necrosis factor ligand superfamily and are known as B-cell activating factor (BAFF) and A proliferation related induced ligand (APRIL). BAFF binds BAFF-receptor (BAFFR), B-cell maturation antigen (BCMA), and transmembrane activator and cyclophilin ligand interactor (TACI); APRIL only binds

BCMA and TACI.[58,59] To add complexity to the field, some proteoglycans have been reported to bind APRIL alone.[60]

In female BALB/c mice with established hyperthyroidism (induced by recombinant A-subunit adenovirus), blockade of BAFF or BAFF plus APRIL with the antagonists BAFFR-Fc and BCMA-Fc, respectively, leads to a dramatic reduction in the degree of hyperthyroidism with significant suppression of serum T4 and TSAb levels.[61,62] These results imply an important role for BAFF and APRIL in the pathogenesis of Graves' disease. A variety of therapeutic approaches with different antagonists for BAFF and APRIL are under clinical trials for rheumatoid arthritis and systemic lupus erythematosus, and their extension to treating Graves' disease and its complications, such as thyroid eye disease, may prove promising.[63]

The development of animal models of Graves' disease together with the successful isolation of monoclonal TSAbs with powerful biologic activity is beginning to allow studies on the variable regions of the heavy (H) and light (L) chain immunoglobulin (Ig) genes. In diseased animals, the complementarity-determining region-3 (CDR3) sequences of the H chains have been studied at a population level, which by statistical analysis indicate elevated transcription of IgHV1 genes.[64] Moreover, an increased frequency of IgHD52, IgHJ1, and IgHJ4 genes was also shown to be associated with disease.[64] With regard to the mAbs with TSAb activities reported thus far, although the V-region gene sequences have not been entirely published, it is clear that the IgHDQ52 and IgHJ2 gene families have critical roles in the TSAb properties, because all three independent groups with TSAbs report on the same family usage[29,34,65] (as do the authors' unpublished findings [J. Paul Banga, PhD, unpublished data, 2009]). A high ratio of replacement and silent mutation in the CDR3 regions is apparent in all of the reported TSAbs, indicating an antigen (possibly TSHR) driven expansion. The extraordinary high affinity of the TSAbs appears to be derived by somatic mutations in the V-region genes of both the H- and L-chain genes[29,34,65] (authors' unpublished findings). It remains a matter of speculation whether the TSAbs derive from non–TSHR-reactive B cells, which through affinity maturation attain the reactivity of the pathogenic antigen (TSHR), or whether the original inciting antigen is the TSHR itself. It is hoped that the improved models will give insights into these fundamental questions on the immunology of Graves' disease, which will lead to a better understanding of the etiology and the underlying disease mechanisms.

## REFERENCES

1. Nagayama Y, Kaufman KD, Seto P, et al. Molecular cloning, sequence and functional expression of the cDNA for the human thyrotropin receptor. Biochem Biophys Res Commun 1989;165(3):1184–90.

2. Libert F, Lefort A, Gerard C, et al. Cloning, sequencing and expression of the human thyrotropin (TSH) receptor: evidence for binding of autoantibodies. Biochem Biophys Res Commun 1989;165(3):1250–5.

3. Misrahi M, Loosfelt H, Atger M, et al. Cloning, sequencing and expression of human TSH receptor. Biochem Biophys Res Commun 1990;166(1):394–403.

4. Frazier AL, Robbins LS, Stork PJ, et al. Isolation of TSH and LH/CG receptor cDNAs from human thyroid: regulation by tissue specific splicing. Mol Endocrinol 1990;4(8):1264–76.

5. Shimojo N, Kohno Y, Yamaguchi K, et al. Induction of Graves'-like disease in mice by immunization with fibroblasts transfected with the thyrotropin receptor and a class II molecule. Proc Natl Acad Sci U S A 1996;93(20):11074–9.

6. Bottazzo GF, Pujol-Borrell R, Hanafusa T, et al. Role of aberrant HLA-DR expression and antigen presentation in induction of thyroid autoimmunity. Lancet 1983; 2(8359):1115–9.
7. Banga JP. The long and winding road for an experimental model of hyperthyroid Graves' disease. In: Wiersinga WM, Drexhage HA, Weetman AP, editors. The thyroid and autoimmunity. Stuttgart: Verlag; 2007. p. 118–25.
8. Kita M, Ahmad L, Marians RC, et al. Regulation and transfer of a murine model of thyrotropin receptor antibody mediated Graves' disease. Endocrinology 1999; 140(3):1392–8.
9. Ando T, Imaizumi M, Graves P, et al. Induction of thyroid stimulating hormone receptor autoimmunity in hamsters. Endocrinology 2003;144(2):671–80.
10. Kaithamana S, Fan J, Osuga Y, et al. Induction of experimental autoimmune Graves' disease in BALB/c mice. J Immunol 1999;163(9):5157–64.
11. Land KJ, Moll JS, Kaplan MH, et al. Signal transducer and activator of transcription (Stat)-6-dependent, but not Stat-4-dependent, immunity is required for the development of autoimmunity in Graves' hyperthyroidism. Endocrinology 2004; 145(8):3724–30.
12. Costagliola S, Rodien P, Many MC, et al. Genetic immunization against the human thyrotropin receptor causes thyroiditis and allows production of monoclonal antibodies recognizing the native receptor. J Immunol 1998;160(3):1458–65.
13. Costagliola S, Many MC, Denef JF, et al. Genetic immunization of outbred mice with thyrotropin receptor cDNA provides a model of Graves' disease. J Clin Invest 2000;105(6):803–11.
14. Barrett K, Liakata E, Rao PV, et al. Induction of hyperthyroidism in mice by intradermal immunization with DNA encoding the thyrotropin receptor. Clin Exp Immunol 2004;136(3):413–22.
15. Pichurin P, Yan XM, Farilla L, et al. Naked TSH receptor DNA vaccination: a Th1 T cell response in which interferon g production rather than antibody dominates the immune response in mice. Endocrinology 2001;142(8):3530–6.
16. Rao PV, Watson PF, Weetman AP, et al. Contrasting activities of thyrotropin receptor antibodies in experimental models of Graves' disease induced by injection of transfected fibroblasts or deoxyribonucleic acid vaccination. Endocrinology 2003;144(1):260–6.
17. Baker G, Mazziotti G, von Ruhland C, et al. Reevaluating thyrotropin receptor induced mouse models of Graves' disease and ophthalmopathy. Endocrinology 2005;146(2):835–44.
18. Kong YM. Recent developments in the relevance of animal models to Hashimoto's thyroiditis and Graves' disease. Curr Opin Endocrinol Diabetes Obes 1997; 4:347–53.
19. Flynn JC, Rao PV, Gora M, et al. Graves' hyperthyroidism induced in HLA-DRB1*0301 (DR3) transgenic mice by immunization with thyrotropin receptor DNA. Clin Exp Immunol 2004;135(1):35–40.
20. Pichurin P, Chen CR, Pichurina O, et al. Thyrotropin receptor-DNA vaccination of transgenic mice expressing HLA-DR3 or HLA-DQ6b. Thyroid 2003;13(10):911–7.
21. Bangari DS, Mittal SK. Current strategies and future directions for eluding adenoviral vector immunity. Curr Gene Ther 2006;6(2):215–26.
22. Nagayama Y, Kita-Furuyama M, Ando T, et al. A novel murine model of Graves' hyperthyroidism with intramuscular injection of adenovirus expressing the thyrotropin receptor. J Immunol 2002;168(6):2789–94.
23. Jaume JC, Rapoport B, McLachlan SM. Lack of female bias in a mouse model of autoimmune hyperthyroidism (Graves' disease). Autoimmunity 1999;29(4):269–72.

24. Cooper DS. Hyperthyroidism. Lancet 2003;362(9382):459–68.
25. Nagayama Y, Rapoport B. The thyrotropin receptor 25 years after its discovery: new insight after its molecular cloning. Mol Endocrinol 1992;6(2):145–56.
26. McLachlan SM, Nagayama Y, Rapoport B. Insight into Graves' hyperthyroidism from animal models. Endocr Rev 2005;26(6):800–32.
27. Chazenbalk GD, Pichurin P, Chen CR, et al. Thyroid stimulating autoantibodies in Graves' disease preferentially recognize the free A subunit, not the thyrotropin receptor holoreceptor. J Clin Invest 2002;110(2):209–17.
28. Chen CR, Pichurin P, Nagayama Y, et al. The thyrotropin receptor autoantigen in Graves' disease is the culprit as well as the victim. J Clin Invest 2003;111(12):1897–904.
29. Gilbert JA, Gianoukakis AG, Salehi S, et al. Monoclonal pathogenic antibodies to the TSH receptor in Graves' disease with potent thyroid stimulating activity, but differential blocking activity activate multiple signaling pathways. J Immunol 2006;176(8):5084–92.
30. Land KJ, Gudapati P, Kaplan MH, et al. Differential requirement of signal transducer and activator of transcription-4 (Stat4) and Stat6 in a thyrotropin receptor-289 adenovirus induced model of Graves' hyperthyroidism. Endocrinology 2006;147(1):111–9.
31. Chen CR, Pichurin P, Chazenbalk GD, et al. Low dose immunization with adenovirus expressing the thyroid stimulating hormone receptor A-subunit deviates the antibody response toward that of autoantibodies in human Graves' disease. Endocrinology 2004;145(1):228–33.
32. Mizutori Y, Saitoh O, Eguchi K, et al. Adenovirus encoding the thyrotropin receptor A-subunit improves the efficacy of dendritic cell-induced Graves' hyperthyroidism in mice. J Autoimmun 2006;26(1):32–6.
33. Ando T, Latif R, Davies TF. Concentration dependent regulation of thyrotropin receptor function by thyroid stimulating antibody. J Clin Invest 2004;113(11):1589–95.
34. Costagliola S, Bonomi M, Morgenthaler N, et al. Delineation of the discontinuous conformational epitope of a monoclonal antibody displaying full in vitro and in vivo thyrotropin activity. Mol Endocrinol 2004;18(12):3020–34.
35. Flynn JC, Gilbert JA, Meroueh C, et al. Chronic exposure in vivo to thyrotropin receptor stimulating monoclonal antibodies sustains high thyroxine levels and thyroid hyperplasia in thyroid autoimmunity-prone HLA-DRB1*0301 transgenic mice. Immunology 2007;122(2):261–7.
36. Rees Smith B, McLachlan SM, Furmaniak J. Autoantibodies to the thyrotropin receptor. Endocr Rev 1988;9(1):106–21.
37. Kaneda T, Honda A, Hakozaki A, et al. An improved Graves' disease model established by using in vivo electroporation exhibited long-term immunity to hyperthyroidism in BALB/c mice. Endocrinology 2007;148(5):2335–44.
38. Rapoport B, Alsabeh R, Aftergood D, et al. Elephantiasic pretibial myxedema: insight into and a hypothesis regarding the pathogenesis of the extrathyroidal manifestations of Graves' disease. Thyroid 2000;10(8):685–92.
39. Many MC, Costagliola S, Detrait M, et al. Development of an animal model of autoimmune thyroid disease. J Immunol 1999;162(8):4966–74.
40. Yamada M, Li AW, West KA, et al. Experimental model for ophthalmopathy in BALB/c and outbred (CD-1) mice genetically immunized with G2s and the thyrotropin receptor. Autoimmunity 2002;35(6):403–13.
41. Smith TJ, Hoa N. Immunoglobulins from patients with Graves' disease induce hyaluronan synthesis in their orbital fibroblasts through the self-antigen, insulin-like growth factor-I receptor. J Clin Endocrinol Metab 2004;89(10):5076–80.

42. Ng HP, Banga JP, Kung AW. Development of a murine model of autoimmune thyroiditis induced with homologous mouse thyroid peroxidase. Endocrinology 2004;145(2):809–16.

43. Saitoh O, Nagayama Y. Regulation of Graves' hyperthyroidism with naturally occurring CD4+CD25+ regulatory T cells in a mouse model. Endocrinology 2006;147(5):2417–22.

44. Saitoh O, Abiru N, Nakahara M, et al. CD8+CD122+ T cells, a newly identified regulatory T subset, negatively regulate Graves' hyperthyroidism in a murine model. Endocrinology 2007;148(12):6040–6.

45. Wei WZ, Jacob JB, Zielinski JF, et al. Concurrent induction of antitumor immunity and autoimmune thyroiditis in CD4+CD25+ regulatory T cell–depleted mice. Cancer Res 2005;65(18):8471–8.

46. McLachlan SM, Nagayama Y, Pichurin PN, et al. The link between Graves' disease and Hashimoto's thyroiditis: a role for regulatory T cells. Endocrinology 2007;148(12):5724–33.

47. Pichurin P, Schwarz-Lauer L, Braley-Mullen H, et al. Peptide scanning for thyrotropin receptor T-cell epitopes in mice vaccinated with naked DNA. Thyroid 2002;12(9):755–64.

48. Martin A, Nakashima M, Zhou A, et al. Detection of major T cell epitopes on human thyroid stimulating hormone receptor by overriding immune heterogeneity in patients with Graves' disease. J Clin Endocrinol Metab 1997;82(10):3361–6.

49. Soliman M, Kaplan E, Yanagawa T, et al. T cells recognize multiple epitopes in the human thyrotropin receptor extracellular domain. J Clin Endocrinol Metab 1995;80(3):905–14.

50. Banga JP, Nielsen CH, Gilbert JA, et al. Application of new therapies in Graves' disease and thyroid associated ophthalmopathy: animal models and translation to human clinical trials. Thyroid 2008;18(9):973–81.

51. Mosmann TR, Coffman RL. Th1 and Th2 cells: different patterns of lymphokine secretion lead to different functional properties. Annu Rev Immunol 1989;7:145–73.

52. Steinman L. A brief history of TH17, the first major revision in the Th1/Th2 hypothesis of T cell mediated tissue damage. Nat Med 2007;13(2):139–45.

53. Morris GP, Brown NK, Kong YC. Naturally existing CD4+CD25+Foxp3+ regulatory T cells are required for tolerance to experimental autoimmune thyroiditis induced by either exogenous or endogenous autoantigen. J Autoimmun, in press.

54. Dogan RN, Vasu C, Holterman MJ, et al. Absence of IL4, and not suppression of Th2 response, prevents development of experimental autoimmune Graves' disease. J Immunol 2003;170(4):2195–204.

55. Nagayama Y, Mizuguchi H, Hayakawa T, et al. Prevention of autoantibody-mediated Graves' like hyperthyroidism in mice with IL4, a Th2 cytokine. J Immunol 2003;170(7):3522–7.

56. Nagayama Y, Watanabe K, Niwa M, et al. Schistosoma mansoni and a-galactosylceramide: prophylactic effect of Th1 immune suppression in a mouse model of Graves' hyperthyroidism. J Immunol 2003;173(3):2167–73.

57. Nagayama Y, Saitoh O, McLachlan SM, et al. TSH receptor adenovirus-induced Graves' hyperthyroidism is attenuated in both interferon-gamma and interleukin-4 knockout mice: implications for the Th1/Th2 paradigm. Clin Exp Immunol 2004;138(3):417–22.

58. Dillon SR, Gross JA, Ansell SM, et al. An APRIL to remember: novel TNF ligands as therapeutic targets. Nat Rev Drug Discov 2006;5(3):235–46.

59. Mackay F, Silveira PA, Brink R. B cells and the BAFF/APRIL axis: fast forward on autoimmunity and signaling. Curr Opin Immunol 2007;19(3):327–36.

60. Ingold K, Zumsteg A, Tardivel A, et al. Identification of proteoglycans as the APRIL-specific binding partners. J Exp Med 2005;201(9):1375–83.

61. Gilbert JA, Kalled SL, Moorhead J, et al. Treatment of autoimmune hyperthyroidism in a murine model of Graves' disease with tumour necrosis factor family ligand inhibitors suggests a key role for B cell activating factor in disease pathology. Endocrinology 2006;147(10):4561–8.

62. Wang SH, Baker JR. Targeting B cells in Graves' disease. Endocrinology 2006; 147(10):4559–60.

63. Stohl W. BlySfulness does not equal BlissFulness in systemic lupus erythematosus: a therapeutic role for BlyS antagonists. Curr Dir Autoimmun 2005;8:289–304.

64. Martinez O, Gangi E, Mordi D, et al. Diversity in the complementarity-determining region 3 (CDR3) of antibodies from mice with evolving anti-thyroid-stimulating hormone receptor antibody responses. Endocrinology 2007;148(2):752–61.

65. Sanders J, Jeffreys J, Depraetere H, et al. Thyroid-stimulating monoclonal antibodies. Thyroid 2002;12(12):1043–50.

# Treatment of Graves' Hyperthyroidism: Evidence-Based and Emerging Modalities

Laszlo Hegedüs, MD, DMSc

**KEYWORDS**

- Graves' disease • Hyperthyroidism • Goiter
- Antithyroid drugs • Radioactive iodine • Thyroidectomy

The etiology of Graves' disease (GD) presently is thought to be based on genetic susceptibility interacting with a number of known and unknown environmental or intrinsic factors.[1,2] Therefore, its treatment optimally would be based on modifying these environmental triggers, of which smoking is best documented.[3,4] Without the potential breakthrough of a novel, biologically modifying class of drugs, such as the B-cell–depleting drug rituximab (RTX),[5] knowledge of the effects and side-effects of the available routine therapeutic options has changed only to a limited degree during the past 50 years. Antithyroid drug (ATD) therapy and radioactive iodine ($^{131}$I; RAI) have been used for more than half a century, and thyroidectomy has been used for more than 100 years. The main advances during the last couple of decades have been the improved knowledge of factors associated with the maximum efficacy of any therapeutic choice, the increased focus on tailoring the therapy to the individual patient, and recognition of the advantages gained by the patient's active participation in the decision-making process. Consequently, congruent phenotypic presentations may not always lead to the same choice of therapy. Besides physician and patient preferences, factors such as the availability of surgical expertise and restrictions in outpatient RAI use may be decisive.

This article discusses the efficacy, side-effects, cost, and influence on quality of life of all the therapeutic options, insofar as data are available. The focus is on the short- and long-term influence of the therapy on thyroid function and size. Special situations such as therapy during pregnancy and during lactation, in childhood and adolescence, in the elderly, and in case of thyroid storm are discussed in passing. A discussion of

This work was supported by grants from the Novo Nordisk Foundation, the Agnes and Knut Mørks Foundation, and the Institute of Clinical Research, Odense University Hospital.

Department of Endocrinology and Metabolism, Odense University Hospital, University of Southern Denmark, Kloevervaenget 6, 3rd floor, DK-5000, Odense, Denmark

*E-mail address:* laszlo.hegedus@ouh.regionsyddanmark.dk

Endocrinol Metab Clin N Am 38 (2009) 355–371
doi:10.1016/j.ecl.2009.01.009
0889-8529/09/$ – see front matter © 2009 Elsevier Inc. All rights reserved.

the treatment of extrathyroidal manifestations of GD, such as Graves' ophthalmopathy or dermopathy (pretibial myxedema), is beyond the scope of this article.

## ANTITHYROID DRUGS
### Clinical Pharmacology

ATDs, known as thionamides, were introduced into clinical practice in the early 1940s. Propylthiouracil (PTU) and methimazole (MMI) are the preferred drugs in the United States, Europe, and Asia; carbimazole, a prodrug of MMI, is the preferred drug in the United Kingdom. Their major action, after active concentration by the thyroid, is to inhibit thyroid hormone synthesis by interfering with thyroid peroxidase (TPOAb)–mediated iodination of tyrosine residues in thyroglobulin.[6] Other effects relate to the blocking of the conversion of thyroxine (T4) to triiodothyronine (T3), but these effects are seen only with PTU and are of limited clinical importance in most cases. Other effects may rely on immunosuppression, as suggested by a decrease in thyrotropin receptor antibodies (TSHRAb), intracellular adhesion molecule, and soluble interleukin-2 and interleukin-6 receptors, as well as decrease in HLA class II expression. Whether these and other changes are caused by the effect of the drug per se on the immune system or by the simultaneous normalization of thyroid function is still a matter of debate.[6,7]

Both PTU and MMI are absorbed rapidly and nearly completely from the gastrointestinal tract. **Table 1** gives the pertinent properties of the two drugs and the differences between them. Importantly, dose adjustment is not necessary in children, in the elderly, or in persons who have impaired liver or kidney function.[6,8]

### Clinical Use of Antithyroid Drugs

ATDs can be used in two ways: either as the primary treatment for hyperthyroidism in an attempt to achieve remission (defined as biochemical euthyroidism for a minimum

**Table 1**
**Comparison of characteristics of the thionamides methimazole and propylthiouracil in the treatment of Graves' disease**

| Characteristic | Methimazole | Propylthiouracil |
|---|---|---|
| Relative potency | 10–50 | 1 |
| Administration | Oral | Oral |
| Absorption | Nearly complete | Nearly complete |
| Binding to serum proteins | Negligible | 80%–90% |
| Serum half-life (hours) | 4–6 | 1–2 |
| Volume of distribution (L) | 40 | 20 |
| Duration of action (hours) | > 24 | 12–24 |
| Metabolism during liver disease | Decreased | Normal |
| Metabolism during kidney disease | Normal | Normal |
| Transplacental passage | Low | Even lower |
| Level in breast milk | Low | Even lower |
| Inhibition of T4/T3 conversion | No | Yes |
| Dosing[a] | 1–2 times daily | 2–3 times daily |

[a] At initial therapy. During titrated ATD therapy, when doses of 5 mg methimazole or 100 propylthiouracil are reached, once-daily dosing is considered prudent and probably secures a higher compliance than the use of divided doses.

of 1 year following cessation of ATD) or to normalize thyroid function as a preparative therapy before ablative treatment with [131]I or thyroid surgery. ATDs often are considered the primary therapy in pregnancy, in children and adolescents, and for patients who have severe Graves' eye disease. Graves' ophthalmopathy has been shown to worsen after the use of [131]I,[9] although this worsening can be prevented by concomitant administration of glucocorticoids.[10]

The choice of ATD is based on custom and personal preference, because few large-scale, randomized clinical trials are available.[11] MMI has the advantages of once- or twice-daily dosing (as opposed dosing two or three times per day with PTU), leading to better compliance; also, thyroid function improves more rapidly with MMI.[11] There is no significant difference in the cost of the drugs. The usual starting dose for MMI is 10 to 40 mg daily, increasing with increasing thyroid size and iodine intake, and taken as one or two daily doses. The usual starting dose for PTU is 300 to 600 mg daily in two to three divided doses. A randomized, controlled trial found little difference in the number of patients achieving euthyroidism within 6 weeks taking 10 mg (85%) or 40 mg (92%) of MMI,[12] suggesting that many patients may do well on relatively small doses of MMI. Initially, thyroid function should be tested every month. After symptom improvement, usually within 1 to 3 months, the drug dose can be tapered, and often 5 to 10 mg MMI or 100 to 200 mg PTU controls the disease. At this point testing every 2 to 3 months suffices. Failure to reduce drug dose adequately can lead to hypothyroidism and goiter growth. During the first 6 months, or even longer, the serum level of thyroid-stimulating hormone (TSH) may remain suppressed despite the normalization of thyroid hormone levels, necessitating the determination of serum thyroid hormone levels in addition to TSH. A subgroup of patients may experience falling serum T4 levels, rising serum T3 levels, and increasing goiter size.[13] This development is seen especially during treatment with PTU and has been ascribed to high levels of type 1 and type 2 deiodinase in thyroid tissue. In such patients a suppressed TSH level and a low serum T4 level does not indicate hypothyroidism, and the ATD dose should not be decreased. Many of patients eventually need treatment with [131]I or surgery.

An alternative to the dose-titration regimen described in the previous paragraph is the block-and-replace regimen, that is, the administration of high doses of ATD and the institution of levothyroxine (LT4) when euthyroidism has been reached to prevent iatrogenic hypothyroidism. Initial reports that the block-and-replace regimen increases the remission rate markedly have not been confirmed subsequently.[12,14,15] An advantage of this combined therapy is the need for less blood testing.

### Factors Associated with Remission

Ideally, the decision to offer remission-inducing ATD therapy should be based on an individualized risk assessment. Key questions are whether the therapy is feasible and whether the choice of ATD, drug dose, therapy length, or the combination of ATD and LT4 influences remission rate. Retrospective studies have suggested that a number of factors are associated with relapse after a course of ATD. These factors include severe hyperthyroidism, a large goiter, thyroid nodularity by imaging, high intrathyroidal blood flow at the termination of ATD therapy, a high serum T3/T4 ratio, high TSHRAb levels initially or at end of therapy, young age, male sex, smoking, presence of ophthalmopathy, long delay from the start of symptoms to initiation of therapy, and problems in coping with daily life (**Box 1**).[6,16] Unfortunately, none of these variables alone is sufficiently sensitive or specific to allow risk stratification. Moreover, a prospective study of more than 300 patients who had GD failed to identify any marker that predicted remission after a 1-year course of ATD.[16] These limitations do not mean that these markers are not useful. In the author's experience, T3-dominated

---

**Box 1**
**Factors thought to be associated with a higher risk of recurrence after treatment with ATD for Graves' disease**

- Recurrence after a previous course of ATD therapy
- Long duration of symptoms pretreatment
- Young age and male sex
- Family history of autoimmune thyroid disease
- Certain genetic markers
- Cigarette smoking
- Presence of clinical ophthalmopathy
- Pronounced hyperthyroidism at presentation
- High serum T3/T4 ratio
- High ATD dose at end of therapy
- Pronounced TSHRAb concentration initially and/or at termination of ATD therapy
- Large goiter size initially and/or at termination of ATD therapy[a]
- Increasing goiter size during therapy[a]
- Nodularity, and/or hypoechogenicity, and/or high intrathyroidal flow (Doppler ultrasound) initially or at termination of therapy[a]

Certain genetic markers are associated with an increased risk of developing Graves' disease (See the article by Pearce and Merriman elsewhere in this issue).[2,21,22]

[a] Size, morphology, and echogenicity determined by high-frequency ultrasound and flow using Doppler ultrasound.

---

hyperthyroidism, increased thyroid size and blood flow, hypoechogenicity on ultrasound, and a markedly elevated TSHRAb—in a variety of combinations—are associated almost invariably with recurrence (author's unpublished observations). Knowledge of these parameters allows a balanced discussion with the patient about the likelihood of success. Based on these criteria, which are facilitated by the increasing availability of ultrasound, many clinicians offer an early choice of ablative therapy, with the aim of limiting futile long-term ATD therapy in many patients. Serial monitoring of the TSHRAb titer already is common practice, and these levels at end of therapy correlate positively with the risk of recurrence.[17,18] The normalization of levels is no guarantee of remission, however, because relapse rates still are 30% to 50%. The observation of Hashizume and colleagues[19] that following ATD plus thyroxine for 1 year by thyroxine alone for 3 years has a beneficial effect on the relapse has not been replicated by others.[20]

Most prospective trials suggest that neither increasing the ATD dose[14] nor prolonging treatment duration beyond 12 months affects relapse rates.[23] Based on the discussion in the previous sections and on a recent evidence-based systematic review,[15] treatment with ATD for 12 to 18 months is recommended. In case of relapse, the patient and the physician may opt for long-term treatment with low-dose ATD as an alternative to ablative therapy. This ATD therapy could, in practice, be life-long. In that case, thyroid function testing need not be performed more than every 4 months or so.

### Long-Term Follow-up

Factors associated with a high risk of relapse of hyperthyroidism have been described earlier in this article. Overall the recurrence rate is 50% to 60%,[14] and most cases of relapse occur within 3 to 6 months of stopping the drug. Most women in remission who become pregnant have a postpartum relapse of GD or develop postpartum thyroiditis.[24] In these women, as in all other patients who have GD, including those in remission, life-long follow-up is recommended, because spontaneous hypothyroidism may develop in a significant number of patients.[25]

### Side Effects of Antithyroid Drugs

The side effects of ATDs are underreported, and the lack of data based on prospective, randomized studies hampers any comparisons of the existing drugs.[11]

Overall, side effects occur in approximately 5% of patients. In most studies, side effects for MMI and PTU are seen with equal frequency,[26,27] although some studies report a higher frequency for side effects with PTU.[6,11] Most side effects are considered minor and include urticaria or other skin rash, pruritus, arthralgia, fever, gastrointestinal complaints, abnormalities of taste and smell, arthritis, and transient granulocytopenia. Side effects of MMI are dose related[6,11] and often are seen within the first weeks or few months of therapy; the side effects of PTU are less clearly related to dose. Most side effects resolve spontaneously or are alleviated by decreasing the drug dose or by taking an antihistamine. It is prudent to switch from one antithyroid drug to the other, but cross-reactivity is around 50%; therefore many patients subsequently need definitive therapy with surgery or [131]I.

Serious side effects that are potentially life threatening, occur in about 3 of 1000 patients.[26] Agranulocytosis (defined as an absolute granulocyte count < 500/mL) is the most feared complication. It often occurs within the first 3 months of therapy and occurs with the same frequency for MMI and PTU ($\sim$ 0.35%); the risk probably is increased in the elderly.[6] There is consensus that a baseline differential white-cell count should be obtained, but most experts do not recommend routine monitoring of granulocyte count during treatment. Patients should be instructed to stop medication and to seek medical attention if they develop a fever or a sore throat (or urinary tract symptoms in women), which are the most common presenting symptoms. If the granulocyte count is less than 1000/mL, the drug should be stopped. In case of sepsis, often associated with *Pseudomonas aeruginosa* in the blood, the patient should be hospitalized, and broad-spectrum antibiotics should be administered intravenously. Although many authorities recommend the use of granulocyte-colony stimulating factor (G-CSF), a prospective, randomized, controlled study showed that G-CSF had no effect on recovery time when used for agranulocytosis caused by ATD.[28] Most patients recover within 2 to 3 weeks, and a fatal outcome is rare. There is cross-reactivity between PTU and MMI; therefore the substitution of one for the other is contraindicated in this situation.

Hepatotoxicity is even rarer than agranulocytosis, with a frequency ranging around 0.1% to 0.2%.[26] Asymptomatic elevation of aminotransferase levels occurs frequently in untreated hyperthyroid patients and can increase slightly after institution of PTU therapy but is not predictive of further increase and usually normalizes during continued therapy. Therefore routine monitoring of liver-function tests is not recommended. Hepatotoxicity, on average, occurs after 3 months of therapy. It is an allergic hepatitis, accompanied by massive hepatic destruction and a marked elevation of aminotransferase levels, which should cause an immediate cessation of PTU therapy. Reported fatality rates of up to 50% probably are the result of publication bias. Liver transplantation may be necessary. Hepatic abnormalities associated with MMI therapy are typical of cholestasis, and complete recovery after drug cessation is the rule. Although the mechanism of hepatotoxicity differs between PTU and MMI, the alternative drug should not be substituted in case of hepatic side effects.

Another very rare major toxic reaction, seen more commonly with PTU than with MMI, is vasculitis. Some patients develop drug-induced systemic lupus erythematosus, but the development of antineutrophil cytoplasmic antibody (ANCA)-positive vasculitis has been reported also, especially in Asians. A recent cross-sectional study from the United Kingdom suggests that around 30% of patients who have present or previous Graves' disease have detectable ANCA, as opposed to around 5% in controls and untreated GD.[29] Other very rare side effects include hypoprothrombinemia, hypoglycemia, and pancreatitis. Based on the evidence, the side-effect profile favors the use of MMI as the ATD of first choice.

### Use of Antithyroid Drugs During Pregnancy and Lactation

Hyperthyroidism occurs in 0.1% to 0.2% of all pregnancies. Untreated it is associated with an increased risk of abortion, preterm delivery, low birth-weight, and neonatal morbidity and mortality. The mother is at increased risk of heart failure, eclampsia, and thyroid storm.[30] ATDs are not contraindicated in pregnancy, and pregnancy is not contraindicated in women who have GD and are taking ATD. The drug should be started at diagnosis and titrated to the lowest possible dose. The block-and-replace regimen should not be used, because it requires using a higher dose of ATD, which passes the placenta and may affect the fetus, causing fetal hypothyroidism and goiter. Maternal freeT4 should be maintained in the upper part of the reference range. Typically, 30% of women are able to discontinue ATD in the second half of pregnancy, but postpartum recurrence is common. Although no prospective trials have compared MMI and PTU, the latter is recommended in North America, based mostly on a lower risk of congenital abnormalities. In particular, aplasia cutis (single or multiple lesions of 0.5–3.0 cm at the vertex or occipital area of the scalp), only seen with MMI, has been thought to occur more frequently in women treated with MMI than in the background population. Population-based data are not available, however.[30] Choanal and esophageal atresia, although very rare, also are reported more frequently in fetuses exposed to MMI than in those exposed to PTU. Nevertheless, in the author's clinic, women who have had no side effects with MMI and become pregnant usually are kept on this drug. This decision is based on a similar fetal transfer of the drugs and on similar fetal outcomes and on the absence of developmental and intellectual impairment if maternal euthyroidism is achieved.[30,31]

Both MMI and PTU appear in low concentrations in breast milk (the former in a higher concentration than the latter) and do not negatively influence infant thyroid function or subsequent intellectual development.[30] Routine monitoring of infant thyroid function is not necessary.

### B-ADRENERGIC ANTAGONIST DRUGS

B-adrenergic antagonist drugs are important in the early management of GD because they ameliorate the symptoms that are caused by increased sympathetic action, such as sweating, anxiety, tremor, palpitation, and tachycardia.[32] The effect commences rapidly. Propranolol, which mildly inhibits the conversion of T4 to T3, or other drugs can be used. They do not affect thyroid hormone synthesis or release, however, and therefore should not be used alone. The usual contraindications should be respected; as an alternative, persons who have asthma can use rate-limiting calcium-channel blockers.

## GLUCOCORTICOIDS

Glucocorticoids, in high doses, block the conversion of T4 to T3 in a similar fashion to beta-blockers. Because of their side effects, however, they should not be used except in patients who have Graves' ophthalmopathy. (See the article by Dickinson and Perros elsewhere in this issue).[10]

## INORGANIC IODIDE

Iodide decreases T4 and T3 synthesis by inhibiting iodide oxidation and organification, the Wolff-Chaikoff effect. It also blocks the release of T4 and T3 by inhibiting thyroglobulin proteolysis. The effect is rapid and pronounced but in most cases lasts only for a few weeks. Subsequently, escape from this phenomenon is seen with rising serum T4 and T3 levels. Additionally, iodide significantly decreases the vascularity of the thyroid. It can be given as Lugol's solution (8 mg iodide per drop) or as a saturated solution of potassium iodide (SSKI, 50 mg iodide per drop); doses typically are 3 to 5 drops, three times a day and 1 drop three times a day, respectively.

Given for 10 days before surgery, iodide reduces thyroid secretion and vascularity, but in a controlled study iodide had no significant influence on blood loss or the perioperative course.[33] It can be administered after RAI but probably has very little effect beyond that of MMI.[34]

## IODINE-CONTAINING COMPOUNDS

Oral cholecystographic agents (eg, sodium iopanoate and sodium ipodate) inhibit T4-deiodinase activity and thereby acutely lower serum T3 levels. Additionally, they block thyroid hormone secretion. They can be used in the situations outlined in a previous section for inorganic iodide. The drugs have few side effects except for the escape from the inhibitory effect on thyroid hormone synthesis, which makes them unsuited for long-term therapy. In the short term, when combined with either MMI or PTU, they lower serum T3 more rapidly than either MMI or PTU given as mono-therapy.[34] Although rarely necessary, these drugs are potentially beneficial in case of thyrotoxic storm or T4 poisoning.

## POTASSIUM PERCHLORATE

Potassium perchlorate is a competitive inhibitor of iodide transport. Because of adverse effects, it rarely is used, except in iodine-induced—specifically amiodarone-induced—thyrotoxicosis. In that situation it has proven effective when combined with an ATD.[35]

## LITHIUM CARBONATE

Lithium acts by inhibiting T4 and T3 release from the thyroid and possibly also by inhibiting their synthesis. Given in a dose of 900 mg daily, it reduces the degree of thyrotoxicosis during the temporary discontinuation of ATD before and in the period after [131]I therapy.[36] It can be used in cases of severe thyrotoxicosis in persons allergic to iodide or when caused by amiodarone.

## NOVEL IMMUNOMODULATORY AGENTS

The relatively low remission rate of GD following ATD therapy and the well-known side effects of ablative therapy with [131]I or surgery justify research into alternative therapies.

### Rituximab

RTX is a monoclonal chimeric human/mouse antibody directed against the surface molecule CD20, which is expressed by pre-B cells but lost upon differentiation into plasma cells.[37] The drug rapidly causes B-cell depletion in the circulation as well as in the target organs of autoimmune diseases, such as the thyroid.[38] The mechanisms of action are thought to comprise (1) decrease of autoantibody production caused by depletion of B lymphocytes, thereby preventing the development of new autoantibody-producing plasma cells, (2) abrogation of B lymphocyte–mediated antigen presentation to T-helper cells, and (3) abrogation of cytokine production from B lymphocytes.[37]

Two studies comprising only 9 patients who had Graves' ophthalmopathy have recently reported promising results.[39,40] These patients had a striking and rapid reduction in both the clinical activity score and the severity score. The effect of RTX on hyperthyroidism in GD is less pronounced,[5,40] but in a controlled study[5] 4 of 10 patients receiving RTX remained in remission for more than 1 year, whereas all 10 control patients, who did not receive RTX, relapsed within the same period. Remission occurred in those who had very low initial TSHRAb values.[5] Ongoing studies aim to clarify whether remission is caused by an alteration of the balance between stimulatory and blocking antibodies. Because of limited experience, its cost, its side-effect profile, and the availability of alternative therapy, RTX currently should not be used in uncomplicated GD.[5,37]

### Other Biologic Drugs

In a murine model of GD, treatment with anti-B-cell maturation factor or anti-B-cell maturation antigen receptor (anti-BAFF) and anti-B-cell maturation antigen (anti-BCMA) has been tested for its influence on BAFF and a proliferation-inducing ligand (APRIL) activity. (See the article by Dagdelen, Kong, and Banga elsewhere in this issue).[41] These entities are involved in B-cell survival, and treatment resulted in a fall in TSHRAb and thyroid hormone levels. Drugs interacting with the BAFF and APRIL systems currently are being tested in humans, albeit not in GD.[41] Other potential targets could be blocking the interaction between B lymphocytes, other antigen-presenting cells, and T lymphocytes. Thus, blockade of the CD40-CD154 (CD40-ligand) interaction has shown promising results in a murine model of autoimmune thyroiditis. Another potential drug is the hybrid molecule abatacept (CTLA-4/Ig); results in early clinical trials of non-GD autoimmune disease are encouraging.[42]

## RADIOACTIVE IODINE

Introduced in the mid-1940s, [131]I has become the most widely used therapy for hyperthyroidism, including GD, although international questionnaire studies show that geographic differences do exist.[43] RAI is considered effective, safe, and relatively inexpensive. The isotope of choice is [131]I. It is given orally (in a capsule or in water) and is absorbed rapidly and completely, after which it is concentrated, oxidized, and organified by follicular thyroid cells. The ionizing effect of $\beta$ particles, with a path length of 1 to 2 mm, destroys the thyroid cells by an early inflammatory response, necrosis of follicular cells, and vascular occlusion. Subsequently chronic inflammation and fibrosis result in a decrease in thyroid size and an impaired ability to secrete thyroid hormone.[44] Ultimately, almost all patients develop hypothyroidism following [131]I. Interpretation of thyroid cytology, at this stage, is complicated by bizarre nuclear changes that may resemble those of thyroid carcinoma; therefore fine-needle aspiration, if necessary, preferably should be done before [131]I therapy.

### Dose Calculation

Ideally, the smallest possible [131]I dose that rapidly renders the patient euthyroid and does not lead to hypothyroidism should be administered. Estimating this dose has proven impossible, and there is no universal consensus concerning the optimal dose and how it should be calculated. Any attempt at individual dose calculation must take into consideration whether the criterion for success is the patient remaining euthyroid or the avoidance of repeat treatment. The latter consideration is increasingly of concern because of the effect of the treatment on quality of life and the increased risk of ophthalmopathy when repeat [131]I treatment is given.[45] There is a positive relation between [131]I dose and the development of hypothyroidism within the first year of therapy; the incidence of hypothyroidism beyond 1 year seems to be largely independent of [131]I dose and is around 2% to 3% annually.[44,46] Thus, the final outcome depends on both the retained thyroid dose, which can be measured, and incompletely understood individual factors that cannot be measured. The dose of [131]I is determined most often according to the following algorithm:

$$\text{Dose (mCi)} = \frac{80-200 \text{ microCi } {}^{131}\text{I/g thyroid} \times \text{estimated thyroid gland weight (g)}}{24-\text{hour radioiodine uptake}}$$

Using dose-calculation algorithms, typical activities are in the range of 5 to 15 mCi [131]I (corresponding to 185–555 MBq), yielding an absorbed radiation dose of 50 to 100 Gy. Retrospective data suggest that those who failed to respond to [131]I therapy were characterized by a young age and had a large thyroid, severe thyrotoxicosis, prior exposure to ATD, or a higher [131]I uptake value.[47,48] In addition to such patients, a higher [131]I dose should be considered in individuals who have a recurrence of GD and those in whom persistence of disease should be minimized (eg, the elderly and patients who have cardiac disease).

Because most patients become euthyroid and eventually develop hypothyroidism, and because determining an individualized dose is costly and time consuming, fixed activities of [131]I are widely used in many health care environments.[49–51] The fact that a fixed dose simplifies and reduces cost of [131]I therapy and the lack of a significant difference in outcome between patients randomized to fixed and calculated [131]I doses[49–51] favor the use of fixed doses.

### Influence on Thyroid Function

Following [131]I therapy, thyroid secretion declines gradually over weeks to months. Around 50% to 70% of patients become euthyroid within 6 to 8 weeks, concomitantly with a marked reduction in thyroid size.[44] During this period symptoms can be controlled with a B-adrenergic antagonist. It may be necessary to start ATD therapy and, extremely rarely, to administer potassium iodide, as mentioned earlier. If so, ATD should be discontinued after a couple of months to determine the efficacy of the [131]I. Because [131]I occasionally acts more slowly, a second dose should not be given for 6 to 12 months. In this situation, also, there is no consensus on dose calculation. Many centers, including the Department of Endocrinology and Metabolism at the Odense University Hospital, choose to give a fixed dose, which is higher than the initial one. In general, receiving either a calculated dose or a fixed dose in the 10 to 15 mCi (370–555 MBq) range, 80% to 90% of patients ultimately become euthyroid or hypothyroid after one dose of [131]I. Ten percent to 20% require a second dose, and only rarely is an additional dose needed. If hypothyroidism develops within the first 6 months of therapy, LT4 should be given in suboptimal doses so that serum TSH can be checked a few months later. Elevation of serum TSH suggests permanent thyroid failure.

The incidence of early hypothyroidism increases with increasing [131]I dose and is higher in those who have high concentrations of autoantibodies to TPOAb,[52] a large gland, and hypoechogenicity using ultrasound of the thyroid.[53] By contrast, pre- and post- [131]I therapy with ATD increases rates of failure and reduces rates of hypothyroidism.[48] In a prospective, randomized study resumption of MMI 7 days after [131]I therapy did not influence final outcome (ie, had no radioprotective effect) but slightly reduced goiter shrinkage.[54] In another randomized study, the investigators demonstrated an increase in failure rate when giving continuous MMI therapy (with no break in treatment around [131]I administration).[55] Finally, in a randomized study, pretreatment with PTU, discontinued 4 days before [131]I therapy and not resumed after therapy, reduced the cure rate compared with no pretreatment.[56] With an understanding of the shortcomings of pooling these and other incongruent studies, a recently performed[57] meta-analysis did not find differences in outcome between MMI and PTU, or according to whether ATD were given before or after [131]I therapy. Thus, the current practice of the author and his colleagues is to discontinue ATD temporarily, independent of type, 4 days before and 1 week after [131]I therapy. This recommendation should take into consideration the fact that the optimal interruption period for avoiding relapse of hyperthyroidism and cardiovascular complications on the one hand, and for limiting the long-term risk of hypothyroidism, on the other hand, is still unclear and needs to be balanced in each patient. Importantly, the radioprotective effect of ATD can be overcome by increasing [131]I dose. The final long-term hypothyroidism rate (beyond 12 months) seems largely independent of these variables and occurs at an incidence of around 2% to 3% annually. Eventually almost all Graves' patients develop hypothyroidism following RAI.

### Influence on Thyroid Size

Surprisingly, the effect of [131]I on thyroid size reduction has received little attention. Nygaard and colleagues[44] studied 117 consecutive patients who had GD treated with a calculated [131]I dose. They demonstrated a 58% decrease (from a median of 33 to14 mL) at 12 months after therapy and no significant further reduction. A highly significant reduction in thyroid size also was seen in patients needing additional therapy and in those developing hypothyroidism. With few exceptions, all achieved normalization of thyroid size within 12 months of therapy.[44] This reduction in thyroid size was uninfluenced by pretreatment with ATD.

### Carcinogenicity and Teratogenicity

A major concern has been the possible carcinogenic effect of ionizing radiation. Although external head and neck irradiation is associated with an increased incidence of thyroid carcinoma, such an association has not been found with [131]I therapy.[58–60] Additionally, with the exception of small bowel cancer in one study,[61] there is no evidence for increased mortality from any other form of cancer. The recent finding of a dose-related increase in cancer incidence, especially of the stomach, kidney, and breast commencing 5 years after [131]I therapy, however, suggests that this issue may not have been laid finally to rest.[62] In large studies focusing exclusively on children, the incidence of thyroid carcinoma or other cancers was not increased,[63,64] nor was there evidence of abnormal reproductive histories in women. The risk for the pediatric population is unclear, because only limited numbers of subjects followed for a limited number of years are available. Data from populations exposed to the radioactive isotopes after the Chernobyl accident indicate that infants and adolescents have a more susceptible thyroid.[65,66] Even if an extrapolation from the Chernobyl data to therapeutic [131]I therapy cannot be made with impunity, many authorities discourage use of [131]I in patients younger than 16 to 18 years of age. The author is hesitant to treat adolescents younger than age 20 years, given that many of them have a post-[131]I life expectancy of 70 to 80 years. Nevertheless, the limited data that are available do not suggest early adverse events in children so treated.[64]

Because of transplacental passage and passage into breast milk, pregnancy and breastfeeding are absolute contraindications to [131]I therapy. Pregnancy should be avoided during the first 4 to 6 months after [131]I therapy, and a pregnancy test should be obtained immediately before therapy in all premenopausal sexually active women. In Denmark, the inadvertent use of any radioactive isotope during early pregnancy leads to an offer to terminate the pregnancy, although exposure at a time when the fetal thyroid cannot yet concentrate iodine (before 10–12 weeks of gestation) has been associated with a normal outcome.[67] Later exposure leads to intrauterine fetal hypothyroidism.

Maximum outpatient [131]I dose as well as radiation regulations vary substantially among countries. Independent of these regulations, unnecessary exposure to RAI, especially of children and pregnant women, should be avoided for several days, depending on [131]I dose and taking into consideration that most of the radioactivity is excreted in the urine.

## SURGERY

Surgery is the oldest but currently the least employed therapy for GD. Indications, apart from patient preference, include children, adolescents, pregnant women, patients who have large goiters (whether causing pressure symptoms or for cosmetic reasons) and suspicion of thyroid malignancy. Because of the ophthalmic risk associated with [131]I therapy, many advocate surgery in patients who have GD and pre-existing ophthalmopathy.[68]

The main aim of surgery in GD is rapid normalization of thyroid function with the lowest possible rate of relapse, while minimizing complication rate. Most surgeons now recommend total or nearly total thyroidectomy rather than subtotal thyroidectomy leaving a few grams of each lobe. Total thyroidectomy invariably leads to hypothyroidism, also requiring long-term follow-up, but no risk of recurrence.[69] The anesthesiologic risk is low, and mortality is nearly zero. Surgical complications depend on numerous factors and increase with increasing patient age, size of the goiter, and degree of hyperthyroidism and, most importantly, are inversely related to the experience of the surgeon. Two distressing complications, permanent damage to the recurrent laryngeal nerve and hypoparathyroidism, occur in at least 1% to 2% of patients, even in the most experienced hands, and figures up to 5% to 10% have been reported.[70,71] Other complications include transient hypocalcemia, postoperative bleeding, wound infections, and the formation of keloids. Hypothyroidism generally is considered a consequence of, rather than a complication from, surgery and occurs in 12% to 80% of patients during the first year and at a rate of 1% to 3% annually thereafter. The risk of hypothyroidism is greater in those who have high concentrations of TPOAb and increases with length of follow-up. Subtotal thyroidectomy decreases the overall complication rate but is associated with recurrent hyperthyroidism in 5%

to 15% of patients[69] and is positively related to the initial TSHRAb level, the presence of ophthalmopathy, and the size of the thyroid remnant. Independent of the type of surgery, lifelong surveillance is needed for control of thyroid and parathyroid function. Stålberg and colleagues,[72] in a current evidence-based review, found support for total thyroidectomy as the surgical technique of choice for GD, if surgery is considered. Available evidence also supports surgery in the presence of Graves' ophthalmopathy. Children who have GD should be treated with ablative therapy, either total thyroidectomy or [131]I. If hyperthyroidism recurs following surgery, RAI is the therapy of choice.

Rarely is preparation of the patient for surgery a problem, because almost all patients are euthyroid on thionamide therapy. Preoperative administration of inorganic iodine for 10 days (one to three drops of a saturated solution of potassium iodide [SSKI] daily) is used frequently. It decreases blood flow significantly but does not alter blood loss significantly. The author and his colleagues do not use it routinely. Another option, in case of side effects to ATD or in case of urgent surgery, is the combination of a B-adrenergic antagonist drug (eg, propranolol) for days to weeks and SSKI for 10 days. The latter regimen is associated with a higher frequency of postoperative problems than seen in euthyroid patients.[73] Alternatively, in case of emergency surgery, oral cholecystographic agents provide the most rapid way of reaching euthyroidism.[74]

**Table 2**
**Advantages and disadvantages of treatment modalities for Graves' disease**

| Treatment Modality | Advantages | Disadvantages |
|---|---|---|
| Thionamides | No radiation hazard<br>No surgical and anesthesiologic risk<br>No permanent hypothyroidism<br>Outpatient therapy | Recurrence rate high (>50%)<br>Frequent testing required<br>Common mild side effects<br>Rare but potentially lethal side effects |
| Radioactive iodine | Definitive treatment of hyperthyroidism<br>No surgical or anesthesiologic risk<br>Outpatient therapy, rapidly performed<br>Rapid control of hyperthyroidism in most<br>Low cost<br>Side effects mild, rare, and transient<br>Normalizes thyroid size within 1 year | Potential radiation hazards<br>Worsening of thyroid eye disease<br>Adherence with radiation regulations<br>Decreasing efficacy with increasing goiter size<br>May need to be repeated<br>Hypothyroidism eventually develops in most cases |
| Thyroidectomy | Definitive treatment of hyperthyroidism<br>No radiation hazard<br>Rapid normalization of thyroid dysfunction<br>Definitive histology<br>Most effective in cases with pressure symptoms | Cost<br>Inpatient therapy<br>Anesthesiologic risk[a]<br>Hypoparathyroidism (1%–2%)[b]<br>Damage to the recurrent laryngeal nerve (1%–2%)[b]<br>Risk of bleeding, infection, unsatisfactory scarring[b]<br>Hypothyroidism in most patients[b] |

[a] Hyperthyroidism at time of surgery increases the risk associated with anesthesia.
[b] The surgical risk generally is higher for total thyroidectomy than for subtotal thyroidectomy. The risk of hypothyroidism and the risk of recurrence are inversely related and depend on the amount of thyroid tissue removed.

If none of the traditional therapeutic options are applicable, however unlikely, an initial report suggests that arterial embolization was able to cure 16 of 22 patients who had GD and concomitantly reduced goiter size by 30% to 50%.[75]

## CHOICE OF THERAPY

From the previous discussion it should be clear that the choice of therapy is rarely indisputable. The final decision often is, and should be, based on the preference and experience of both patient and physician. Local practice and the availability of expertise, as well as regulations and legislation that may vary considerably, may influence and even limit the options. A number of surveys focusing on an index case in which these limitations did not apply and the patient had no part in the decision[43] indicate that there is no consensus, and that factors related solely to the physician have a great influence. It therefore is important to inform the patient as objectively as possible about advantages and disadvantages of the therapeutic options (**Table 2**) to reach a mutual agreement regarding the choice of therapy.

It is recognized increasingly that the choice of therapy also should be based on an evaluation of cost and quality of life. A number of studies suggest that most thyroid disorders, not only Graves' ophthalmopathy, significantly affect the everyday life of these patients.[76–78] A prospective, randomized study suggested, whether or not relapse costs were included, that overall costs were a bit higher for surgical than for medical therapy, and were higher for $^{131}$I therapy than for ATD.[79] The study could not detect a difference among the three therapeutic options in quality of life.[80] Although studies have focused on these issues, a recent evidence-based review concluded that no recommendation stating a preference for ATD, surgery, or $^{131}$I could be based on any grade of evidence.[72]

## REFERENCES

1. Brix TH, Kyvik KO, Christensen K, et al. The importance of genetic versus environmental factors in the etiology of Graves' disease: a population based study of female Danish twins. J Clin Endocrinol Metab 2001;86(2):930–4.
2. Tomer Y, Davies TF. Searching for the autoimmune thyroid disease susceptibility genes: from gene mapping to gene function. Endocr Rev 2003;24(5):694–717.
3. Brix TH, Hansen PS, Kyvik KO, et al. Cigarette smoking and the risk of clinically overt thyroid disease: a population based twin case-control study. Arch Intern Med 2000;160(5):661–6.
4. Bartalena L, Marcocci C, Tanda ML, et al. Cigarette smoking and treatment outcomes in Graves' ophthalmopathy. Ann Intern Med 1998;129(8):632–5.
5. El Fassi D, Nielsen CH, Bonnema SJ, et al. B lymphocyte depletion with the monoclonal antibody rituximab in Graves' disease: a controlled pilot study. J Clin Endocrinol Metab 2007;92(5):1769–72.
6. Cooper DS. Antithyroid drugs. N Engl J Med 2005;352(9):905–17.
7. Laurberg P. Remission of Graves' disease during anti-thyroid drug therapy. Time to reconsider the mechanism? Eur J Endocrinol 2006;155(6):783–6.
8. Cooper DS, Steigerwalt S, Migdal S. Pharmacology of propylthiouracil in thyrotoxicosis and chronic renal failure. Arch Intern Med 1987;147(4):785–6.
9. Tallstedt L, Lundell G, Torring O, et al. Occurrence of ophthalmopathy after treatment for Graves' hyperthyroidism. N Engl J Med 1992;326(26):1733–8.
10. Bartalena L, Marcocci C, Bogazzi F, et al. Relation between therapy for hyperthyroidism and the course of Graves' ophthalmopathy. N Engl J Med 1998;338(2):73–8.

11. Nakamura H, Noh JY, Itoh K, et al. Comparison of methimazole and propylthiour-acil in patients with hyperthyroidism caused by Graves' disease. J Clin Endocrinol Metab 2007;92(6):2157–62.

12. Reinwein D, Benker G, Lazarus JH, et al. A prospective randomized trial of anti-thyroid drug dose in Graves' disease therapy. European Multicenter Study Group on Antithyroid Drug Treatment. J Clin Endocrinol Metab 1993;76(6):1516–21.

13. Bliddal H, Hegedüs L, Hansen JM, et al. The relationship between serum T3 index, thyroid volume, and thyroid stimulating, TSH receptor binding and thyroid growth stimulating antibodies in Graves' disease. Clin Endocrinol (Oxf) 1987; 27(1):75–84.

14. Benker G, Reinwein D, Kahaly G, et al. Is there a methimazole dose effect on remission rate in graves' disease? Results from a long-term prospective study. The European Multicenter Trial Group of the Treatment of Hyperthyroidism with Antithyroid Drugs. Clin Endocrinol (Oxf) 1998;49(4):451–7.

15. Abraham P, Avenell A, Watson WA, et al. Antithyroid drug regimen for treating Graves' hyperthyroidism. Cochrane Database Syst Rev 2004;(2):CD003420.

16. Vitti P, Rago T, Chiovato L, et al. Clinical features of patients with Graves' disease undergoing remission after antithyroid drug treatment. Thyroid 1997;7(3):369–75.

17. Schott M, Eckstein A, Willenberg HS, et al. Improved prediction of relapse of Graves' thyrotoxicosis by combined determination of TSH receptor and thyroperoxidase antibodies. Horm Metab Res 2007;39(1):56–61.

18. Feldt-Rasmussen U, Schleusener H, Carayon P. Meta-analysis evaluation of the impact of thyrotropin receptor antibodies on long-term remission after medical therapy of Graves' disease. J Clin Endocrinol Metab 1994;78(1):98–102.

19. Hashizume K, Ichikawa K, Sakurai A, et al. Administration of thyroxine in treated Graves' disease. Effects on the level of antibodies to thyroid stimulating hormone receptors and on the risk of recurrence of hyperthyroidism. N Engl J Med 1991; 324(14):947–53.

20. McIver B, Rae P, Beckett G, et al. Lack of effect of thyroxine in patients with Graves' hyperthyroidism who are treated with an antithyroid drug. N Engl J Med 1996;334(4):220–4.

21. Jacobson EM, Tomer Y. The genetic basis of thyroid autoimmunity. Thyroid 2007; 17(10):949–61.

22. Wang PW, Chen IY, Liu RT, et al. Cytotoxic T-lymphocyte-associated molecule-4 gene polymorphism and hyperthyroid Graves' disease relapse after antithyroid drug withdrawal: a follow-up study. J Clin Endocrinol Metab 2007;92(7): 2513–8.

23. Maugendre D, Gatel A, Campion L, et al. Antithyroid drugs and Graves' disease-prospective randomized assessment of long-term treatment. Clin Endocrinol (Oxf) 1999;50(1):127–32.

24. Amino N, Tanizawa O, Mori H, et al. Aggravation of thyrotoxicosis in early pregnancy and after delivery in Graves' disease. J Clin Endocrinol Metab 1982; 55(1):108–12.

25. Wood LC, Ingbar SH. Hypothyroidism as a late sequela in patient with Graves' disease treated with antithyroid agents. J Clin Invest 1979;64(5):1429–36.

26. Cooper DS. The side effects of antithyroid drugs. Endocrinologist 1999;9:457–76.

27. Pearce SH. Spontaneous reporting of adverse reactions to carbimazole and pro-pylthiouracil in the UK. Clin Endocrinol (Oxf) 2004;61(5):589–94.

28. Fukata S, Kuma K, Sugawara M. Granulocyte colony-stimulating factor (G-CSF) does not improve recovery from antithyroid drug-induced agranulocytosis: a prospective study. Thyroid 1999;9(1):29–31.

29. Harper L, Chin L, Daykin J, et al. Propylthiouracil and carbimazole-associated antineutrophil cytoplasmatic antibodies (ANCA) in patients with Graves' disease. Clin Endocrinol (Oxf) 2004;60(6):671–5.
30. Mandel S, Cooper DS. The use of antithyroid drugs in pregnancy and lactation. J Clin Endocrinol Metab 2001;86(6):2354–9.
31. Mortimer RH, Cannell GR, Addison RS, et al. Methimazole and propylthiouracil equally cross the perfused human term placental lobule. J Clin Endocrinol Metab 1997;82(9):3099–102.
32. Geffner DL, Hershman JM. Beta-adrenergic blockade for the treatment of hyperthyroidism. Am J Med 1992;93(1):61–8.
33. Coyle PJ, Mitchell JE. Thyroidectomy: is Lugol's iodine necessary? Ann R Coll Surg Engl 1982;64(5):344–5.
34. Roti E, Robuschi G, Gardini E, et al. Comparison of methimazole, methimazole and sodium ipodate, and methimazole and saturated solution of potassium iodide in the early treatment of hyperthyroid Graves' disease. Clin Endocrinol (Oxf) 1988;28(3):305–14.
35. Martino E, Bartalena L, Bogazzi F, et al. The effects of amiodarone on the thyroid. Endocr Rev 2001;22(2):240–54.
36. Bogazzi F, Bartalena L, Campomori A, et al. Treatment with lithium prevents serum thyroid hormone increase after thionamide withdrawal and radioiodine therapy in patients with Graves' disease. J Clin Endocrinol Metab 2002;87(10):4490–5.
37. Nielsen CH, El Fassi D, Hasselbalch HC, et al. B-cell depletion with rituximab in the treatment of autoimmune diseases. Graves' ophthalmopathy the latest addition to an expanding family. Expert Opin Biol Ther 2007;7(7):1061–78.
38. El Fassi D, Clemmensen O, Nielsen CH, et al. Evidence of intrathyroidal B-lymphocyte depletion after rituximab therapy in a patient with Graves' disease. J Clin Endocrinol Metab 2007;92(10):3762–3.
39. El Fassi D, Nielsen CH, Hasselbalch HC, et al. Treatment resistant severe active Graves' ophthalmopathy successfully treated with B lymphocyte depletion. Thyroid 2006;16(7):709–10.
40. Salvi M, Vannucchi G, Campi I, et al. Treatment of Graves' disease and associated ophthalmopathy with the anti-CD20 monoclonal antibody rituximab: an open study. Eur J Endocrinol 2007;156(1):33–40.
41. Gilbert JA, Kalled SL, Moorhead J, et al. Treatment of autoimmune hyperthyroidism in a murine model of Graves' disease with tumor necrosis factor-family ligand inhibitors suggest a key role for B cell activating factor in disease pathology. Endocrinology 2006;147(10):4561–8.
42. Banga JP, Nielsen CH, Gilbert JA, et al. Application of new therapies in Graves' disease and thyroid associated ophthalmopathy: animal models and translation to human clinical trials. Thyroid 2008;18(9):973–81.
43. Wartofsky L, Glinoer D, Solomon B, et al. Differences and similarities in the diagnosis and treatment of Graves' disease in Europe, Japan, and the United States. Thyroid 1991;1(2):129–35.
44. Nygaard B, Hegedüs L, Gervil M, et al. Influence of compensated radioiodine therapy on thyroid volume and incidence of hypothyroidism in Graves' disease. J Intern Med 1995;238(6):491–7.
45. Wiersinga WM. Management of Graves' ophthalmopathy. Nat Clin Pract Endocrinol Metab 2007;3(5):396–404.
46. Sridama V, McCormick M, Kaplan EL, et al. Long-term follow-up study of compensated low-dose 131I therapy for Graves' disease. N Engl J Med 1984;311(7):426–32.

47. Allahabadia A, Daykin J, Sheppard MC, et al. Radioiodine treatment of hyperthyroidism–prognostic factors for outcome. J Clin Endocrinol Metab 2001;86(8): 3611–7.
48. Alexander EK, Larsen PR. High dose of (131) I therapy for the treatment of hyperthyroidism caused by Graves' disease. J Clin Endocrinol Metab 2002;87(3): 1073–7.
49. Jarløv AE, Hegedüs L, Kristensen LO, et al. Is calculation of the dose in radioiodine therapy of hyperthyroidism worth while? Clin Endocrinol (Oxf) 1995;43(3): 325–9.
50. Peters H, Fischer C, Bogner U, et al. Radioiodine therapy of Graves' hyperthyroidism: standard vs. calculated 131I activity. Results from a prospective, randomized, multicentre study. Eur J Clin Invest 1995;25(3):186–93.
51. Leslie WD, Ward L, Salamon EA, et al. A randomized comparison of radioiodine doses in Graves' hyperthyroidism. J Clin Endocrinol Metab 2003;88(3):978–83.
52. Ahmad AM, Ahmad M, Young ET. Objective estimates of the probability of developing hypothyroidism following radioactive iodine treatment of thyrotoxicosis. Eur J Endocrinol 2002;146(6):767–75.
53. Markovic V, Eterovic D. Thyroid echogenicity predicts outcome of radioiodine therapy in patients with Graves' disease. J Clin Endocrinol Metab 2007;92(9): 3547–52.
54. Bonnema SJ, Bennedbaek FN, Gram J, et al. Resumption of methimazole after 131I therapy of hyperthyroid diseases: effect on thyroid function and volume evaluated by a randomized clinical trial. Eur J Endocrinol 2003;149(6):485–92.
55. Bonnema SJ, Bennedbaek FN, Veje A, et al. Continuous methimazole therapy and its effect on the cure rate of hyperthyroidism using radioactive iodine: an evaluation by a randomized trial. J Clin Endocrinol Metab 2006;91(8):2946–51.
56. Bonnema SJ, Bennedbaek FN, Veje A, et al. Propylthiouracil before 131I therapy of hyperthyroid diseases: effect on cure rate evaluated by a randomized clinical trial. J Clin Endocrinol Metab 2004;89(9):4439–44.
57. Walter MA, Briel M, Christ-Crain M, et al. Effects of antithyroid drugs on radioiodine treatment: systematic review and meta-analysis of randomized controlled trials. BMJ 2007;334(7592):514–20.
58. Holm LE, Dahlqvist I, Israelsson A, et al. Malignant thyroid tumors after iodine-131 therapy: a retrospective cohort study. N Engl J Med 1980;303(4):188–91.
59. Ron E, Doody MM, Becker DV, et al. Cancer mortality following treatment for adult hyperthyroidism. Cooperative thyrotoxicosis therapy follow-up study group. JAMA 1998;280(4):347–55.
60. Angusti T, Codegone A, Pellerito R, et al. Thyroid cancer prevalence after radioiodine treatment of hyperthyroidism. J Nucl Med 2000;41(6):1006–9.
61. Franklyn JA, Maisonneuve P, Sheppard M, et al. Cancer incidence and mortality after radioiodine treatment for hyperthyroidism: a population-based cohort study. Lancet 1999;353(9170):2111–5.
62. Metso S, Auvinen A, Huhtala H, et al. Increased cancer incidence after radioiodine treatment for hyperthyroidism. Cancer 2007;109(10):1972–9.
63. Hayek A, Chapman EM, Crawford JD. Long-term results of treatment of thyrotoxicosis in children and adolescents with radioactive iodine. N Engl J Med 1970; 283(18):947–53.
64. Rivkees SA, Dinauer C. An optimal treatment for pediatric Graves' disease is radioiodine. J Clin Endocrinol Metab 2007;92(3):797–800.
65. Baverstock K, Egloff B, Pinchera a, et al. Thyroid cancer after Chernobyl. Nature 1992;359(6390):21–2.

66. Pacini F, Vorontsova T, Demidchik EP, et al. Post-Chernobyl thyroid carcinoma in Belarus children and adolescents: comparison with naturally occurring thyroid carcinoma in Italy and France. J Clin Endocrinol Metab 1997;82(11):3563–9.

67. Stoffer SS, Hamburger JI. Inadvertent 131I therapy for hyperthyroidism in the first trimester of pregnancy. J Nucl Med 1976;17(2):146–9.

68. Perros P, Baldeschi L, Boboridis K, et al. A questionnaire survey on the management of Graves' orbitopathy in Europe. Eur J Endocrinol 2006;155(2):207–11.

69. Palit TK, Miller CC III, Miltenburg DM. The efficacy of thyroidectomy for Graves' disease: a meta-analysis. J Surg Res 2000;90(2):161–5.

70. Sosa JA, Bowman HM, Tielsch JM, et al. The importance of surgeon experience for clinical and economic outcomes from thyroidectomy. Ann Surg 1998;228(3):320–30.

71. Pattou F, Combemale F, Fabre S, et al. Hypocalcemia following thyroid surgery: incidence and prediction of outcome. World J Surg 1998;22(7):718–24.

72. Stålberg P, Svensson A, Hessman O, et al. Surgical treatment of Graves' disease: evidence-based approach. World J Surg 2008;32(7):1269–77.

73. Lennquist S, Jortso E, Anderberg BO, et al. Beta blockers compared with antithyroid drugs as preoperative treatment in hyperthyroidism: drug tolerance, complications, and postoperative thyroid function. Surgery 1985;98(6):1141–7.

74. Baeza A, Aguayo J, Barria M, et al. Rapid preoperative preparation in hyperthyroidism. Clin Endocrinol (Oxf) 1991;35(5):439–42.

75. Xiao H, Zhuang W, Wang S, et al. Arterial embolization: a novel approach to thyroid ablative therapy for Graves' disease. J Clin Endocrinol Metab 2002;87(8):3583–9.

76. Watt T, Groenvold M, Rasmussen AK, et al. Quality of life in patients with benign thyroid disorders. A review. Eur J Endocrinol 2006;154(4):501–10.

77. Watt T, Hegedüs L, Rasmussen AK, et al. Which domains of thyroid-related quality of life are most relevant? Patients and clinicians provide complementary perspectives. Thyroid 2007;17(7):647–54.

78. Terwee CB, Wiersinga WM. Graves' quality of life. Ophthalmology 2007;114(7):1416–7.

79. Ljunggren JG, Törring O, Wallin G, et al. Quality of life aspects and costs in treatment of Graves' hyperthyroidism with antithyroid drugs, surgery, or radioiodine: results from a prospective, randomized study. Thyroid 1998;8(8):653–9.

80. Abraham-Nordling M, Törring O, Hamberger B, et al. Graves' disease: a long-term quality-of-life follow up of patients randomized to treatment with antithyroid drugs, radioiodine, or surgery. Thyroid 2005;15(11):1279–86.

# Thyroid-Associated Orbitopathy: Who and How to Treat

Jane Dickinson, MBChB, FRCP, FRCOphth[a],*, Petros Perros, MBBS, MD, FRCP[b]

**KEYWORDS**

- Orbitopathy • Ophthalmopathy • Graves' disease • Thyroid

The goals of management in thyroid-associated orbitopathy (TAO) are to support patients, alleviate symptoms, to prevent disease progression and therefore more serious ocular sequelae, and to rehabilitate the patient both functionally and cosmetically to as near to their premorbid state as possible. The aim of this article is to provide guidance on who to treat and how to treat them, and is designed to assist both internists and ophthalmologists who manage TAO.

## WHO TO TREAT

When a patient presents for the first time with a possible diagnosis of TAO, there are three mandatory objectives. First, the diagnosis of TAO must be verified, which sometimes requires imaging. Once the diagnosis is established, the second objective is to identify the disease phase, which guides the options for treatment. The third is to assess disease severity, hence whether intervention is required and, if so, how quickly. Within this third objective is the necessity to identify sight-threatening features that may be insidious in their onset, but that warrant aggressive intervention if visual loss is to be prevented. Although they are discussed sequentially, diagnosis and the assessment of disease phase and severity take place concurrently in practice.

### Diagnosis

The presentation of TAO is heterogeneous, in that not all features of TAO are present in every patient, however the following features are so typical that in the context of an abnormality of thyroid regulation there is usually little doubt about the diagnosis:[1]

[a] Department of Ophthalmology, Newcastle upon Tyne Hospitals NHS Trust, Queen Victoria Road, Newcastle upon Tyne NE1 4LP UK
[b] Department of Endocrinology, Newcastle upon Tyne Hospitals NHS Trust, Queen Victoria Road, Newcastle upon Tyne NE1 4LP UK
* Corresponding author. Department of Ophthalmology, Newcastle upon Tyne Hospitals NHS Trust, Queen Victoria Road, Newcastle upon Tyne NE1 4LP UK.
*E-mail address:* jane.dickinson@ncl.ac.uk (J. Dickinson).

Endocrinol Metab Clin N Am 38 (2009) 373–388
doi:10.1016/j.ecl.2009.01.004
0889-8529/09/$ – see front matter © 2009 Elsevier Inc. All rights reserved.
endo.theclinics.com

soft tissue swelling and inflammation, upper eyelid retraction (often with lateral flare),[2] proptosis (exophthalmos), and restricted ocular motility. Other presentations are more unusual and should prompt the exclusion of other pathologies, in particular orbital malignancy or other inflammatory conditions. The absence of upper eyelid retraction (normally present in >90% TAO)[1] or the presence of a divergent strabismus or of unilateral disease should ring alarm bells. Asymmetrical disease is relatively common,[3,4] however truly unilateral disease is rare. Any one of these three scenarios should prompt orbital imaging, as should more typical TAO features if there is no demonstrable thyroid abnormality. Once the diagnosis is established, then indications for treatment will be determined by the severity of TAO, whereas options for such treatment will be determined by disease phase.

### Disease Phase

TAO has a predictable natural history, whereby there is an early phase of increasing severity, which eventually plateaus, followed by a gradual improvement, before reaching a steady state where no further spontaneous change takes place.[5,6] In the 1990s this led on to the concepts of activity and severity, with the changeable phases of TAO being recognized to reflect active disease and the final stable phase to reflect inactive disease.[7] Hence, activity denotes the inflammatory phase and therefore the potential for disease modulation with medical treatments.[2,8] Just as importantly, inflammation resolves to leave the disease inactive, and therefore there is no potential for disease modulation with medical treatments during this final phase. Instead, this is the optimal phase for surgical rehabilitation, as spontaneous change has ceased and the tissues are no longer inflamed. From this it follows that in order to determine which patients should be considered for which therapies, it is first essential to determine disease phase. This can reliably be assessed clinically in the vast majority of patients, although a few will require alternative strategies or further investigation.

#### Clinical assessment of disease phase

**Symptoms** Patients with active disease are much more likely to be symptomatic than those with inactive disease. Forty percent of patients with active disease develop symptoms of ocular surface irritation, which include tearing, light sensitivity, and a gritty feeling.[2,9,10] Light sensitivity and grittiness tend to resolve with improvement of inflammation, regardless of lid retraction. Their presence thus helps to clarify disease phase. Orbital ache is much less common but also strongly suggestive of active disease.[11] Other symptoms such as altered appearance and double vision are not specific for active disease unless clearly changing; however, intermittent diplopia that worsens on waking and is associated with gaze-evoked aching is strongly suggestive of active TAO.[2,7,9] Uncorrectable alterations in visual function (patchy or generalized blurring or altered color appreciation) are potential markers of dysthyroid optic neuropathy (DON) but are not always volunteered by patients.[2,9,10,12,13] DON is associated with active disease so may help determine disease phase, however the corollary is that these symptoms should be specifically sought from all patients suspected of having active disease, as treatment for DON is mandatory.

**Signs** No single clinical sign can directly identify the degree of orbital inflammation, ie, activity; therefore, visible evidence of external inflammation is used as a surrogate marker. The classical signs of inflammation have been incorporated into a clinical activity score (CAS).[7] Change in disease features that denote *severity* rather than *activity* of TAO, eg, proptosis (see assessment of severity below), over a several-month period, implies that the orbitopathy is active.

**CAS score** The clinical activity score was devised in 1989[7] and allows most patients to be categorized as having either active or inactive disease. On first presentation, patients are scored for two symptoms of pain and five soft tissue inflammatory signs, totaling seven points. Thereafter, any progression in three features of severity, namely proptosis, restriction of eye movements, or deterioration in visual acuity also adds to the activity score giving it a possible total of 10 points. It is easier to clarify the presence or absence of both symptoms and signs if a strict protocol is used together with a comparative atlas to score the soft tissue signs.[2,14] The European Group on Graves' Orbitopathy (EUGOGO) atlas is one such tool and is freely available at www.eugogo.org.[15] The validity of the CAS has come from studies showing a correlation between pretreatment CAS and response to immunomodulation. The positive predictive value (PPV) for a treatment response for a CAS of 3/7 (or 4/10) is 80%, whereas the negative predictive value (NPV) is 64%.[16] Although the CAS is extremely useful for assessment of activity, its binary scoring makes it much less useful for monitoring change over time.[2]

**Assessment of soft tissue signs** The five important signs are eyelid swelling, eyelid redness, conjunctival swelling (chemosis), conjunctival redness, and inflammation of the plica or caruncle, which both lie at the inner corner of the eye medial to the conjunctiva.[2,15] It is important to distinguish fat prolapse, which is common and seen as discreet bulges through the orbital septum (**Fig. 1**A), from inflammatory *eyelid swelling*, which is more diffuse horizontally (see **Fig. 1**B). They may coexist, but fat prolapse is not a marker for activity. *Eyelid redness* more often affects the area anterior to the septum (**Fig. 2**) than the area closer to the eyelid margin. The latter is a site where redness is more likely to be caused by the very common condition of blepharitis. In the absence of a slit lamp, significant *chemosis* (**Fig. 3**A) can still be identified by placing a finger on the skin of the lower eyelid lateral to the cornea and gently nudging

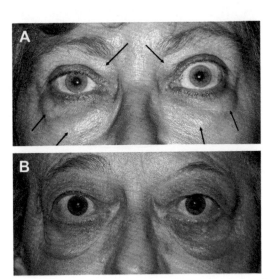

**Fig. 1.** (*A*) Fat prolapse causing discreet bulges in eyelids in inactive TAO (*arrows*). (*B*) Diffuse upper and lower eyelid edema in active TAO.

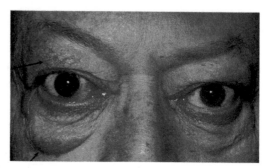

Fig. 2. Eyelid erythema anterior to the orbital septum in active TAO (*arrows*).

the eyelid upward (see **Fig. 3**B). Chemosis is then seen as a bulge moving over the deeper layers of the bulbar tissue. *Inflammation of the caruncle and plica* are relatively less common signs, even in active disease, but are identified by significant redness and prominence (**Fig. 4**), which may make them visible even with the eyelids closed. A more detailed description of precisely what constitutes presence or absence of these important signs can be found at www.eugogo.org.

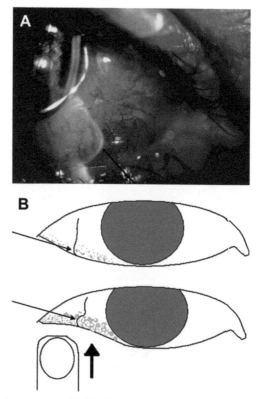

Fig. 3. (*A*) Chemosis in active TAO highlighted by slit-beam (*arrow*). (*B*) Accentuating chemosis (*arrows*) by nudging the lower eyelid upward.

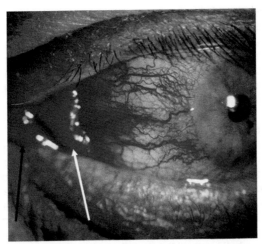

**Fig. 4.** Inflammation and swelling of both the caruncle (*black arrow*) and the plica (*white arrow*) in active TAO.

### Laboratory and imaging assessment of disease phase

Over the past 10 years there have been many attempts to identify active disease with greater accuracy. Parameters studied include thyrotropin receptor antibodies, glycos-aminoglycans (GAG) in serum and urine, a wide range of cytokines in serum, quantitative MRI, and scintigraphy. However, to date, no single laboratory or imaging parameter is able to reliably detect activity and predict response to treatment. A recent study[17] integrated all previously identified laboratory parameters with quantitative data from A-mode ultrasonography, MRI T2 imaging, and octreoscan scintigraphy to develop a multivariate prediction model that determined response to radiotherapy. Although its negative and positive predictive values for determining response to treatment were higher than any previous study, clinical assessment and duration of TAO of less than16 months still identified disease phase in most patients. Therefore, the value of ancillary assessment tools in routine practice remains undetermined. Their use will depend on availability, cost, and whether they will influence management. Hence, they are unnecessary in patients with high CAS and severe disease, or low CAS and mild disease; however, they may guide intervention in patients with moderately severe TAO but low CAS. Where unavailable, an alternative approach is simply to give a short trial of treatment, provided the anticipated morbidity for that patient is acceptable.

## Disease Severity

### How severe is the orbitopathy?

There is widespread agreement that sight-threatening orbitopathy represents the most severe form of TAO; however, many non–sight-threatening features may be considered "severe," especially by the affected individual, and categorizing severity then becomes more controversial. For the purpose of describing appropriate management strategies for different groups of patients, this discussion separates patients into the following categories: (1) sight-threatening TAO, (2) moderate-severe but non–sight-threatening TAO, and (3) mild TAO. Sight-threatening TAO occurs most commonly in the context of DON, but may reflect corneal breakdown, or occasionally globe subluxation. Urgent treatment is mandatory. In line with a recent EUGOGO consensus statement,[18] moderate-to-severe non–sight-threatening TAO is defined as orbitopathy with sufficient impact on daily life to justify the risks of immunosuppression (if active) or surgical intervention (if inactive). Mild TAO denotes disease with only minor impact on daily life, insufficient to justify immunosuppressive or surgical treatment. Such patients usually have only one or more of the following: minor lid retraction (<2 mm), mild soft tissue involvement, exophthalmos less than 3 mm above normal for race and gender, transient or no diplopia, and corneal exposure symptoms responsive to lubricants.

### Clinical assessment of severity

Severity describes the degree of functional or cosmetic deficit experienced by the patient at any point in time. Apart from the "severity" of the soft tissue signs, some of which can be broadly graded, the following features are measured: eyelid aperture, proptosis, restriction in ocular motility including loss of binocular field and the development of diplopia, corneal exposure including a risk of ulceration, and impairment of visual function. Visual function is measured subjectively by acuity and color vision, and objectively to record any relative afferent pupil defect. If there is a suspicion of DON, then ancillary tests including visual fields and visual evoked potentials may be helpful. As with activity scoring, consistency is paramount for accurate sequential assessment of severity, and a detailed methodology is available at www.eugogo.org. It is described briefly here. *Eyelid apertures* are measured in the mid-pupil line with each eye in primary fixation and without an abnormal head posture. Upper and lower eyelid retraction is similarly measured with reference to either the normal lid position or the respective limbus. *Proptosis* is ideally measured by the same observer, using the same instrument, set to the same snug intercanthal diameter. *Extra-ocular muscle function* can be assessed subjectively and objectively, and both are useful. Subjective diplopia can be scored as grade I, intermittent fatigue-related diplopia; grade II, inconstant diplopia evoked by lateral or upward gaze; grade III, constant diplopia correctable by prisms; and grade IV, constant uncorrectable diplopia.[19] Additional objective assessments are extremely useful for further establishing severity of restriction and monitoring change. The most useful of these are the prism cover test, the uniocular fields of fixation (excursions) and the binocular field of vision.[2] Although eyelid retraction can give symptoms and signs of mild exposure, sight-threatening *corneal exposure* relates to incomplete eyelid closure where the cornea remains visible. This constitutes an emergency if ulceration and perforation are to be avoided.

### How to assess for dysthyroid optic neuropathy

Assessment of visual function is mandatory for any patient who might have DON. This applies to all patients with active disease where there is significant muscle swelling at the orbital apex to compress the optic nerve. There is potentially a greater risk of compression in the non-proptosed eye showing signs of restricted eye movements, and such patients should be examined very carefully. Rarely, DON results from extreme proptosis stretching the nerve. Particular care should be taken to exclude DON in any patient with visual symptoms unrelieved by spectacle correction; those at particular risk are individuals who are smokers, elderly, male, or diabetic. Most patients with DON have reasonably good vision at presentation and, as it is frequently bilateral, they may not show a relative afferent pupil defect. Optic disc swelling is found in fewer than 50% of cases. Subtle evidence of color impairment should be taken very seriously and should prompt additional testing with perimetry and visual evoked potentials, although neither is specific for DON. An orbital CT will show either apical crowding, or rarely optic nerve stretch from extreme proptosis. Despite all of these assessments, it can sometimes be difficult to decide whether a patient does or does not have DON.[13] This is particularly true when there are confounding factors such as diabetic retinopathy and cataract, both more common in high-risk patients. However, diagnostic criteria for DON have yet to be agreed. A practical approach to this problem is to diagnose DON on disc swelling alone, but when it is absent, to diagnose DON only if there are abnormalities in at least two of the following features: acuity, pupil responses, color vision, perimetry, or visual evoked potentials.[20] Additionally, there should be imaging evidence of likely DON.

## HOW TO TREAT
### Indications for Treatment

Some simple interventions are applicable to all patients with TAO and can be instituted without delay (see the next section, Supportive Measures). The remaining options are: (1) no other intervention, (2) medical treatments, and (3) surgical treatments. Sight-threatening TAO needs to be treated urgently and aggressively (see Management of DON, later in this article). Treatments need to be tailored to disease phase, disease severity, and to the individual. A strategy of "no intervention" is appropriate when there is no sight-threatening TAO, and symptoms are well controlled or tolerated. Such patients need to be monitored to ensure their disease does not progress. Medical treatments are useful only during the active phase of the disease. Use of such treatments in patients with burnt-out TAO is ineffective and carries risks of side effects. The use of medical treatments in patients with active disease needs to take into account whether potential benefits outweigh the risks of side effects, bearing in mind that most patients will improve spontaneously with time. Surgical treatments may be used at two stages: either for sight-threatening disease when it is not controlled by medical treatments, or for restoring function and appearance during the inactive phase if that is desired by the patient.

### Supportive Measures

People with TAO are one of the most psychologically fragile groups of patients in both endocrine and ophthalmic practice. This is not surprising, as their journey often includes misdiagnosis ("conjunctivitis"), experience of worrying symptoms (weight loss as a result of thyrotoxicosis, leading to a suspicion of more sinister causes), visual disturbance (fear of blindness) and not least, change in facial appearance. Once the diagnosis is made, patients face uncertainty about the future, the prospect of treatments associated with significant side effects, and usually many months of waiting before symptoms settle spontaneously or rehabilitative surgery can take place. The psychological morbidity associated with TAO is substantial.[21] Although the value of formal psychological intervention is unknown, an important part of managing these patients is for clinicians to use a listening, sympathetic approach and impart appropriate information about their disease, prognosis, and potential treatments. Patient-led organizations also have an important role in supporting patients. Cigarette use is particularly prevalent among patients with TAO, and is associated with severe disease, and with less favorable response to treatment than in nonsmokers.[22] Giving up smoking almost certainly has a beneficial effect in terms of the course of TAO. Smoking cessation should therefore be part of the management plan for patients with TAO who are smokers. Dysthyroidism, especially hypothyroidism, has an adverse effect on the course of TAO.[23–25] Euthyroidism therefore should be restored as rapidly as possible and maintained. The modality of treatment (anti-thyroid drugs, radioiodine, or thyroidectomy) is probably less important than restoration of euthyroidism. A small detrimental effect of radioiodine on TAO is well documented,[26] although this was not observed in patients with stable inactive disease.[27] A number of distressing symptoms can be addressed to some extent immediately and with relative ease, before more definitive treatments are used. Lubricants are effective in most cases in relieving grittiness, photophobia, and excessive lacrimation and help protect the cornea from ulceration. Eye drops or gels are useful during the day, whereas nocturnal ointments are of value for those with persistent conjunctival exposure when their eyes are closed. Excessive use of preservative-containing topical treatments can confound symptoms and specific advice about frequency of use should be given. Some patients with significant periorbital edema may benefit from raising the head of the bed. Sunglasses can relieve photophobia and other symptoms of exposure. Prisms may restore binocular vision. Botulinum toxin can temporarily improve upper lid retraction and dysmotility[28,29] and may be very useful for patients whose orbitopathy is active and therefore unsuitable for definite rehabilitative surgery.

### Medical Intervention in Active Thyroid-Associated Orbitopathy

Steroids remain the most useful medical treatment for active TAO.[30] Having considered which patients to treat and when, the next decision is route of administration and dose. Oral, intravenous, retrobulbar, and subconjunctival administration of steroids are the available options. Topical steroid drops have no role in the management of TAO. Retrobulbar and subconjunctival steroids are no more efficacious nor do they avoid systemic side effects and therefore are rarely justified. Numerous regimens of oral and intravenous steroids have been described. Oral steroids need to be given in relatively high doses to be effective (generally greater than 40 mg of prednisolone daily). Pulses of intravenous steroids given at one or two weekly cycles have been shown in randomized trials to be more effective than oral steroids (response rates ~80% versus ~60%) and are associated with fewer side effects.[31,32] A further advantage of pulses of intravenous steroids is that a clinical response can be detected within 1 to 2 weeks of treatment, which is predictive of longer-term response. This allows nonresponders to be identified early and alternative treatments to be considered before the development of Cushingoid side effects.[33] High-dose intravenous steroids have been associated with hepatic failure,[34] although this is fortunately rare and only observed in patients who received more than 8 g of methylprednisolone. The optimal intravenous steroid regimen is unknown, although on the basis of available data, the cumulative dose of methylprednisolone should not exceed 8 g.[35] The principal limitations of steroids are the frequent Cushingoid side effects, and the tendency of the disease to relapse when they are withdrawn. The combination of oral steroids and cyclosporine has been shown to be more effective than oral steroids alone; this treatment may have a role in a small proportion of patients with TAO who are resistant to oral prednisolone alone.[36,37] Numerous other drugs have been reported to be effective in uncontrolled studies but subsequently shown not to be so in controlled trials, and will not be discussed further.[38] Orbital irradiation has been shown in two randomized controlled trials (RCTs)[39,40] to be moderately useful as monotherapy, while this was not observed in a third RCT.[41] The main benefit is improvement in motility. The effects of orbital irradiation are slow in onset and maximal about 6 months after treatment. The main risk is earlier onset of cataract. Tumorigenesis is a theoretical concern, but sufficient to withhold this treatment in patients younger than 35 years. Orbital irradiation may exacerbate microvascular retinopathy; diabetes and hypertension are regarded as contraindications.[18] The combination of oral steroids and orbital irradiation is more efficacious than either therapy alone.[42,43]

T cells, B cells, macrophages, cytokines, and possibly antibodies are implicated in the pathogenesis of TAO.[44] Adipogenesis in the orbit is also an important contributor to expansion of intaorbital volume. Insulin-like Growth Factor 1 and its receptor and oxidative stress are also thought to be involved. There are, therefore, numerous potential specific therapeutic targets. Several novel biological agents employed in other autoimmune diseases or in transplantation medicine are already available and may prove to have a role in the management of TAO. Etanercept has been reported to improve TAO in a small uncontrolled study.[45] Rituximab (a monoclonal antibody that causes depletion of activated B cells) appears to be most promising.[46] Antioxidants have been reported to be helpful in uncontrolled studies, but need to be evaluated in properly randomized controlled studies, the attraction being safety if efficacy is proven.

### Treatment of Sight-Threatening Thyroid-Associated Orbitopathy Including Dysthyroid Optic Neuropathy

DON is an ophthalmological emergency. The optimal initial treatment is high-dose systemic steroids, which leads to improvement within days in about 80% of cases.[33] Response to treatment needs to be monitored closely, as a suboptimal response mandates urgent surgical decompression. If decompression is chosen as first-line treatment for DON, most patients will still require steroids; whereas less than half of patients treated initially with steroids will require decompression,[47] including some who initially respond well to steroids but then require high doses to maintain optic nerve function.

The treatment of sight-threatening corneal ulceration may include both local and systemic treatments. It is paramount that eyelid closure is improved and this may require high-dose intravenous steroids to improve levator function, emergency upper lid lengthening (either with Botulinum toxin or surgically), or emergency orbital decompression. Tarsorrhaphy alone is never sufficient, although it may have a place in emergency corneal protection.

### Surgical Rehabilitation of Inactive Thyroid-Associated Orbitopathy

Quality-of-life studies clearly demonstrate the enormous negative impact of TAO on patients. While functional problems impact significantly on well-being, the overall impact of disfigurement is even more profound.[48] This highlights the vital role of rehabilitative surgery.[49,50] Rehabilitation can safely commence about 6 months after all symptoms and signs have stabilized, but there is no clinical detriment to waiting longer.[51] Surgery must follow a strict sequence determined by potential side effects of each step. Thus, orbital decompression precedes strabismus surgery, which precedes eyelid surgery, first to lengthen and finally to debulk the eyelids/brows and remove excess skin. Premorbid photographs are extremely useful in helping the patient and surgeon agree on the aims of any intervention and may, for example, influence whether a decompression procedure is done.

### Decompression

Decompression involves either enlarging the bony orbit or removing orbital fat, or commonly both. General anesthesia is generally required. The end result is a reduction in proptosis, usually with reduced lower and upper eyelid retraction,[52] and a significant positive impact on quality of life.[53,54] Numerous bone removal techniques are described and the reduction in proptosis will depend on which walls are removed,[54–56] how many are removed,[57,58] and whether fat is also removed. If the indication for decompression is compressive optic neuropathy, then decompression of the medial wall in the region of the posterior ethmoid is generally performed[55]—either via a transconjunctival, transcaruncular, or transnasal approach. However for rehabilitation, the trend has altered in an attempt to reduce the risk of induced diplopia, the most debilitating frequent complication.[56,59] Several studies suggest that induced diplopia is less frequent with deep lateral wall decompression[54] or balanced lateral and medial wall decompression,[60,61] than with older inferomedial decompression techniques. However, there is currently no standardized reporting of preoperative motility restriction to allow true comparison of procedures, and very few studies have addressed this.[58] This important question therefore remains to be answered. What is generally accepted is that there is no place for decompression of the roof, which adds little to the orbital volume while risking additional complications including pulsatile proptosis. There has also been a trend away from coronal approach decompression toward approaches that leave minimal or no visible scarring. Hence an orbital surgeon will tailor the surgery to an individual patient, which is particularly important for ameliorating asymmetrical proptosis. The place of fat only decompression is difficult to evaluate as the excellent results reported by Richter and colleagues[62] have not been matched by others.[56] Apart from diplopia, other complications of decompression include periorbital paresthesia, sinusitis, cerebrospinal fluid leak, and hypoglobus, whereas serious ocular, vascular, infective, or cerebral events are extremely rare. However short- and long-term outcomes strongly support the immense value of decompression in rehabilitation of TAO, and should be considered for all patients with disfiguring proptosis.

### Strabismus

Strabismus surgery follows decompression. The usual indication is diplopia in the primary or reading position. Occasionally surgery is indicated for compensatory head posture, usually because of bilaterally tight inferior recti. Surgery most commonly involves recession of one or more tight muscles, either with nonadjustable sutures or with sutures that are adjusted peri- or postoperatively.[63] Outcomes are broadly similar in experienced hands with late overcorrection being the most frequent complication. Prior decompression may influence outcomes,[63–65] and revision surgery is fairly common. Nevertheless up to 90% of patients eventually achieve a useful field of binocular single vision with or without the use of spectacle prisms; a minority resort to monocular occlusion.[64,65] Timing of surgery is important, particularly for those patients who cannot be helped by prisms, usually because of too large a deviation. The deviation must be stable before surgery and whereas most surgeons wait 6 months to verify this, some proceed earlier, particularly after decompression or where there is evidence of inactivity on imaging.[66,67] Vertical muscle recessions can influence the position of both the upper and lower eyelids. Although the upper eyelid is often helpfully lowered, increased lower lid retraction is a troublesome side effect. Although techniques have been described to try to prevent this,[68–70] it remains a frequent problem.

### Eyelid surgery

Most patients feel much disfigured by eyelid swelling and retraction, and these final stages of rehabilitation may involve adjustment of eyelid positions, cautious removal of excess orbital fat and eyelid skin, and/or repositioning of a prolapsed lachrymal gland. A small lateral tarsorrhaphy occasionally supplements the aesthetic appearance during upper eyelid lengthening, but is never helpful as a stand-alone procedure, as it is much more likely to disfigure the eyelid contours.[71] Eyelid lengthening frequently improves exposure symptoms. Upper eyelids can be lengthened via an anterior or posterior approach and are best done under local anesthetic to allow intraoperative adjustment. The posterior approach allows recession or extirpation of Mullers muscle; extirpation being ideal for correcting retraction when it is grossly variable during normal conversation but only mild at rest.[72] The anterior approach is normally chosen for moderate to severe retraction. There are numerous techniques for upper lid lengthening, most showing success rates of 77% to 100%.[71,73,74] Spacers appear to be unnecessary and associated with more complications.[75] Blepharotomy is one of the simplest and most effective procedures and appears particularly good for eliminating the lateral contour disturbance known as lateral flare;[76,77] however, true comparisons of outcomes are hard to come by. The main complications are under- or overcorrection and contour abnormalities, but there is a small risk of dry eye from damage to the lacrimal ductules. Lengthening can be combined with blepharoplasty, although this may be safer as a second procedure after the eyelid position has been corrected.[71,74] Lower eyelid lengthening is indicated for inferior scleral show. Any proptosis should first have been addressed by decompression, as there is otherwise a risk of creating an eyelid that bulges anterior to the plane of the cheek (negative orbital vector) and will never look natural. In contrast to upper lid lengthening, the effect of gravity necessitates a spacer for lengthening the lower lid; several materials are in common use. Sclera is now avoided in some parts of the world owing to the risk of transmissible encephalopathies, but hard palate, auricular cartilage, and tarsal struts are suitable alternatives. Synthetic materials such as expanded polyethylene have been used, but carry a higher risk of complications. Lower lid blepharoplasty should be considered only after lower lid lengthening and should remain cautious.

## Why Treat Patients with Thyroid-Associated Orbitopathy?

Nobody would question the merits of treating patients with sight-threatening orbitopathy. Such cases however constitute a very small minority. Ultimately, clinicians must be guided by the potential impact on their patients' quality of life. Patients with TAO have been shown to have a poor quality of life comparable to patients with diabetes and other chronic diseases.[21] This may persist and become chronic. Visual impairment, discomfort, and disfigurement are important determinants of poor quality of life in patients with TAO.[21] A disease-specific quality-of-life questionnaire has been developed and validated. Using this tool, improvements in quality of life after orbital decompression, orbital irradiation, strabismus surgery, and lid surgery have been demonstrated.[78] The relationship however between the impact of treatment on quality of life is complex and sometimes unpredictable, illustrating the importance of including quality-of-life assessments as outcome measures in interventional studies.

## Who Should Treat Patients with Thyroid-Associated Orbitopathy?

It is apparent[79] that many patients with TAO receive suboptimal treatment for a variety of reasons. A common scenario is too much use of steroid for too long, and too little surgery too late. There is now a consensus of opinion to suggest that patients with TAO should ideally be treated in a multidisciplinary clinic with expertise in its management.[18] Such clinics are becoming more widespread, at least in Europe; however, they are rare in North America, and most patients worldwide never reach one. Too often this leaves the patient without the dual management of both their thyroid and their eye disease, or without a clinician skilled in assessment of TAO and therefore unable to make timely and appropriate therapeutic choices, or without access to an appropriately experienced surgeon, or frequently without any of these. As a consequence they may suffer unnecessary side effects from too much corticosteroid, or permanent unnecessary disfigurement and/or functional visual problems; at worst blindness.

## SUMMARY

The available treatments are far from perfect, but appropriate selection of treatments to the individual and timely intervention can lead to very satisfactory outcomes, with restoration of visual function, appearance, and improved quality of life. An important part of managing these patients is "damage limitation." Hyper- or hypothyroidism must be avoided, smoking must cease, the cornea must be protected with lubricants, and steroids must be abandoned in favor of other treatment modalities if the response is unsatisfactory. For these reasons TAO should be managed in specialist centers.

## REFERENCES

1. Bartley GB, Gorman CA. Diagnostic criteria for Graves' ophthalmopathy. Am J Ophthalmol 1995;119(6):792–5.
2. Dickinson AJ, Perros P. Controversies in the clinical evaluation of active thyroid-associated orbitopathy: use of detailed protocol with comparative photographs for objective assessment. Clin Endocrinol (Oxf) 2001;55(3):283–303.
3. Soroudi AE, Goldberg RA, McCann JD. Prevalence of asymmetric exophthalmos in Graves orbitopathy. Ophthal Plast Reconstr Surg 2004;20(3):224–5.
4. Von Arx G. Atypical manifestations. In: Wiersinga WM, Kahaly GJ, editors. Graves' orbitopathy: a multidisciplinary approach. Basel (Switzerland): S Karger AG; 2007. p. 212–20.
5. Rundle FF, Wilson CW. Development and course of exophthalmos and ophthalmoplegia in Graves' disease with special reference to the effect of thyroidectomy. Clin Sci 1944;5:177–94.
6. Perros P, Kendall-Taylor P. Natural history of thyroid eye disease. Thyroid 1998; 8(5):423–5.
7. Mourits MP, Koornneef L, Wiersinga WM, et al. Clinical criteria for the assessment of disease activity in Graves' ophthalmopathy: a novel approach. Br J Ophthalmol 1989;73(8):639–44.
8. Prummel MF, Wiersinga WM, Mourits MP. Assessment of disease activity of Graves' ophthalmopathy. In: Prummel MF, editor. Recent developments in Graves' ophthalmopathy. London: Kluwer Academic Publishers; 2000. p. 59–80.
9. Kendler DL, Lippa J, Rootman J. The initial clinical characteristics of Graves' orbitopathy vary with age and sex. Arch Ophthalmol 1993;111(2):197–201.
10. Bartley GB, Fatourechi V, Kadrmas EF, et al. Clinical features of Graves' ophthalmopathy in an incidence cohort. Am J Ophthalmol 1996;121(3):284–90.
11. Khan JA, Doane JF, Whitacre MM. Does decompression diminish the discomfort of severe dysthyroid orbitopathy? Ophthal Plast Reconstr Surg 1995;11(2): 109–12.
12. Wiersinga WM, Perros P, Kahaly GJ, et al. Clinical assessment of patients with Graves' orbitopathy: the European Group on Graves' Orbitopathy recommendations to generalists, specialists and clinical researchers. Eur J Endocrinol 2006; 155(3):387–9.
13. McKeag D, Lane CM, Lazarus JH, et al. Clinical features of dysthyroid optic neuropathy: a European Group on Graves' Orbitopathy (EUGOGO) survey. Br J Ophthalmol 2007;91(4):455–8.
14. Gerding MN, Prummel MF, Kalmann R, et al. The use of colour slides in the assessment of changes in soft-tissue involvement in Graves' ophthalmopathy. J Endocrinol Invest 1998;21(7):459–62.
15. Available at: www.eugogo.org.

16. Mourits MP, Prummel MF, Wiersinga WM, et al. Clinical activity score as a guide in the management of patients with Graves' ophthalmopathy. Clin Endocrinol (Oxf) 1997;47(1):9–14.

17. Terwee CB, Prummel MF, Gerding MN, et al. Measuring disease activity to predict therapeutic outcome in Graves' ophthalmopathy. Clin Endocrinol 2005;62: 145–55.

18. Bartalena L, Baldeschi L, Dickinson A, et al. European Group on Graves' Orbitopathy (EUGOGO). Consensus statement of the European Group on Graves' orbitopathy (EUGOGO) on management of GO. Eur J Endocrinol 2008;158(3): 273–85.

19. Bahn RS, Gorman CA. Choice of therapy and criteria for assessing treatment outcome in thyroid-associated ophthalmopathy. Endocrinol Metab Clin North Am 1987;16(2):391–407.

20. Dickinson AJ. Clinical manifestations. In: Wiersinga WM, Kahaly GJ, editors. Graves' orbitopathy: a multidisciplinary approach. Basel (Switzerland): S Karger AG; 2007. p. 1–26.

21. Coulter I, Frewin S, Krassas GE, et al. Psychological implications of Graves' orbitopathy. Eur J Endocrinol 2007;157(2):127–31.

22. Thornton J, Kelly SP, Harrison RA, et al. Cigarette smoking and thyroid eye disease: a systematic review. Eye 2007;21(9):1135–45.

23. Prummel MF, Wiersinga WM, Mourits MP, et al. Amelioration of eye changes of Graves' ophthalmopathy by achieving euthyroidism. Acta Endocrinol (Copenh) 1989;121(Suppl 2):185–9.

24. Prummel MF, Wiersinga WM, Mourits MP, et al. Effect of abnormal thyroid function on the severity of Graves' ophthalmopathy. Arch Intern Med 1990;150(5): 1098–101.

25. Tallstedt L, Lundell G, Blomgren H, et al. Does early administration of thyroxine reduce the development of Graves' ophthalmopathy after radioiodine therapy? Eur J Endocrinol 1990;130(5):494–7.

26. Bartalena L, Marcocci C, Bogazzi F, et al. Relation between therapy for hyperthyroidism and the course of Graves' ophthalmopathy. N Engl J Med 1998;338(2): 73–8.

27. Perros P, Kendall-Taylor P, Neoh C, et al. A prospective study of the effects of radioiodine therapy for hyperthyroidism in patients with minimally active Graves' ophthalmopathy. J Clin Endocrinol Metab 2005;90(9):5321–3.

28. Uddin JM, Davies PD. Treatment of upper eyelid retraction associated with thyroid eye disease with subconjunctival botulinum toxin injection. Ophthalmology 2002;109(6):1183–7.

29. Kikkawa DO, Cruz RC Jr, Christian WK, et al. Botulinum A toxin injection for restrictive myopathy of thyroid-related orbitopathy: effects on intraocular pressure. Am J Ophthalmol 2003;135(4):427–31.

30. Hart RH, Perros P. Glucocorticoids in the medical management of Graves' ophthalmopathy. Minerva Endocrinol 2003;28(3):223–31.

31. Marcocci C, Bartalena L, Tanda ML, et al. Comparison of the effectiveness and tolerability of intravenous or oral glucocorticoids associated with orbital radiotherapy in the management of severe Graves' ophthalmopathy: results of a prospective, single-blind, randomized study. J Clin Endocrinol Metab 2001; 86(8):3562–7.

32. Kahaly GJ, Pitz S, Hommel G, et al. Randomized, single-blind trial of intravenous versus oral steroid monotherapy in Graves' orbitopathy. J Clin Endocrinol Metab 2005;90(90):5234–40.

33. Hart RH, Kendall-Taylor P, Crombie A, et al. Early response to intravenous gluco-corticoids for severe thyroid-associated ophthalmopathy predicts treatment outcome. J Ocul Pharmacol Ther 2005;21(4):328–36.

34. Marinò M, Morabito E, Brunetto MR, et al. Acute and severe liver damage associated with intravenous glucocorticoid pulse therapy in patients with Graves' ophthalmopathy. Thyroid 2004;14(5):403–6.

35. Le Moli R, Baldeschi L, Saeed P, et al. Determinants of liver damage associated with intravenous methylprednisolone pulse therapy in Graves' ophthalmopathy. Thyroid 2007;17(4):357–62.

36. Kahaly G, Schrezenmeir J, Krause U, et al. Ciclosporin and prednisone vs. prednisone in treatment of Graves' ophthalmopathy: a controlled, randomized and prospective study. Eur J Clin Invest 1986;16(5):415–22.

37. Prummel MF, Mourits MP, Berghout A, et al. Prednisone and cyclosporine in the treatment of severe Graves' ophthalmopathy. N Engl J Med 1989;321(20):1353–9.

38. Wiersinga WM. Management of Graves' ophthalmopathy. Nat Clin Pract Endocrinol Metab 2007;3(5):396–404.

39. Mourits MP, van Kempen-Harteveld ML, Garcia MB, et al. Radiotherapy for Graves' orbitopathy: randomised placebo-controlled study. Lancet 2000;355(9214):1505–9.

40. Prummel MF, Terwee CB, Gerding MN, et al. A randomized controlled trial of orbital radiotherapy versus sham irradiation in patients with mild Graves' ophthalmopathy. J Clin Endocrinol Metab 2004;89(1):15–20.

41. Gorman CA, Garrity JA, Fatourechi V, et al. A prospective, randomized, double-blind, placebo-controlled study of orbital radiotherapy for Graves' orbitopathy. Ophthalmology 2001;108(9):1523–34.

42. Bartalena L, Marcocci C, Chiovato L, et al. Orbital cobalt irradiation combined with systemic corticosteroids for Graves' ophthalmopathy: comparison with systemic corticosteroids alone. J Clin Endocrinol Metab 1983;56(6):1139–44.

43. Marcocci C, Bartalena L, Bogazzi F, et al. Orbital radiotherapy combined with high-dose systemic glucocorticoids for Graves' ophthalmopathy is more effective than orbital radiotherapy alone: results of a prospective study. J Endocrinol Invest 1991;14(10):853–60.

44. Garrity JA, Bahn RS. Pathogenesis of Graves ophthalmopathy: implications for prediction, prevention, and treatment. Am J Ophthalmol 2006;142(1):147–53.

45. Paridaens D, van den Bosch WA, van der Loos TL, et al. The effect of etanercept on Graves' ophthalmopathy: a pilot study. Eye 2005;19(12):1286–9.

46. Salvi M, Vannucchi G, Campi I, et al. Treatment of Graves' disease and associated ophthalmopathy with the anti-CD20 monoclonal antibody rituximab: an open study. Eur J Endocrinol 2007;156(1):33–40.

47. Wakelkamp IM, Baldeschi L, Saeed P, et al. Surgical or medical decompression as a first-line treatment of optic neuropathy in Graves' ophthalmopathy? A randomized controlled trial. Clin Endocrinol (Oxf) 2005;63(3):323–8.

48. Farid M, Roch-Levecq AC, Levi L, et al. Psychological disturbance in Graves ophthalmopathy. Arch Ophthalmol 2005;123(4):491–6.

49. Tehrani M, Krummenauer F, Mann WJ, et al. Disease-specific assessment of quality of life after decompression surgery for Graves' ophthalmopathy. Eur J Ophthalmol 2004;14(3):193–9.

50. Schotthoefer EO, Wallace DK. Strabismus associated with thyroid eye disease. Curr Opin Ophthalmol 2007;18(5):361–5.

51. Baldeschi L, Wakelkamp IM, Lindeboom R, et al. Early versus late orbital decompression in Graves' orbitopathy: a retrospective study in 125 patients. Ophthalmology 2006;113(5):874–8.
52. Ben Simon GJ, Mansury AM, Schwarcz RM, et al. Simultaneous orbital decompression and correction of upper eyelid retraction versus staged procedures in thyroid-related orbitopathy. Ophthalmology 2005;112(5):923–32.
53. Bahn RS. Is orbital decompression a safe and effective treatment for Graves' orbitopathy? Nat Clin Pract Endocrinol Metab 2007;3(12):796–7.
54. Baldeschi L, MacAndie K, Hintschich C, et al. The removal of the deep lateral wall in orbital decompression: its contribution to exophthalmos reduction and influence on consecutive diplopia. Am J Ophthalmol 2005;140(4):642–7.
55. McCann JD, Goldberg RA, Anderson RL, et al. Medial wall decompression for optic neuropathy but lateral wall decompression with fat removal for non vision-threatening indications. Am J Ophthalmol 2006;141(5):916–7.
56. Baldeschi L. Orbital decompression. In: Wiersinga WM, Kahaly GJ, editors. Graves' orbitopathy: a multidisciplinary approach. Basel (Switzerland): S Karger AG; 2007. p. 163–75.
57. Kikkawa DO, Pornpanich K, Cruz RC Jr, et al. Graded orbital decompression based on severity of proptosis. Ophthalmology 2002;109(7):1219–24.
58. Paridaens D, Lie A, Grootendorst RJ, et al. Efficacy and side effects of 'swinging eyelid' orbital decompression in Graves' orbitopathy: a proposal for standardized evaluation of diplopia. Eye 2006;20(2):154–62.
59. Abramoff MD, Kalman R, de Graaf MEL, et al. Rectus extraocular muscle paths and decompression surgery for Graves' orbitopathy: mechanism of motility disturbances. Invest Ophthalmol Vis Sci 2002;43(2):300–7.
60. Goldberg RA, Perry JD, Hortaleza V, et al. Strabismus after balanced medial plus lateral wall versus lateral wall only orbital decompression for dysthyroid orbitopathy. Ophthal Plast Reconstr Surg 2000;16(4):271–7.
61. Kacker A, Kazim M, Murphy M, et al. "Balanced" orbital decompression for severe Graves' orbitopathy: technique with treatment algorithm. Otolaryngol Head Neck Surg 2003;128:228–35.
62. Richter DF, Stoff A, Olivari N. Transpalpebral decompression of endocrine ophthalmopathy by intraorbital fat removal (Olivari technique): experience and progression after more than 3000 operations over 20 years. Plast Reconstr Surg 2007;120(1):109–23.
63. Pitz S, Esch A, Müller-Forell WS, et al. Is there a relationship between the degree of preoperative motility impairment or the muscle thickness and the outcome of strabismus surgery in patients with Graves' orbitopathy after decompression surgery? Orbit 2005;24(3):173–6.
64. Mourits MP, Koornneef L, van Mourik-Noordenbos AM, et al. Extraocular muscle surgery for Graves' ophthalmopathy: does prior treatment influence surgical outcome? Br J Ophthalmol 1990;74(8):481–3.
65. Mocan MC, Ament C, Azar NF. The characteristics and surgical outcomes of medial rectus recessions in Graves' ophthalmopathy. J Pediatr Ophthalmol Strabismus 2007;44(2):93–100.
66. Coats D, Paysee E, Plager D, et al. Early strabismus surgery for thyroid ophthalmopathy. Ophthalmology 1999;106(2):324–9.
67. Yolar M, Oguz V, Pazarli H, et al. Early surgery for dysthyroid orbitomyopathy based on magnetic resonance imaging findings. J Pediatr Ophthalmol Strabismus 2002;39(6):336–9.

68. Kushner B. A surgical procedure to minimize lower-eyelid retraction with inferior rectus recession. Arch Ophthalmol 1992;110(7):1011–4.

69. Pacheco M, Guyton D, Repka M. Changes in eyelid position accompanying vertical rectus muscle surgery and prevention of lower lid retraction with adjustable suture. J Pediatr Ophthalmol Strabismus 1992;29(5):265–72.

70. Liao S, Shih M, Lin A. A procedure to minimize lower lid retraction during large inferior rectus recession in Graves ophthalmopathy. Am J Ophthalmol 2006; 141(3):340–5.

71. Neoh C, Eckstein A. Eyelid surgery. In: Wiersinga WM, Kahaly GJ, editors. Graves' orbitopathy: a multidisciplinary approach. Basel (Switzerland): S Karger AG; 2007. p. 188–200.

72. Velasco e Cruz AA, Vagner de Oliveira M. The effect of Müllerectomy on Kocher sign. Ophthal Plast Reconstr Surg 2001;17(5):309–15.

73. Harvey JT, Corin S, Nixon D, et al. Modified levator aponeurosis recession for upper eyelid retraction in Graves' disease. Ophthalmic Surg 1991;22(6):313–7.

74. Mourits MP, Sasim IV. A single technique to correct various degrees of upper lid retraction in patients with Graves' orbitopathy. Br J Ophthalmol 1999;83(1):81–4.

75. Mourits MP, Koornneef L. Lid lengthening by sclera interposition for eyelid retraction in Graves' ophthalmopathy. Br J Ophthalmol 1991;75(6):344–7.

76. Elner VM, Hassan AS, Frueh BR. Graded full-thickness anterior blepharotomy for upper eyelid retraction. Arch Ophthalmol 2004;122(1):55–60.

77. Hintschich C, Haritoglou C. Full thickness eyelid transsection (blepharotomy) for upper eyelid lengthening in lid retraction associated with Graves' disease. Br J Ophthalmol 2005;89(4):413–6.

78. Terwee CB, Dekker FW, Mourits MP, et al. Interpretation and validity of changes in scores on the Graves' ophthalmopathy quality of life questionnaire (GO-QOL) after different treatments. Clin Endocrinol (Oxf) 2001;54(3):391–8.

79. Perros P, Baldeschi L, Boboridis K, et al. A questionnaire survey on the management of Graves' orbitopathy in Europe. Eur J Endocrinol 2006;155(2):207–11.

# Immunology of Addison's Disease and Premature Ovarian Failure

Eystein S. Husebye, MD, PhD[a,b,*], Kristian Løvås, MD, PhD[a,b]

KEYWORDS

- Adrenal • Addison's disease • Ovary • Autoimmune
- Autoantibodies • 21-hydroxylase

Primary adrenal insufficiency (Addison's disease) is a condition with many causes. In industrialized countries it is most often provoked by an autoimmune destruction of the adrenal cortex, whereas in developing countries tuberculosis is common, often in combination with AIDS.[1] Other rare causes are enzymatic failure (congenital adrenal hyperplasia) and mutations in transcription factors, such as steroidogenic factor 1 and dosage-sensitive sex reversal adrenal hypoplasia region-1 (DAX-1).[1,2] In several of these conditions, gonadal function is also affected. In patients with adrenoleuko-dystrophy and DAX-1 mutations, gonadal failure is the rule, but with autoimmune adrenalitis, an immune-mediated destruction of the gonads is also seen as a component of autoimmune polyglandular failure.[3]

## AUTOIMMUNE ADDISON'S DISEASE

The clinical features of adrenal failure were first described by Thomas Addison[4] in 1855. He showed that the general weakness, debility, and hyperpigmentation of the skin was caused by disease in the adrenal glands. Even if tuberculous adrenalitis was common in the days of Addison, there were cases in his selection that were clearly autoimmune. No therapy was available before adrenal extracts containing steroids were tried in the 1930s, followed by deoxycorticosterone in 1937 and eventually cortisone, which was synthesized in 1949. After establishment of hydrocortisone (cortisol) and fludrocortisone therapy in the 1950s, the therapy has been virtually unchanged.

A typical feature of autoimmune Addison's disease is the high prevalence of other autoimmune manifestations.[5-9] In cross-sectional studies, approximately 50% of

[a] Section of Endocrinology, Institute of Medicine, University of Bergen, N-5021 Bergen, Norway
[b] Department of Medicine, Haukeland University Hospital, N-5021 Bergen, Norway
* Corresponding author.
E-mail address: eyhu@helse-bergen.no (E.S. Husebye).

Endocrinol Metab Clin N Am 38 (2009) 389–405
doi:10.1016/j.ecl.2009.01.010
0889-8529/09/$ – see front matter © 2009 Elsevier Inc. All rights reserved.
endo.theclinics.com

the patients have other autoimmune entities, most commonly autoimmune thyroid disease and type 1 diabetes mellitus.[5–7,9,10] Premature ovarian failure, celiac disease, and autoimmune gastritis are common in these patients. Such polyendocrine involvement was recognized as early as 1924, when Schmidt described Addison's disease in combination with chronic lymphocytic thyroiditis.[11] In the ensuing years, multiple reports followed about polyendocrine failure, including in patients with type 1 diabetes,[12] tetany, and stomatitis.[13] Later, several polyendocrine syndromes were defined.[8] Autoimmune polyendocrine syndrome type 1 (APS-1) is defined as the combination of two of the following three components: Addison's disease, hypoparathyroidism, and chronic mucocutanous candidiasis (see article by author elsewhere in this issue).[14,15] It commonly presents in childhood and is an autosomal recessive trait caused by mutations in the autoimmune regulator (AIRE) gene.[16,17] Even if it is rare, it has proven useful as a model disease of autoimmunity (see later discussion).[18] Autoimmune polyendocrine syndrome type 2 (APS-2) denotes the cluster of organ-specific autoimmune diseases of polygenetic origin. The more common combinations are Addison's disease with either autoimmune thyroid disease or type 1 diabetes; most commonly it occurs with hypothyroidism, but Graves' disease is also seen.[5,9]

Autoimmune Addison's disease can start at virtually any age but commonly presents in young and middle aged individuals. Women are more often affected than men, but below the age of 30 years, there is no gender difference.[5,6] The principal symptoms are tiredness, fatigue, reduced appetite, and weight loss. Many patients experience salt craving, orthostatism, and, as the disease progresses, a characteristic hyperpigmentation caused by high adrenocorticotropic hormone (ACTH) levels.[2] In retrospect, many patients have symptoms for years before diagnosis, whereas others progress more rapidly to adrenal insufficiency. Many cases are diagnosed only after acute life-threatening adrenal failure develops.[5] The challenge for physicians is to consider adrenal failure as a differential diagnosis. Once suspected, the diagnosis in most cases is easily confirmed by the measurement of adrenal steroid hormones. Typically, ACTH values are elevated, whereas serum cortisol levels are low; likewise, plasma renin levels are high and serum aldosterone levels are low.[1] In cases in which adrenal function is already virtually abolished, the diagnosis may be made with suitably timed serum cortisol estimations without the need for an ACTH stimulation test.

The highest prevalence of Addison's disease was found in Western Norway and was estimated at 14 per 100,000 inhabitants.[19] A slightly lower prevalence was found in Italy[20] and in the United Kingdom[21] at about 10 per 100,000. There is evidence of increasing incidence, similar to the situation with type 1 diabetes,[22] which indicates important environmental factors that contribute to the development of these diseases.

Standard replacement therapy is unphysiologic in the sense that the diurnal cortisol rhythm cannot be reconstituted. Hydrocortisone and cortisone acetate have short half-lives, and intake typically gives periods with supraphysiological levels and periods with inadequately low values over the course of a day. Patients experience reduced quality of life and impaired working capacity.[23–25] Our hypothesis is that this aberrant cortisol rhythm reduces quality of life in treated patients. Few studies have addressed the efficacy of different replacement regimens and more physiologic treatment strategies to substitute glucocorticoids, but studies are ongoing to evaluate the efficacy of novel slow-release hydrocortisone preparations[26] and continuous subcutaneous infusion of hydrocortisone using a standard insulin pump (reviewed in detail by authors elsewhere in this issue).[27]

The first report on autoantibodies in Addison's disease came in 1957 in an article by Anderson and colleagues,[28] but it was not until 1992 that Winqvist and coworkers[29] identified the steroidogenic enzyme 21-hydroxylase (CYP21) as the main target of autoantibodies in patients who have Addison's disease. Assay of 21-hydroxylase anti-bodies has since become established medical practice in the diagnostic evaluation of adrenal insufficiency. Much is still unknown about the genetics and environmental trig-gers that underlie the pathogenesis of the disease, the current knowledge of which is reviewed in this issue.

## Humoral Autoimmunity in Addison's Disease

Autoantibodies against 21-hydroxylase are considered diagnostic of autoimmune Ad-dison's disease and are found in approximately 80% of patients in cross-sectional studies.[5,30–32] In newly diagnosed patients, the proportion is even higher, at approx-imately 95%.[5] The titer of anti–21-hydroxylase antibodies is stable over years, but the number of patients with positivity against 21-hydroxylase tends to decrease over time, reaching approximately 50% after 20 years.[5,33] The frequency of these anti-bodies in the general population is usually below 0.5%. In first-degree relatives of patients with Addison's disease or other organ-specific autoimmune diseases, however, approximately 1% are anti–21-hydroxylase antibody positive. Of these persons, approximately 15% develop overt Addison's disease during an observation period of 6 years.[34]

The presence of anti–21-hydroxylase antibodies predicts the development of adrenal failure. The prediction can be improved by including genetic risk alleles in the calculation (ie, human leukocyte antigen [HLA] type determination) (see later discussion). Because therapeutic intervention to prevent the development of adrenal failure is not available, however, assaying 21-hydroxylase autoantibodies in individuals without adrenal failure is not advisable, but individuals should be informed about the risks and symptoms of adrenal failure. Early treatment with glucocorticoids may slow and prevent the progression to overt adrenal failure,[35] but controlled trials are needed to test this treatment strategy. Before the discovery of 21-hydroxylase as the principal autoantigen in Addison's disease, immunofluorescence assay was performed using frozen adrenal tissue and patient serum. The assay is difficult to standardize, is inves-tigator-dependent, and has lower sensitivity than the radioimmunoassay based on re-combinant 21-hydroxylase.[5] Reactivity toward 21-hydroxylase accounts for most of the immunoreactivity, but antibodies directed toward side-chain cleavage enzyme also contribute. In a minority of patients, positive immunofluorescence is seen without detection of either of these antibodies.[5] Previously unknown antigens may still be present.

The antibodies are of IgG1 and, to a lesser extent IgG3, class, indicating participa-tion in a Th1-mediated immune response.[36] Human autoantibodies have shown to inhibit 21-hydroxylase enzymatic activity in vitro.[37] Several groups have performed epitope mapping of 21-hydroxylase,[38–40] showing that autoantibodies target mainly the carboxy-terminal part of the protein. The mechanism of enzyme inhibition seems to be inhibition of the interaction between 21-hydroxylase and the adenine dinucleo-tide phosphate reduced cytochrome P450 reductase with which it interacts.[37] There is no evidence that the autoantibodies actually inhibit the enzyme in vivo,[41] however, and the autoantibodies should be looked upon as markers of an ongoing immune process.

## Cellular Autoimmunity in Addison's Disease

In contrast to the extensive knowledge about 21-hydroxylase antibodies, little is known about the cellular immune components taking part in the destruction of the adrenal cortex. It is known from autopsy studies that the adrenal cortices of patients who have Addison's disease are atrophic and contain enlarged eosinophilic cortex cells and a prominent lymphocytic infiltration.[42] Lymphocytic infiltration also can be seen in the adrenals of apparently healthy older individuals, however.[43] This picture of cellular infiltration is reminiscent of the insulinitis seen in animal models and patients who have type 1 diabetes. These finding are consistent with the early work by Nerup and coworkers,[44] who showed that patients with Addison's disease had reactive T cells when exposed to fetal adrenal extracts or to a mitochondrial fraction from adrenals.[45] Recently, patients with APS-2—but not individuals with isolated Addison's disease—were found to have CD4 + CD25+ regulatory T cells with defective suppressive capacity,[46] further pointing at a pathogenetic role of T cells in autoimmune adrenal failure.

Assuming that B and T cells react with the same proteins, as is the case for insulin in type 1 diabetes,[47] we recently identified an immunodominant epitope that encompasses the substrate-binding domain of 21-hydroxylase in autoimmunity-prone SJL mice.[48] Whether patients with Addison's disease have T-cell reactivity toward 21-hydroxylase is currently not known. An obstacle in human studies is that analysis is restricted to peripheral polymorphonuclear cells and not those of the adrenal gland or lymph nodes draining the adrenals. An experimental animal model of Addison's disease is lacking. Fujii and coworkers[49] reported that immunization of mice with adrenal extracts with klebsiella O3 lipopolysaccharide as adjuvant lead to infiltration of immune cells in the adrenal glands that could be transferred to other mice by spleen cells. No adrenal insufficiency was reported, however. Since then, no Addison's disease mouse models have been reported.

### Genes Associated with Addison's Disease

Autoimmune Addison's disease and APS-2 are inherited as complex genetic traits with multiple genetic factors interacting with environmental factors to confer disease susceptibility. While data on genes are starting to emerge, nothing is known about environmental factors; their implication is based on increase in incidence. It has been known for a long time that autoimmune Addison's disease has been associated with certain HLA haplotypes (**Table 1**), particularly DR3-DQ2 and DR4-DQ8,[50] but

**Table 1**
**Genes associated with Addison's disease**

|  | Gene | Variant/Allele | Reference |
|---|---|---|---|
| HLA region | *DR3-DQ2* | — | 5,52 |
|  | *DR4-DQ8* | DRB*0404 | 5,53,54 |
|  | *MICA* | 5.1A | 59,60 |
| Genes related to the immune system | CTLA-4 | 4A/G polymorphism in exon 1 | 67 |
|  |  | Dinucleotide (AT)$_n$ repeat in the 3' untranslated region of exon 3 | 66 |
|  |  | JO30G | 71 |
|  | PTPN22 | 1858T | 75,77 |
|  |  | Rare mutations | 77 |
|  | MHC2TA | −168G | 62 |
| Vitamin D metabolism | 1α-hydroxylase | −1260C | 83,84 |
|  |  | −1918 | 84 |
|  |  | −1077 | 84 |

*Abbreviations:* CTLA-4, Cytotoxic T lymphocyte antigen-4; HLA, Human leucocyte antigen; MHC, Major histocompatibility complex; MICA, MHC class I chain-related genes A; MHC2TA, MCH class II transactivator gene; PTPN22, protein tyrosine phosphatase nonreceptor type 22.

genetic association studies have been greatly impeded by lack of power because of small patient samples. Most studies have been performed with cohorts of fewer than 100 patients, and few studies have included more than 200 patients. These studies are often too small to identify susceptibility genes with odds ratios in the range of 1.25 to 2.0.

The association to HLA class II molecules is the best established. An association to the autoimmune HLA haplotypes DR3 and DR4 was reported 20 years ago,[51] although the association to DR4-DQ8 was confined to patients with Addison disease and type 1 diabetes.[52] Several consecutive studies have confirmed and extended these findings and shown an association of Addison's disease with DR4 alleles, particularly with the subtype DRB1*0404,[5,53,54] although this was not seen in Italians.[55] This finding is in contrast to type 1 diabetes in which DRB1*0401 is most associated with disease.[56] The association to DRB1*0404 holds also among patients with Addison's disease and type 1 diabetes combined.[5] Recently, association to DRB1*0403 was shown in Russian patients with Addison's disease.[54] The low frequency of this haplotype in other populations may explain why such an association was not noted before. The genotype DR3-DQ2/DR4 (DRB1*0404)-DQ8 gives the highest risk for Addison's disease (odds ratio of 36.7).[5] Conversely, DRB1*01-DQA1*01-DQB1*0501 (DQ5) confers protection against Addison's disease.[5] Analyses of larger patient cohorts should enable more confident and detailed HLA class II associations and possibly unravel other genes in the HLA region that increase or decrease disease susceptibility.

HLA class I genes have not been systematically studied in relation to Addison's disease. Dittmar and Kahaly[57] reported associations to a number of HLA-A and HLA-B alleles in 126 patients with autoimmune polyendocrine syndromes, of whom 28 had Addison's disease. Recent data from the Wellcome Trust Case Control Consortium implicated HLA-B and HLA-A, particularly HLA-B*29 in the etiology of type 1 diabetes.[58] Whether a similar association is valid for autoimmune Addison's disease remains to be shown.

HLA class II haplotypes cannot explain all heritability linked to the HLA region, and searches for other genes are being conducted. Among the candidates are the MHC class I chain-related genes A and B (MICA and MICB).[59] The MICA-A5.1/A5.1 genotype gives an odd ratio of 18.0 and an absolute risk of 1 per 1131 for Addison's disease.[59] It was found in 28 of 46 (60%) patients who have Addison's disease but only 4 of 72 (6%) controls.[60] Whether MICA is an independent risk gene or reflects the effect of neighboring genes is currently uncertain. Although the matching of DR3-DQ2/DR4-DQ8 patients and controls indicates that MICA is an independent risk gene,[60] this was recently challenged in a large-scale genotype analysis of MIC-A and MIC-B in patients with type 1 diabetes.[61] The MHC2TA gene on chromosome 16p13, which controls the constitutive MHC class II expression on antigen-presenting cells, was shown to confer risk of Addison's disease independent of HLA class II genotype.[62] Similar associations have been shown for other autoimmune diseases.[63]

Cytotoxic T lymphocyte antigen-4 (CTLA-4) is an important down-regulator of the T-cell response. The interaction between the T-cell receptor and HLA molecule with peptide on antigen-presenting cells is not sufficient to activate T cells. A co-stimulatory interaction between CD28 on T cells and B7/B7.1 on antigen-presenting cells is also required. CTLA-4 is expressed on the surface of activated T cells and competes with CD28 for the interaction with B7 and B7.1, thereby inhibiting T-cell activation. The first report on association between CTLA-4 polymorphisms and Graves' disease was published in 1995.[64] Since then, the risk of several autoimmune diseases, including celiac disease, rheumatoid arthritis, multiple sclerosis, primary biliary sclerosis, and type 1 diabetes,[65] has been associated with CTLA-4 polymorphisms. Initial studies of autoimmune Addison's disease looked at the CTLA-4A/G polymorphism in exon 1 or the variant lengths of a dinucleotide $(AT)_n$ repeat in the 3′ untranslated region of exon 3 of the CTLA-4 gene, showing association to Addison's disease in English patients.[66,67] Other researchers were unable to confirm these results, however.[68,69] In addition to the problem of insufficient power, population differences may be present.[66]

Ueda and coworkers[70] performed an extensive linkage disequilibrium mapping of the CTLA-4 gene region and showed that susceptibility to type 1 diabetes, Graves' disease, and autoimmune hypothyroidism mapped to a 6.1 kb region 3′ of the CTLA-4 gene; the polymorphisms possibly determined the relative amount of soluble CTLA-4 and full-length CTLA-4 produced.[70] Surprisingly, the CTLA-4A/G polymorphism in exon 1 was not associated. Using the same polymorphisms as Ueda and coworkers, Blomhoff and coworkers[71] confirmed the association between the CTLA-4 gene region and Addison's disease in Norwegian and English patients. Taken together, CTLA-4 seems to be a disease susceptibility gene in Addison's disease and several other autoimmune diseases. Interestingly, a locus syntenic with CTLA-4 was shown to associate with Addison's disease in Portuguese Water Dogs,[72] emphasizing a possible similarity between Addison's disease in humans and dogs (see later discussion).

Another extensively studied immune gene, protein tyrosine phosphatase nonreceptor type 22 (PTPN22) encoding lymphoid tyrosine phosphatase, which is involved in the intracellular T-cell receptor signaling. A PTPN22 polymorphism has been identified as an important genetic susceptibility factor in several autoimmune diseases, including type 1 diabetes.[73] Most of the increased risk can be explained by the 1858 T-allele considered to be an activation mutation of lymphoid tyrosine phosphatase eventually leading to the survival of more autoreative T cells during thymic selection.[74] Again, earlier studies in small cohorts revealed conflicting results in relation to Addison's disease.[75,76] In a recent study by Skinningsrud and coworkers,[77] an association with the 1858 T-allele was seen in Norwegian patients who have Addison's disease and in a meta-analysis of Norwegian, German, and English patients. Several rare mutations were detected in the PTPN22 gene, many of which were predicted to reduce or disrupt gene function.[77] The functional consequences of these rare mutations remain to be elucidated, however. PTPN22 seems to be one of the important immune genes involved in susceptibility to Addison's disease and other autoimmune diseases, alongside HLA and CTLA-4.

Great interest has been dedicated to the role of vitamin D status and vitamin D receptor variants for susceptibility to autoimmune diseases. Observational but not prospective studies have shown that vitamin D supplementation reduces the risk of type 1 diabetes.[78] Vitamin D treatment ameliorates experimental autoimmune diseases in animal models.[79] One report showed association between Addison's disease and polymorphisms in the vitamin D receptor;[80] however, the finding has not been corroborated by studies in other populations and larger cohorts. Similar findings of associations in Graves' disease and type 1 diabetes were not replicated in comprehensive well-powered studies.[81,82] A stronger case has been made for the association with variations in 1α-hydroxylase (CYP27B1), the enzyme that hydroxylates 25-hydroxyvitamin D3 to form the active hormone. Associations with polymorphisms in the 1α-hydroxylase promoter region were shown in German[83] and British patients who have Addison's disease.[84] A similar association was also found in a large cohort of patients who have type 1 patients.[85]

Associations with the genes responsible for the two major monogenic autoimmune polyendocrine diseases also have been studied (ie, the *AIRE* [APS-1] and FOXP3 [immune dysregulation, polyendocrinopathy, enteropathy, X-linked syndrome] genes), indicating no associations with autoimmune Addison's disease.[86,87] Most of the genes studied in Addison pathogenesis are in some way involved in the adaptive immune system. Recently, however, a polymorphism—the NACHT leucine-rich repeat protein 1 (NALP1) gene—was linked to risk of vitiligo and complex autoimmune diseases (ie, multiorgan autoimmunity), including Addison's disease.[88] The same association was confirmed in Romanian patients with generalized vitiligo.[89] NALP1 is thought to be involved in the innate immune system, activating the proinflammatory cytokine interleukin 1β. Whether NALP-1 is specifically involved in the pathogenesis of other autoimmune diseases is currently not known.

A recent genome-wide screening project of type 1 diabetes identified several new genes that may impact on susceptibility of Addison's disease,[90] including HLA class I molecules.[58] Undoubtedly, reports on how these genes and allelic variants relate to autoimmune Addison's disease will appear in the near future.

### Addison's Disease in Dogs

Addison's disease is a well-known disease in dogs. It occurs typically in young and middle-aged females, and dogs experience many of the same symptoms as humans (lethargy, anorexia, vomiting, and weakness). Hyponatremia, hyperkalemia, and high ACTH levels are also found.[91] Diagnosis and treatment follows similar principles as for humans. Prednisolone and fludrocortisone in near physiologic doses are commonly used, and most dogs respond well to treatment.[92] The combination of Addison's disease and autoimmune thyroiditis has been reported, equivalent to APS-2 in humans.[93] Certain purebred dogs have a disproportionately high prevalence of Addison's disease, mainly Portuguese Water Dogs, Standard Poodles, Rottweilers, Great Danes, West Highland White Terriers, and Wheaton Terriers.[72]

The recent sequencing of the canine genome[94] opens new avenues into genetics of canine disease, with potential to shed light on the corresponding human disease. Because inbred strains are often generated from a small pool of individuals, there are long haplotype stretches with high linkage disequilibrium within breeds,but short stretches between breeds, which may facilitate the identification of new genes.[95] Evidence from studies of Portuguese Water Dogs suggests that Addison's disease is inherited under the control of a single, autosomal recessive locus.[96] Recently, disease-associated loci were found on *Canis familiaris* (CFA) chromosomes CFA12 and 37, which correspond to HLA-DRB1*04 and DRB1*0301 and to a locus for immunosuppression syntenic with CTLA-4.[72] As in humans, lymphocytic infiltration has been observed in the adrenals of diseased dogs,[93] but nothing is known about the targets of cellular and humoral autoimmunity. Sera from Portuguese Water Dogs have been checked for anti–21-hydroxylase with negative results (E.S. Husebye and colleagues, unpublished data, 2007). Because it is easier to access the adrenals of diseased dogs than humans, dogs may provide a useful model to study cellular autoimmunity in Addison's disease.

### Autoimmune Regulator Deficiency in Mouse and Man: A Model of Autoimmunity

Monogenic diseases have proved to be powerful models for more common polygenic variants of various disorders and have characterized new physiologic pathways. APS-1 is such a disease. It is rare, with a prevalence of approximately 1:80,000 in most populations,[97] but numbers are higher in certain cohorts, such as Finns (1:25,000),[14] Iranian Jews (1:9000),[98] and Sardinians (1:14,000).[99] It usually presents in childhood, and the main components are primary hypoparathyroidism, Addison's disease, and chronic mucocutaneous candidiasis. A range of other manifestations are also seen, such as type 1 diabetes, ovarian failure, pernicious anemia, malabsorption, and autoimmune hepatitis (reviewed by author elsewhere in this issue). Several ectodermal components occur, such as enamel hypoplasia, vitiligo, keratitis, and nail dystrophy.[15] In 1997, two independent groups cloned the disease-causing gene named autoimmune regulator (AIRE).[16,17] Subsequent studies on AIRE knockout mouse models have shown that AIRE is an important transcriptional regulator in the thymus because it regulates and facilitates the expression of tissue-specific proteins in thymic medullary epithelial cells.[100] AIRE orchestrates the exposure of immature T cells to a "shadow of self" protein array so that autoreative clones can be deleted from the immunological repertoire (see article by author elsewhere in this issue). If AIRE is defective, autoreactive clones escape to the periphery, where they are predisposed to autoimmune disease.[18]

Patients with APS-1 have circulating autoantibodies against several tissue-specific autoantigens.[101,102] Most patients have antibodies against 21-hydroxylase, as do other patients with Addison's disease and APS-2.[101] Many patients also display autoantibodies with reactivity to the steroidogenic enzymes side-chain cleavage and 17$\alpha$-hydroxylase that are also expressed in gonadal tissue; the presence of both autoantibodies correlates with ovarian failure.[101] Findings in APS-1 underpin the principle that the organ targeted by the immune system is that which expresses the autoantigen. Even if the animal models have been useful for elucidating the mechanism of AIRE in APS-1, there are important differences between the disease in mice and humans. As far as we know, the main components of APS-1 are not found in the knockout mouse models, although they have some manifestations in common, such as gastritis, oophoritis, and hepatitis.[103] These differences may be caused by HLA types and other genes predisposing to autoimmunity. Jiang and coworkers[103] beautifully demonstrated the diversity in phenotype of Aire knockout mice dependent on the background mouse strain onto which the AIRE knockout is crossed. Interactive studies of AIRE in humans and mouse models should have the potential to further unravel the mechanisms of autoimmunity in Addison's disease and other diseases and to test novel treatment modalities.

## AUTOIMMUNE OVARIAN FAILURE

Premature ovarian failure is defined as menopause before the age of 40 years. An alternative and scientifically more accurate notation is primary ovarian insufficiency.[104] That term usually denotes amenorrhea of more than 4 months' duration in women with elevated follicle-stimulating hormone and low estradiol levels, although follicle-stimulating hormone values may initially wax and wane with periods of normal ovarian function and even pregnancies.[105] Several causes have been implicated, including chromosomal abnormalities, defects in gonadotrophin secretion, irradiation, chemotherapy, infection, and autoimmunity, but in most cases the cause remains unknown.[104,105] The prevalence is approximately 1%, and the most frequent causes are chromosome anomalies, fragile X permutations, and autoimmunity.[104,105] Autoimmune ovarian failure can be separated into two categories: cases associated with Addison's disease and cases associated with other autoimmune diseases, the former being best characterized.

### Autoimmune Ovarian Failure

Autoimmune etiology constitutes approximately 5% of the total cases of premature ovarian insufficiency[105] and occurs in approximately 10% of patients who have Addison's disease.[106] In patients with APS-1, the frequency is much higher—in the range of

50% to 60%.[15] A typical feature is the association to other autoimmune diseases (eg, Addison's disease, autoimmune thyroid disease, rheumatoid arthritis, and vitiligo). Menopause occurs any time between menarche and 40 years but tends to be earlier among patients with APS-1. The presence of circulating autoantibodies against targets in steroid-producing cells and lymphocytic infiltration in ovarian tissue are the hallmarks of autoimmune ovarian insufficiency.[105,106] Initially, the theca cells seems to be the primary target of the autoimmune attack, resulting in multifollicular development, decreased estradiol secretion, and increased inhibin levels.[107] This disproportionate elevation of inhibin levels facilitates the distinction of autoimmune cases from other forms of ovarian failure at early stages of disease development.[108]

### Autoantibodies in Ovarian Autoimmunity

The best characterized autoantibodies associated with autoimmune premature ovarian insufficiency are steroid-producing cell antibodies and antibodies against the steroidogenic enzymes 21-hydroxylase, side-chain cleavage enzyme, and 17$\alpha$-hydroxylase. Among patients who have Addison's disease and premature ovarian insufficiency, these autoantibodies are found in more than 90% of cases,[31,109] in contrast to approximately 10% of patients with nonadrenal autoimmunity and isolated premature ovarian failure.[109] Virtually all patients with anti–side-chain cleavage enzyme and anti–17$\alpha$-hydroxylase antibodies also have anti–21-hydroxylase antibodies.[110] A comparable percentage of patients also has antibodies against a forth steroidogenic enzyme, 3$\beta$-hydroxysteroid dehydrogenase,[111,112] but others have found lower frequency and an association to APS-1.[113] The presence of autoantibodies correlates with lymphocytic infiltration in ovarian tissue as analyzed in ovarian biopsies.[105] Immunofluorescence assays are difficult to standardize and positivity varies a lot among studies, which illustrates the low specificity of these assays.

Screening of an ovarian cDNA library with sera from neonatally thymectomized mice that subsequently developed autoimmune ovarian failure (see later discussion) identified an autoantigen called Mater (ie, maternal antigen that embryos require).[114] The expression of Mater is necessary for development past the earliest stages of cell division.[115] The human ortholog of Mater, NALP5, was recently identified as an autoantigen in the parathyroid gland; the presence of autoantibodies against NALP5 was associated to hypoparathyroidism and ovarian insufficiency in APS-1.[102] NALP5 is expressed almost exclusively in parathyroid and ovarian cells.[102]

### Immunogenetics of Ovarian Insufficiency

Genes involved in autoimmune premature ovarian insufficiency have not been studied systematically, although it is plausible that many of the same immunoregulatory genes involved in Addison's disease also confer susceptibility to autoimmune ovarian failure, at least the subtype associated with Addison's disease. More is known about the genetic predisposition for nonautoimmune, nonsyndromic premature ovarian failure, in which bone morphogenetic protein 15, follicle-stimulating hormone and luteinizing hormone receptors, and members of the fork-head family of transcriptions factors are involved.[116]

### Animal Models of Ovarian Insufficiency

In contrast to Addison's disease, there are several animal models of autoimmune ovarian insufficiency. One of the most interesting is the neonatally thymectomized Balb/c and C57BL/6, which develop an autoimmune polyglandular syndrome with severe autoimmune oophoritis and autoimmune disorders of the thyroid, gut, parotid gland, and lacrimal gland.[117] One of the targets of the immune response in this model is Mater.[114] Whether non–APS-1 human patients with autoimmune ovarian failure have autoantibodies against the human Mater ortholog NALP5 remains to be shown.

Another illustrative model of premature ovarian insufficiency is experimental oophoritis induced by inhibin-α.[118] Immunization of SWXJ mice with a peptide derived from mouse inhibin-α induces a unique biphasic phenotype that is characterized by an initial phase of increased fertility followed by delayed stage of premature ovarian failure. The model features two important elements of the human disease: autoreactivity against an ovarian target combined with elevation of follicle-stimulating hormone.[118] This model should be useful for further studies related to human autoimmune ovarian failure.

## SUMMARY

Autoimmune Addison's disease and autoimmune ovarian insufficiency are caused by selective targeting by T and B lymphocytes of structures in these organs. Addison's disease is characterized by a high frequency of polyendocrine failure and associated autoimmunity, notably autoimmune thyroid disease, type 1 diabetes, and ovarian insufficiency. Detection of autoantibodies against 21-hydroxylase is a clinically useful diagnostic marker. Notwithstanding their instrumental role in the destruction of the adrenal cortex, little is known about T-cell autoimmunity. The susceptibility genes are steadily being unraveled; MHC class II genes seem to be most important, but CTLA-4, PTPN22, MIC-A, and MHC2TA also contribute. In the wake of large genome-wide screening projects, new susceptibility genes probably will be identified in the imminent future. It is hoped that exciting developments in canine genetics—together with studies of Addison's disease in dogs—will advance the understanding of the human disease. The development of an experimental animal model of Addison's disease is also needed to advance our understanding of the pathogenesis of the disease.

Autoimmune primary ovarian insufficiency is often related to Addison's disease but can occur alone. Autoantibodies are also present in this condition, typically against 21-hydroxylase but also against other steroid-producing enzymes, such as side-chain cleavage enzyme and 17α-hydroxylase. T-lymphocyte infiltration parallels the generation of autoantibodies and primarily targets the theca cells and yields elevated concentrations of inhibin, which seems useful as a diagnostic marker of autoimmune etiology. There is a lack of knowledge about immunogenetics, but most likely many of the same susceptibility genes that are involved in Addison's disease also predispose patients to autoimmune ovarian failure. In contrast to Addison's disease, several experimental animal models are available for study of immunopathogenesis.

It is hoped that increased understanding of autoimmune adrenal and ovarian failure will pave the way for novel treatment strategies to prevent autoimmune destruction of these organs.

## REFERENCES

1. Arlt W, Allolio B. Adrenal insufficiency. Lancet 2003;361(9372):1881–93.
2. Betterle C, Dal Pra C, Mantero F, et al. Autoimmune adrenal insufficiency and autoimmune polyendocrine syndromes: autoantibodies, autoantigens, and their applicability in diagnosis and disease prediction. Endocr Rev 2002;23(3): 327–64.
3. Eisenbarth GS. Autoimmune polyendocrine syndromes. Adv Exp Med Biol 2004; 55:2204–18.

4. Addison T. On the constitutional and local effects of disease of the suprarenal capsules. London: Warren & Son; 1855.

5. Myhre AG, Undlien DE, Lovas K, et al. Autoimmune adrenocortical failure in Norway autoantibodies and human leukocyte antigen class II associations related to clinical features. J Clin Endocrinol Metab 2002;87(2):618–23.

6. Nerup J. Addison's disease: clinical studies. A report of 108 cases. Acta Endocrinol (Copenh) 1974;76(1):127–41.

7. Kong MF, Jeffcoate W. Eighty-six cases of Addison's disease. Clin Endocrinol (Oxf) 1994;41(6):757–61.

8. Neufeld M, Maclaren NK, Blizzard RM. Two types of autoimmune Addison's disease associated with different polyglandular autoimmune (PGA) syndromes. Medicine (Baltimore) 1981;60(5):355–62.

9. Falorni A, Laureti S, De Bellis A, et al. Italian Addison network study: update of diagnostic criteria for the etiological classification of primary adrenal insufficiency. J Clin Endocrinol Metab 2004;89(4):1598–604.

10. Kasperlik-Zaluska AA, Migdalska B, Czarnocka B, et al. Association of Addison's disease with autoimmune disorders: a long-term observation of 180 patients. Postgrad Med J 1991;67(793):984–7.

11. Schmidt MB. Eine biglandulare erkrankung (Nebennieren und Schilddrüse) bei Morbus Adisonii. Verh Dtsch Ges Pathol 1926;21:212–21 [in German].

12. Rowntree LG, Snell AM. A clinical study of Addison's disease. Mayo Clinic monographs. Philadelphia: WB Saunders Co; 1931.

13. Torpe ES, Handley HE. Chronic tetany and chronic mycelial stomatitis in a child aged 4 and a half years. Am J Dis Child 1929;38:328–38.

14. Ahonen P, Myllarniemi S, Sipila I, et al. Clinical variation of autoimmune polyendocrinopathy-candidiasis-ectodermal dystrophy (APECED) in a series of 68 patients. N Engl J Med 1990;322(26):1829–36.

15. Perheentupa J. Autoimmune polyendocrinopathy-candidiasis-ectodermal dystrophy. J Clin Endocrinol Metab 2006;91(8):2843–50.

16. Fininish-German APECED Consortium. An autoimmune disease, APECED, caused by mutations in a novel gene featuring two PHD-type zinc-finger domains. Nat Genet 1997;17(4):399–403.

17. Nagamine K, Peterson P, Scott HS, et al. Positional cloning of the APECED gene. Nat Genet 1997;17(4):393–8.

18. Mathis D, Benoist C. A decade of AIRE. Nat Rev Immunol 2007;7(8):645–50.

19. Lovas K, Husebye ES. High prevalence and increasing incidence of Addison's disease in western Norway. Clin Endocrinol (Oxf) 2002;56(6):787–91.

20. Laureti S, Vecchi L, Santeusanio F, et al. Is the prevalence of Addison's disease underestimated? J Clin Endocrinol Metab 1999;84(5):1762.

21. Willis AC, Vince FP. The prevalence of Addison's disease in Coventry, UK. Postgrad Med J 1997;73(859):286–8.

22. Aamodt G, Stene LC, Njolstad PR, et al. Spatiotemporal trends and age-period-cohort modeling of the incidence of type 1 diabetes among children aged <15 years in Norway 1973–1982 and 1989–2003. Diabetes Care 2007; 30(4):884–9.

23. Lovas K, Loge JH, Husebye ES. Subjective health status in Norwegian patients with Addison's disease. Clin Endocrinol (Oxf) 2002;56(5):581–8.

24. Hahner S, Loeffler M, Fassnacht M, et al. Impaired subjective health status in 256 patients with adrenal insufficiency on standard therapy based on cross-sectional analysis. J Clin Endocrinol Metab 2007;92(10):3912–22.

25. Gurnell EM, Hunt PJ, Curran SE, et al. Long-term DHEA replacement in primary adrenal insufficiency: a randomized, controlled trial. J Clin Endocrinol Metab 2008;93(2):400–9.
26. Newell-Price J, Whiteman M, Rostami-Hodjegan A, et al. Modified-release hydrocortisone for circadian therapy: a proof-of-principle study in dexamethasone-suppressed normal volunteers. Clin Endocrinol (Oxf) 2008;68(1):130–5.
27. Lovas K, Husebye ES. Continuous subcutaneous hydrocortisone infusion in Addison's disease. Eur J Endocrinol 2007;157(1):109–12.
28. Anderson JR, Goudie RB, Gray KG, et al. Auto-antibodies in Addison's disease. Lancet 1957;272(6979):1123–4.
29. Winqvist O, Karlsson FA, Kampe O. 21-Hydroxylase, a major autoantigen in idiopathic Addison's disease. Lancet 1992;339(8809):1559–62.
30. Soderbergh A, Winqvist O, Norheim I, et al. Adrenal autoantibodies and organ-specific autoimmunity in patients with Addison's disease. Clin Endocrinol (Oxf) 1996;45(4):453–60.
31. Chen S, Sawicka J, Betterle C, et al. Autoantibodies to steroidogenic enzymes in autoimmune polyglandular syndrome, Addison's disease, and premature ovarian failure. J Clin Endocrinol Metab 1996;81(5):1871–6.
32. Falorni A, Laureti S, Nikoshkov A, et al. 21-hydroxylase autoantibodies in adult patients with endocrine autoimmune diseases are highly specific for Addison's disease. Belgian Diabetes Registry. Clin Exp Immunol 1997;107(2):341–6.
33. Laureti S, Aubourg P, Calcinaro F, et al. Etiological diagnosis of primary adrenal insufficiency using an original flowchart of immune and biochemical markers. J Clin Endocrinol Metab 1998;83(9):3163–8.
34. Coco G, Dal Pra C, Presotto F, et al. Estimated risk for developing autoimmune Addison's disease in patients with adrenal cortex autoantibodies. J Clin Endocrinol Metab 2006;91(5):1637–45.
35. De Bellis AA, Falorni A, Laureti S, et al. Time course of 21-hydroxylase antibodies and long-term remission of subclinical autoimmune adrenalitis after corticosteroid therapy: case report. J Clin Endocrinol Metab 2001;86(2):675–8.
36. Boe AS, Bredholt G, Knappskog PM, et al. Autoantibodies against 21-hydroxylase and side-chain cleavage enzyme in autoimmune Addison's disease are mainly immunoglobulin G1. Eur J Endocrinol 2004;150(1):49–56.
37. Nikfarjam L, Kominami S, Yamazaki T, et al. Mechanism of inhibition of cytochrome P450 C21 enzyme activity by autoantibodies from patients with Addison's disease. Eur J Endocrinol 2005;152(1):95–101.
38. Nikoshkov A, Falorni A, Lajic S, et al. A conformation-dependent epitope in Addison's disease and other endocrinological autoimmune diseases maps to a carboxyl-terminal functional domain of human steroid 21-hydroxylase. J Immunol 1999;162(4):2422–6.
39. Volpato M, Prentice L, Chen S, et al. A study of the epitopes on steroid 21-hydroxylase recognized by autoantibodies in patients with or without Addison's disease. Clin Exp Immunol 1998;111(2):422–8.
40. Wedlock N, Asawa T, Baumann-Antczak A, et al. Autoimmune Addison's disease: analysis of autoantibody binding sites on human steroid 21-hydroxylase. FEBS Lett 1993;332(1–2):123–6.
41. Boscaro M, Betterle C, Volpato M, et al. Hormonal responses during various phases of autoimmune adrenal failure: no evidence for 21-hydroxylase enzyme activity inhibition in vivo. J Clin Endocrinol Metab 1996;81(8):2801–4.

42. al Sabri AM, Smith N, Busuttil A. Sudden death due to auto-immune Addison's disease in a 12-year-old girl. Int J Legal Med 1997;110(5):278–80.
43. Hayashi Y, Hiyoshi T, Takemura T, et al. Focal lymphocytic infiltration in the adrenal cortex of the elderly: immunohistological analysis of infiltrating lymphocytes. Clin Exp Immunol 1989;77(1):101–5.
44. Nerup J, Andersen V, Bendixen G. Anti-adrenal, cellular hypersensitivity in Addison's disease. Clin Exp Immunol 1969;4(4):355–63.
45. Nerup J, Andersen V, Bendixen G. Anti-adrenal cellular hypersensitivity in Addison's disease. IV. In vivo and in vitro investigations on the mitochondrial fraction. Clin Exp Immunol 1970;6(5):733–9.
46. Kriegel MA, Lohmann T, Gabler C, et al. Defective suppressor function of human CD4 + CD25+ regulatory T cells in autoimmune polyglandular syndrome type II. J Exp Med 2004;199(9):1285–91.
47. Mallone R, Martinuzzi E, Blancou P, et al. CD8 + T-cell responses identify beta-cell autoimmunity in human type 1 diabetes. Diabetes 2007;56(3): 613–21.
48. Husebye ES, Bratland E, Bredholt G, et al. The substrate-binding domain of 21-hydroxylase, the main autoantigen in autoimmune Addison's disease, is an immunodominant T cell epitope. Endocrinology 2006;147(5):2411–6.
49. Fujii Y, Kato N, Kito J, et al. Experimental autoimmune adrenalitis: a murine model for Addison's disease. Autoimmunity 1992;12(1):47–52.
50. Robles DT, Fain PR, Gottlieb PA, et al. The genetics of autoimmune polyendocrine syndrome type II. Endocrinol Metab Clin North Am 2002;31(2): 353–68.
51. Maclaren NK, Riley WJ. Inherited susceptibility to autoimmune Addison's disease is linked to human leukocyte antigens-DR3 and/or DR4, except when associated with type I autoimmune polyglandular syndrome. J Clin Endocrinol Metab 1986;62(3):455–9.
52. Huang W, Connor E, Rosa TD, et al. Although DR3-DQB1*0201 may be associated with multiple component diseases of the autoimmune polyglandular syndromes, the human leukocyte antigen DR4-DQB1*0302 haplotype is implicated only in beta-cell autoimmunity. J Clin Endocrinol Metab 1996;81(7): 2559–63.
53. Yu L, Brewer KW, Gates S, et al. DRB1*04 and DQ alleles: expression of 21-hydroxylase autoantibodies and risk of progression to Addison's disease. J Clin Endocrinol Metab 1999;84(1):328–35.
54. Gombos Z, Hermann R, Kiviniemi M, et al. Analysis of extended human leukocyte antigen haplotype association with Addison's disease in three populations. Eur J Endocrinol 2007;157(6):757–61.
55. Gambelunghe G, Kockum I, Bini V, et al. Retrovirus-like long-terminal repeat DQ-LTR13 and genetic susceptibility to type 1 diabetes and autoimmune Addison's disease. Diabetes 2005;54(3):900–5.
56. Undlien DE, Friede T, Rammensee HG, et al. HLA-encoded genetic predisposition in IDDM: DR4 subtypes may be associated with different degrees of protection. Diabetes 1997;46(1):143–9.
57. Dittmar M, Kahaly GJ. Polyglandular autoimmune syndromes: immunogenetics and long-term follow-up. J Clin Endocrinol Metab 2003;88(7):2983–92.
58. Nejentsev S, Howson JM, Walker NM, et al. Localization of type 1 diabetes susceptibility to the MHC class I genes HLA-B and HLA-A. Nature 2007; 450(7171):887–92.

59. Gambelunghe G, Falorni A, Ghaderi M, et al. Microsatellite polymorphism of the MHC class I chain-related (MIC-A and MIC-B) genes marks the risk for autoimmune Addison's disease. J Clin Endocrinol Metab 1999;84(10):3701–7.

60. Park YS, Sanjeevi CB, Robles D, et al. Additional association of intra-MHC genes, MICA and D6S273, with Addison's disease. Tissue Antigens 2002; 60(2):155–63.

61. Field SF, Nejentsev S, Walker NM, et al. Sequencing-based genotyping and association analysis of the MICA and MICB genes in type 1 diabetes. Diabetes 2008;57(6):1753–6.

62. Ghaderi M, Gambelunghe G, Tortoioli C, et al. MHC2TA single nucleotide polymorphism and genetic risk for autoimmune adrenal insufficiency. J Clin Endocrinol Metab 2006;91(10):4107–11.

63. Swanberg M, Lidman O, Padyukov L, et al. MHC2TA is associated with differential MHC molecule expression and susceptibility to rheumatoid arthritis, multiple sclerosis and myocardial infarction. Nat Genet 2005;37(5):486–94.

64. Yanagawa T, Hidaka Y, Guimaraes V, et al. CTLA-4 gene polymorphism associated with Graves' disease in a Caucasian population. J Clin Endocrinol Metab 1995;80(1):41–5.

65. Vaidya B, Pearce S. The emerging role of the CTLA-4 gene in autoimmune endocrinopathies. Eur J Endocrinol 2004;150(5):619–26.

66. Kemp EH, Ajjan RA, Husebye ES, et al. A cytotoxic T lymphocyte antigen-4 (CTLA-4) gene polymorphism is associated with autoimmune Addison's disease in English patients. Clin Endocrinol (Oxf) 1998;49(5):609–13.

67. Vaidya B, Imrie H, Geatch DR, et al. Association analysis of the cytotoxic T lymphocyte antigen-4 (CTLA-4) and autoimmune regulator-1 (AIRE-1) genes in sporadic autoimmune Addison's disease. J Clin Endocrinol Metab 2000; 85(2):688–91.

68. Perez de Nanclares G, Martin-Pagola A, Ramon Bilbao J, et al. No evidence of association of CTLA4 polymorphisms with Addison's disease. Autoimmunity 2004;37(6–7):453–6.

69. Donner H, Braun J, Seidl C, et al. Codon 17 polymorphism of the cytotoxic T lymphocyte antigen 4 gene in Hashimoto's thyroiditis and Addison's disease. J Clin Endocrinol Metab 1997;82(12):4130–2.

70. Ueda H, Howson JM, Esposito L, et al. Association of the T-cell regulatory gene CTLA4 with susceptibility to autoimmune disease. Nature 2003;423(6939): 506–11.

71. Blomhoff A, Lie BA, Kemp EH, et al. Polymorphisms in the CTLA4 gene region confer susceptibility to Addison's disease. J Clin Endocrinol Metab 2004; 89(7):3474–6.

72. Chase K, Sargan D, Miller K, et al. Understanding the genetics of autoimmune disease: two loci that regulate late onset Addison's disease in Portuguese Water Dogs. Int J Immunogenet 2006;33(3):179–84.

73. Bottini N, Musumeci L, Alonso A, et al. A functional variant of lymphoid tyrosine phosphatase is associated with type I diabetes. Nat Genet 2004;36(4):337–8.

74. Vang T, Miletic AV, Bottini N, et al. Protein tyrosine phosphatase PTPN22 in human autoimmunity. Autoimmunity 2007;40(6):453–61.

75. Velaga MR, Wilson V, Jennings CE, et al. The codon 620 tryptophan allele of the lymphoid tyrosine phosphatase (LYP) gene is a major determinant of Graves' disease. J Clin Endocrinol Metab 2004;89(11):5862–5.

76. Kahles H, Ramos-Lopez E, Lange B, et al. Sex-specific association of PTPN22 1858T with type 1 diabetes but not with Hashimoto's thyroiditis or Addison's disease in the German population. Eur J Endocrinol 2005;153(6):895–9.

77. Skinningsrud B, Husebye ES, Gervin K, et al. Mutation screening of PTPN22: association of the 1858T-allele with Addison's disease. Eur J Hum Genet 2008; 16(8):977–82.

78. Zipitis CS, Akobeng AK. Vitamin D supplementation in early childhood and risk of type 1 diabetes: a systematic review and meta-analysis. Arch Dis Child 2008; 93(6):512–7.

79. Mathieu C, Waer M, Laureys J, et al. Prevention of autoimmune diabetes in NOD mice by 1,25 dihydroxyvitamin D3. Diabetologia 1994;37(6):552–8.

80. Pani MA, Seissler J, Usadel KH, et al. Vitamin D receptor genotype is associated with Addison's disease. Eur J Endocrinol 2002;147(5):635–40.

81. Collins JE, Heward JM, Nithiyananthan R, et al. Lack of association of the vitamin D receptor gene with Graves' disease in UK Caucasians. Clin Endocrinol (Oxf) 2004;60(5):618–24.

82. Nejentsev S, Cooper JD, Godfrey L, et al. Analysis of the vitamin D receptor gene sequence variants in type 1 diabetes. Diabetes 2004; 53(10):2709–12.

83. Lopez ER, Zwermann O, Segni M, et al. A promoter polymorphism of the CYP27B1 gene is associated with Addison's disease, Hashimoto's thyroiditis, Graves' disease and type 1 diabetes mellitus in Germans. Eur J Endocrinol 2004;151(2):193–7.

84. Jennings CE, Owen CJ, Wilson V, et al. A haplotype of the CYP27B1 promoter is associated with autoimmune Addison's disease but not with Graves' disease in a UK population. J Mol Endocrinol 2005;34(3):859–63.

85. Bailey R, Cooper JD, Zeitels L, et al. Association of the vitamin D metabolism gene CYP27B1 with type 1 diabetes. Diabetes 2007;56(10):2616–21.

86. Owen CJ, Eden JA, Jennings CE, et al. Genetic association studies of the FOXP3 gene in Graves' disease and autoimmune Addison's disease in the United Kingdom population. J Mol Endocrinol 2006;37(1):97–104.

87. Boe Wolff AS, Oftedal B, Johansson S, et al. AIRE variations in Addison's disease and autoimmune polyendocrine syndromes (APS): partial gene deletions contribute to APS I. Genes Immun 2008;9(2):130–6.

88. Jin Y, Mailloux CM, Gowan K, et al. NALP1 in vitiligo-associated multiple autoimmune disease. N Engl J Med 2007;356(12):1216–25.

89. Jin Y, Birlea SA, Fain PR, et al. Genetic variations in NALP1 are associated with generalized vitiligo in a Romanian population. J Invest Dermatol 2007;127(11): 2558–62.

90. Todd JA, Walker NM, Cooper JD, et al. Robust associations of four new chromosome regions from genome-wide analyses of type 1 diabetes. Nat Genet 2007; 39(7):857–64.

91. Kintzer PP, Peterson ME. Primary and secondary canine hypoadrenocorticism. Vet Clin North Am Small Anim Pract 1997;27(2):349–57.

92. Kintzer PP, Peterson ME. Treatment and long-term follow-up of 205 dogs with hypoadrenocorticism. J Vet Intern Med 1997;11(2):43–9.

93. Kooistra HS, Rijnberk A, van den Ingh TS. Polyglandular deficiency syndrome in a boxer dog: thyroid hormone and glucocorticoid deficiency. Vet Q 1995;17(2): 59–63.

94. Lindblad-Toh K, Wade CM, Mikkelsen TS, et al. Genome sequence, comparative analysis and haplotype structure of the domestic dog. Nature 2005;438(7069): 803–19.

95. Karlsson EK, Baranowska I, Wade CM, et al. Efficient mapping of mendelian traits in dogs through genome-wide association. Nat Genet 2007;39(11): 1321–8.

96. Oberbauer AM, Bell JS, Belanger JM, et al. Genetic evaluation of Addison's disease in the Portuguese Water Dog. BMC Vet Res 2006;2(5):15.

97. Myhre AG, Halonen M, Eskelin P, et al. Autoimmune polyendocrine syndrome type 1 (APS I) in Norway. Clin Endocrinol (Oxf) 2001;54(2):211–7.

98. Zlotogora J, Shapiro MS. Polyglandular autoimmune syndrome type I among Iranian Jews. J Med Genet 1992;29(11):824–6.

99. Rosatelli MC, Meloni A, Devoto M, et al. A common mutation in Sardinian autoimmune polyendocrinopathy-candidiasis-ectodermal dystrophy patients. Hum Genet 1998;103(4):428–34.

100. Anderson MS, Venanzi ES, Klein L, et al. Projection of an immunological self shadow within the thymus by the AIRE protein. Science 2002;298(5597): 1395–401.

101. Soderbergh A, Myhre AG, Ekwall O, et al. Prevalence and clinical associations of 10 defined autoantibodies in autoimmune polyendocrine syndrome type I. J Clin Endocrinol Metab 2004;89(2):557–62.

102. Alimohammadi M, Bjorklund P, Hallgren A, et al. Autoimmune polyendocrine syndrome type 1 and NALP5, a parathyroid autoantigen. N Engl J Med 2008; 358(10):1018–28.

103. Jiang W, Anderson MS, Bronson R, et al. Modifier loci condition autoimmunity provoked by AIRE deficiency. J Exp Med 2005;202(6):805–15.

104. Welt CK. Primary ovarian insufficiency: a more accurate term for premature ovarian failure. Clin Endocrinol (Oxf) 2008;68(4):499–509.

105. Hoek A, Schoemaker J, Drexhage HA. Premature ovarian failure and ovarian autoimmunity. Endocr Rev 1997;18(1):107–34.

106. Betterle C, Rossi A, Dalla Pria S, et al. Premature ovarian failure: autoimmunity and natural history. Clin Endocrinol (Oxf) 1993;39(1):35–43.

107. Welt CK, Falorni A, Taylor AE, et al. Selective theca cell dysfunction in autoimmune oophoritis results in multifollicular development, decreased estradiol, and elevated inhibin B levels. J Clin Endocrinol Metab 2005;90(5):3069–76.

108. Tsigkou A, Marzotti S, Borges L, et al. High serum inhibin concentration discriminates autoimmune oophoritis from other forms of primary ovarian insufficiency. J Clin Endocrinol Metab 2008;93:1263–9.

109. Dal Pra C, Chen S, Furmaniak J, et al. Autoantibodies to steroidogenic enzymes in patients with premature ovarian failure with and without Addison's disease. Eur J Endocrinol 2003;148(5):565–70.

110. Falorni A, Laureti S, Candeloro P, et al. Steroid-cell autoantibodies are preferentially expressed in women with premature ovarian failure who have adrenal autoimmunity. Fertil Steril 2002;78(2):270–9.

111. Arif S, Vallian S, Farzaneh F, et al. Identification of 3 beta-hydroxysteroid dehydrogenase as a novel target of steroid cell autoantibodies: association of autoantibodies with endocrine autoimmune disease. J Clin Endocrinol Metab 1996; 81(12):4439–45.

112. Arif S, Varela-Calvino R, Conway GS, et al. 3 beta hydroxysteroid dehydrogenase autoantibodies in patients with idiopathic premature ovarian failure target N- and C-terminal epitopes. J Clin Endocrinol Metab 2001;86(12):5892–7.

113. Reimand K, Peterson P, Hyoty H, et al. 3beta-hydroxysteroid dehydrogenase autoantibodies are rare in premature ovarian failure. J Clin Endocrinol Metab 2000;85(6):2324–6.

114. Tong ZB, Nelson LM. A mouse gene encoding an oocyte antigen associated with autoimmune premature ovarian failure. Endocrinology 1999;140(8):3720–6.

115. Tong ZB, Gold L, Pfeifer KE, et al. Mater, a maternal effect gene required for early embryonic development in mice. Nat Genet 2000;26(3):267–8.

116. Laissue P, Vinci G, Veitia RA, et al. Recent advances in the study of genes involved in non-syndromic premature ovarian failure. Mol Cell Endocrinol 2008;282(1–2):101–11.

117. Taguchi O, Nishizuka Y, Sakakura T, et al. Autoimmune oophoritis in thymectomized mice: detection of circulating antibodies against oocytes. Clin Exp Immunol 1980;40(3):540–53.

118. Altuntas CZ, Johnson JM, Tuohy VK. Autoimmune targeted disruption of the pituitary-ovarian axis causes premature ovarian failure. J Immunol 2006; 177(3):1988–96.

# Fine Tuning for Quality of Life: 21st Century Approach to Treatment of Addison's Disease

Nicole Reisch, MD, Wiebke Arlt, MD, DSc, FRCP*

**KEYWORDS**

- Adrenal insufficiency • Addison's disease
- Cortisol • Aldosterone • Dehydroepiandrosterone
- Quality of life • Mortality

In 1855, when Thomas Addison[1] first described a disease characterized by salt wasting and hyperpigmentation as the result of adrenal gland destruction, adrenal insufficiency was a fatal condition. The landmark achievement of the synthesis of cortisone in the late 1940s and its introduction into therapeutic use in the early 1950s quickly led to widespread availability of life-saving glucocorticoid replacement therapy. Currently, survival in patients who have adrenal insufficiency is routinely achieved; however, our current treatment regimens may not facilitate a normal quality of life or even a normal life expectancy. Recent data demonstrated an increased mortality not only in patients who have secondary adrenal insufficiency caused by hypopituitarism[2] but also in primary adrenal insufficiency (ie, Addison's disease),[3] a finding still valid when the influence of comorbidities is excluded. The causes underlying this increased mortality remain unclear, but we need to consider the possible impact of current replacement regimens on the observed increased cardiovascular and cerebrovascular mortality and the high number of patients with adrenal insufficiency succumbing to respiratory infections.[2,3] Similarly, quality of life seems to be significantly impaired in patients who have adrenal insufficiency,[4,5] and they show an increased rate of disablement pensions and a reduced capacity for full-time employment—or any work at all.[4–7]

Optimization of corticosteroid replacement therapy in adrenal insufficiency remains a continuous challenge that is not made any easier by the lack of objective biomarkers of glucocorticoid action and the nonphysiologic pharmacokinetic properties of currently available hydrocortisone preparations. Despite these limitations, clinicians

Division of Medical Sciences, Institute of Biomedical Research, Rm 225, University of Birmingham, Birmingham, B15 2TT, UK
* Corresponding author.
*E-mail address:* w.arlt@bham.ac.uk (W. Arlt).

Endocrinol Metab Clin N Am 38 (2009) 407–418
doi:10.1016/j.ecl.2009.01.008
0889-8529/09/$ – see front matter © 2009 Elsevier Inc. All rights reserved.

endo.theclinics.com

and researchers in the field are facing the challenge; recent improvements include the introduction of dehydroepiandrosterone (DHEA) replacement, and we look forward to the introduction of delayed- and controlled-release (long-acting) hydrocortisone formulations. This article focuses on the current state of the art regarding corticosteroid replacement in adrenal insufficiency but also covers promising emerging approaches.

## CORTICOSTEROID REPLACEMENT IN CHRONIC ADRENAL INSUFFICIENCY

Destruction of the adrenal gland (eg, by autoimmune adrenalitis), the classic Addison's disease, results in loss of production of adrenal corticosteroids (ie, cortisol, aldosterone, and the sex steroid precursor DHEA), which are produced by the adrenal zonae fasciculata, glomerulosa, and reticularis, respectively. Life-saving treatment for primary adrenal insufficiency consists of glucocorticoid and mineralocorticoid replacement; the latter is not required in patients who have secondary adrenal insufficiency and an intact regulation of aldosterone release by the renin-angiotensin-aldosterone system. Although DHEA replacement is not yet part of routine replacement regimens, over the last 10 years several studies have reported beneficial effects of DHEA and sex steroid replacement on mood- and health-related subjective health status in patients who have adrenal insufficiency.[8–14]

### Glucocorticoid Replacement

We currently consider hydrocortisone (ie, cortisol) the glucocorticoid of choice for replacement therapy in cases of adrenal insufficiency. As demonstrated by seminal work in the early 1990s, daily cortisol production rates in normal subjects vary between 5 and 10 mg/m$^2$ body surface area.[15,16] Because the oral bioavailability of hydrocortisone is close to 100%,[17] a daily oral dose of hydrocortisone of 15 to 25 mg seems sufficient for replacement, with slightly higher doses for primary than secondary adrenal insufficiency (20–25 mg versus 15–20 mg). Previously used replacement doses of 30 mg or more of hydrocortisone daily must be considered supraphysiologic and come with a high likelihood of undesirable excess exposure to glucocorticoid activity. Body weight–adjusted glucocorticoid doses have been suggested[18] and seem to generate a smoother pharmacokinetic profile, but data demonstrating superiority of such a regimen are lacking. Body surface area–adjusted glucocorticoid dosing is commonly used for guiding glucocorticoid replacement in children.

When deciding on the glucocorticoid dose, it is important to consider concurrent medication, particularly any drugs known to increase glucocorticoid inactivation by induction of CYP3A4 in the liver (eg, rifampicin and mitotane).[19] Such medication invariably requires adjustment (ie, increase of hydrocortisone replacement doses). Similarly, thyroid hormone excess caused by hyperthyroidism or the initiation or increase in dosage of exogenous L-thyroxine replacement increases hydrocortisone/cortisol turnover and may require glucocorticoid dose adjustment. For the same reason, initiation of glucocorticoid replacement in newly diagnosed patients with hypopituitarism always should precede the start of L-thyroxine replacement; choosing the reverse order might precipitate an adrenal crisis.

Although current glucocorticoid replacement regimens aim to mimic the physiologic circadian rhythm of cortisol secretion, they invariably fail because the available hydrocortisone preparations have an unfavorable pharmacokinetic profile with a steep increase to supraphysiologic maximum serum concentrations within 1 to 2 hours of administration followed by a rapid decline to undetectable levels 5 to 7 hours after ingestion. Current preparations also do not allow the mimicking of the physiologic early morning rise in serum cortisol. In general, glucocorticoid replacement is administered in two or three daily doses, with one half to two thirds of the daily dose administered in the morning. Subsequent doses should be administered during lunchtime and in the afternoon. Routine administration of the second replacement dose with the evening meal is at least debatable, because physiologic serum cortisol concentrations in the evening hours are low. Using a twice-daily replacement regimen, with administration of the second dose at 6 PM, would invariably lead to low glucocorticoid levels in the afternoon, which may increase fatigue. Glucocorticoids should not be administered immediately before going to bed, because sleep may be disrupted by high serum cortisol levels.

The evidence base for the superiority of thrice-daily over twice-daily hydrocortisone administration is scarce, with only one small, uncontrolled, open label trial reporting on six patients who switched from thrice- to twice-daily administration and one patient who switched from twice- to thrice-daily administration. The study design, however, prevented valid conclusions.[20] A double-blind, placebo-controlled randomized cross-over design compared twice-daily administration (20 to 10 mg) to two single-dose regimens (30 mg in the morning or 30 mg in the evening). Results of health-related quality of life testing clearly indicated superiority of twice-daily over once-daily administration of hydrocortisone.[21] The decision to choose thrice-daily over twice-daily hydrocortisone administration or vice versa depends on individual preference and the specific circumstances of the patient in question. On the same note, shift work has to be taken into consideration, and replacement regimens clearly should follow the diurnal rhythm of a patient's activity, not clock time (ie, the first dose should be taken upon rising and not necessarily in the morning).

Although hydrocortisone is considered the glucocorticoid of choice for replacement in the context of adrenal insufficiency, in some countries only cortisone acetate is available, which requires activation to cortisol by hepatic 11β-hydroxysteroid dehydrogenase type 1 activity. This yields a greater interindividual variability in pharmacokinetic availability; 15 to 25 mg hydrocortisone are equivalent to 25 to 37.5 mg cortisone acetate.[19]

Synthetic, long-acting glucocorticoids also can be used for replacement therapy. Estimated equipotency doses are as follows: 10 mg hydrocortisone = 2 mg prednisolone = 0.25 mg dexamethasone. Similar to cortisone acetate, prednisone requires activation by hepatic 11β- hydroxysteroid dehydrogenase type 1 activity to prednisolone, so the latter should be preferred. There is a paucity of data on the biologic activity of different glucocorticoids, and equipotency doses are estimated rather than calculated. The data on which these estimations are based mostly refer to the anti-inflammatory activity of different glucocorticoids, which clearly represents only one aspect of glucocorticoid action. Chronic glucocorticoid replacement with long-acting synthetic glucocorticoids is less desirable, mainly because of unfavorable nighttime glucocorticoid activity as a consequence of the longer biologic half-lives of these preparations and the limited options for dose titration. Hydrocortisone also exerts potent mineralocorticoid action, whereas synthetic glucocorticoids only have reduced mineralocorticoid activity (prednisolone) or none at all (dexamethasone), which is an issue of considerable importance for the replacement strategy in patients with primary adrenal insufficiency.

Because there is no reliable and convenient marker of glucocorticoid action, monitoring of glucocorticoid replacement therapy is mainly based on clinical judgment and careful assessment of clinical signs and symptoms potentially suggestive of over- or underreplacement.[19] One general caveat is the lack of specificity of such signs and symptoms; follow-up monitoring of adrenal insufficiency patients requires an experienced physician. Fatigue, nausea, myalgia, lack of energy, and weight loss may indicate underreplacement, whereas weight gain, central obesity, osteoporosis, impaired glucose tolerance, and hypertension may suggest overreplacement. Only patients who receive supraphysiologic daily glucocorticoid replacement doses of 30 mg hydrocortisone or higher have been shown to have an increased risk of osteoporosis.[22] Patients who receive appropriate glucocorticoid replacement doses (ie, 15–25 mg hydrocortisone daily) do not require regular monitoring with bone mineral density measurements.

Serum cortisol day curves are of limited value and cannot be used to assess replacement quality, with a recent publication nicely demonstrating complete overlap of serum cortisol levels by comparing patients who were clinically assessed to have good replacement or under- or overreplacement.[23] Timed serum cortisol measurements can be of some value in selected patients (eg, in cases of suspected noncompliance or malabsorption); however, serum cortisol measurements without concurrent availability of information on the time of the last hydrocortisone administration before blood sampling are not informative.

In patients with primary adrenal insufficiency, levels of plasma adrenocorticotropin (ACTH) are invariably high before administration of hydrocortisone, which is followed by a quick drop in ACTH levels.[24–27] In patients with hypopituitarism, ACTH levels are low and do not change after glucocorticoid administration. Plasma ACTH levels cannot be used as a monitoring tool of glucocorticoid replacement either in primary or secondary adrenal insufficiency. Plasma ACTH levels are only useful in selected cases (ie, increasing hyperpigmentation in patients with bilateral adrenal insufficiency after failure of surgical cure of Cushing's disease). In such cases, Nelson's syndrome, which involves an invasive ACTH-producing pituitary tumor, may need to be excluded or monitored. For this purpose, an ACTH day profile with measurements before and after hydrocortisone administration is of some value in differentiating autonomous ACTH hypersecretion from endogenous ACTH up-regulation caused by low circulating cortisol levels.

Urinary free cortisol has been advocated for monitoring glucocorticoid replacement;[28,29] however, cortisol excretion after exogenous hydrocortisone administration shows considerable interindividual variability.[27] Most importantly, cortisol-binding globulin is rapidly saturated after oral ingestion of hydrocortisone, resulting in transient but pronounced increases in cortisol excretion. Urinary free cortisol results in patients on hydrocortisone replacement not being judged referring to urinary cortisol excretion in healthy volunteers, and aiming at the latter reference range might result in underreplacement. The currently recommended treatment and monitoring concept in patients with chronic adrenal insufficiency is summarized in **Box 1**.

### Mineralocorticoid Replacement

Mineralocorticoids are replaced by oral administration of 9α-fludrocortisone; fluorination at the 9α-position ensures selective binding to the mineralocorticoid receptor and exclusive mineralocorticoid action (ie, a biologic activity resembling that of aldosterone). By contrast, cortisol binds with equal affinity to the glucocorticoid and mineralocorticoid receptors. Oelkers coined the term "mineralocorticoid unit," determining that 100 mineralocorticoid units is equivalent to 100 μg fludrocortisone and 40 mg hydrocortisone.[30] The mineralocorticoid receptor in the kidney is prevented from being swamped by circulating cortisol via the activity of 11β-hydroxysteroid dehydrogenase type 2, which efficiently inactivates cortisol to cortisone. In the newly diagnosed adult patient, mineralocorticoid replacement is initiated at 0.1 mg once daily,

---

**Box 1**
**Current treatment and monitoring concept in chronic adrenal insufficiency**

*Glucocorticoid replacement*

Hydrocortisone 20–25 mg/d in primary (adrenal) insufficiency and 15–20 mg/d in secondary (hypothalamic-pituitary) adrenal insufficiency should be administered in two or three doses, with half to two thirds of the daily dose given in the morning (immediately upon rising)

*Monitoring*

- Detailed history asking for clinical signs and symptoms suggestive of glucocorticoid over- or underreplacement and the ability to cope with daily stress
- Detailed account of stress-related glucocorticoid dose self-adjustments since last visit, potential adverse events, including emergency treatment, and/or hospitalization
- Verification of emergency bracelet/steroid card
- Re-instruction regarding stress-related glucocorticoid dose adjustment and emergency guidelines (involve partners/family members); consider prescription of emergency injection kit
- Body weight

*Mineralocorticoid replacement (only in primary adrenal insufficiency)*

Fludrocortisone 0.1 (0.05–0.25) mg/d taken as a single dose in the morning

Monitoring

- Blood pressure (supine/erect)
- Check for peripheral edema
- Serum sodium, serum potassium
- Plasma renin activity (target: upper normal reference range)

*DHEA replacement (optional)*

DHEA 25–50 mg/d taken as a single dose in the morning

*Monitoring*

- Serum DHEAs, in women also androstenedione, testosterone, sex hormone binding globulin; blood sampling at trough (24 h after last administration); aim for levels within the normal reference range

*Additional monitoring requirements*

- Primary adrenal insufficiency caused by autoimmune adrenalitis: serum thyroid-stimulating hormone
- In women, check for regularity of menstrual cycle; check serum $B_{12}$ levels if lack of well-being is apparent despite apparently adequate corticosteroid replacement
- Secondary adrenal insufficiency: monitor underlying hypothalamic-pituitary disease, including replacement of other axes
- Regular follow-up visits in specialized center (every 6–12 months)

---

and usual replacement doses vary between 0.05 and 0.25 mg daily. Children, particularly neonates and infants, have considerably higher mineralocorticoid dose requirements and often need additional salt supplementation. Among individuals of comparable age, however, there is also a good degree of interindividual variability in mineralocorticoid dose requirements.

Daily salt intake matters, with a high intake slightly reducing mineralocorticoid requirements. An important additional factor is the temperature and humidity. For example, individuals who live in Mediterranean summer or tropical climatic conditions require an increase of up to 50% of their usual fludrocortisone dose because of increased salt loss via sweating. The glucocorticoid chosen for replacement is an important factor, with 20 mg hydrocortisone being equivalent to 0.05 mg fludrocortisones. Reductions in the hydrocortisone impact to a certain degree on mineralocorticoid activity. Prednisolone has reduced mineralocorticoid activity, whereas dexamethasone does not bind to the mineralocorticoid receptor at all. Monitoring of fludrocortisone replacement includes measurement of seated and erect blood pressure to exclude postural hypotension caused by hypovolemia, as indicated by a systolic drop of 20 mm Hg or more when erect. Serum sodium and potassium levels should be monitored and plasma renin activity or concentration should be determined in regular intervals, aiming at values within the upper normal reference range.[30]

### Prevention and Management of Adrenal Crisis

Adrenal crisis is life threatening and may present with severe hypotension or even hypovolemic shock, abdominal pain and tension, fever, and—in some cases—even coma. The risk of adrenal crisis has been reported as varying between 3.3 crises requiring hospital admission per 100 years (53 patients, 511 replacement years)[19] and 6.8 crises requiring emergency glucocorticoid administration per 100 years (440 patients, 6092 patient years).[31] In both series, patients who had primary adrenal insufficiency were at slightly higher risk of suffering an adrenal crisis.[19,31] In a UK-wide survey of 982 patients, 74 of 178 respondents reported that they required hospital treatment with administration of emergency glucocorticoid doses and intravenous fluids.[32] Patients older than age 60 seem to be at higher risk of adrenal crisis.[33] In 45%[31] to 60%[32] of cases, the adrenal crisis was triggered by an acute, mostly gastrointestinal infection. One of the most important factors is failure to increase the glucocorticoid dose in case of illness.[19]

The most important component of crisis prevention is "sick day rules" training for the patient and partners (or parents). This training should be repeated during all outpatient reviews, including review and updating of steroid emergency cards and emergency bracelets. The Addison Self Help Group UK (www.addisons.org.uk) and the Pituitary Foundation UK (www.pituitary.org.uk) distributed patient information leaflets on the emergency administration of hydrocortisone and requirements for stress-related glucocorticoid dose adjustments. Ideally, patients should have a hydrocortisone emergency self-injection kit (eg, 100 mg Solu-Cortef) for intramuscular self-injection in case of an emergency, particularly if they have restricted access to acute medical care (eg, live in isolated or rural areas) or travel to other countries.

Intercurrent illness, such as respiratory infection associated with fever, requires doubling of the daily glucocorticoid dose until recovery. In the event of vomiting or diarrhea, the hydrocortisone dose should be doubled; if the medication is vomited, glucocorticoids should be administered parenterally. For major stress events, such as surgery, trauma, or childbirth, 100 to 200 mg hydrocortisone should be administered over 24 hours. For acute adrenal crisis, an immediate intravenous bolus injection of 100 mg hydrocortisone should be followed by 100 to 200 mg/hydrocortisone over 24 hours, preferably as continuous infusion in glucose 5%, accompanied by infusion of physiologic saline at the initial rate of 1 L/h under cardiac monitoring conditions.

Various routes of administration and doses of hydrocortisone between 100 and 400 mg daily are currently being recommended for major stress events. Reliable studies that address the pharmacokinetics of hydrocortisone under these circumstances and compare it to cortisol levels found in control patients without adrenal insufficiency are lacking. Current recommendations are empirically pragmatic rather than evidence based. The seminal observation that adrenal insufficiency requires increased doses of glucocorticoids during surgical stress was first made in the early 1950s, as reported by Nicholas and colleagues.[34] That report included the description of the famous patient 3, John F. Kennedy, who survived sacroiliac fusion surgery because of increased preoperative glucocorticoid doses.

Using a fluorimetric method to estimate plasma cortisol levels, Plumpton and colleagues[35] reported cortisol levels around 600 nmol/L (normal morning levels) during minor surgery and levels of 1200 nmol/L during major surgery. In a series of 181 patients with septic shock, median cortisol levels of 1284 nmol/L (interquartile range 820–2016 nmol/L) have been reported.[36] Limited pharmacokinetic data suggest that the injection of 25 mg hydrocortisone yields values of approximately 400 nmol/L[17], whereas the infusion of 10 mg hydrocortisone per hour (240 mg/24 h) yields serum cortisol levels ranging between 2800 and 5400 nmol/L,[37] which are five times above levels measured in patients who have septic shock. Thorough studies of the pharmacokinetics of hydrocortisone using different doses and different modes of administration are urgently needed.

## QUALITY OF LIFE, DISABILITY, AND MORTALITY ISSUES

Recent data demonstrated that the current standard therapy of glucocorticoid and mineralocorticoid replacement fails to restore quality of life in patients who have adrenal insufficiency. Predominant complaints are fatigue, lack of energy, depression, anxiety, and reduced ability to cope with daily demands. Many female patients complain about reduced libido. In the Netherlands, a study showed that 50% of patients ($n = 91$) who had Addison's disease considered themselves unfit to work and 30% needed household help. A Norwegian study showed reduced health perception and vitality in patients who had Addison's disease and were receiving conventional treatment with cortisone acetate and mineralocorticoids.[4] The same survey in Norway also revealed that the proportion of patients ($n = 88$) receiving disability pensions was two to three times higher compared with the general population.

Thomsen and colleagues[38] investigated 989 patients who had chronic adrenal insufficiency and found a higher rate of affective and depressive disorders compared with a control group with osteoarthritis. Recently, Hahner and colleagues[5] revealed impaired subjective health status in 256 patients who had adrenal insufficiency on standard therapy. Theirs was the first study to demonstrate that this finding applies similarly to patients with primary and secondary adrenal insufficiency. The same study also demonstrated that the impairment of health-related quality of life remains valid when analyzing patients without any comorbidity. The impairment is most pronounced in younger patients, but patients of all age groups differ significantly from sex- and age-matched controls. Overall, the adverse impact of chronic adrenal insufficiency on health-related quality of life is substantial and comparable to that of congestive heart failure, diabetic foot ulcer, or chronic hemodialysis.[4,5] A large, population-based cohort study from Sweden ($n = 1675$) demonstrated that patients who have primary adrenal insufficiency have a higher mortality rate because of a higher prevalence of cardiovascular, respiratory, and infectious disease,[3] even after correcting for the influence of any comorbidity. These data undoubtedly demonstrate that current replacement strategies in adrenal insufficiency require further optimization.

## Dehydroepiandrosterone Replacement

The introduction of DHEA replacement represents a substantial advance in replacement therapy for adrenal insufficiency. Although glucocorticoids and mineralocorticoids are routinely replaced, the third major steroid produced by the adrenal gland, DHEA, has not been generally considered worthy of replacement. Adrenal DHEA production is the major androgen source in women, and DHEA deficiency results in significant androgen deficiency in affected female patients,[8,39] which is likely to impact energy levels, particularly libido.[40] Arlt and colleagues[8] were the first to demonstrate that DHEA replacement in women with adrenal insufficiency results in significant improvements in mood, quality of life, and libido. Their finding was confirmed by subsequent studies in women with hypopituitarism[11] and male and female patients with primary adrenal insufficiency.[9,10] The effects of DHEA beyond its impact on mood, well-being, and libido remain the subject of current investigations.

Coles and colleagues[41] demonstrated that the number of circulating regulatory T cells in patients who have Addison's disease are decreased at baseline and can be restored to the levels of healthy controls after 12 weeks of oral DHEA replacement. No data on the functional consequences of DHEA deficiency on immune function in adrenal insufficiency patients have been published, however. A recent study in 106 patients (44 men, 62 women) who have Addison's disease indicated positive effects of long-term DHEA replacement.[9] In that trial, patients were randomized to 50 mg daily micronized DHEA or placebo for 12 months. Use of DHEA led to enhanced total body and truncal lean mass, although no change in fat mass was observed. Use of DHEA also reversed loss of bone mineral density at the femoral neck but not at other sites. Compared with baseline data, psychological well-being measured via SF-36 improved significantly during DHEA replacement; however, no effect on fatigue or cognitive or sexual function was observed.

Currently, no licensed preparation of DHEA is available, and the US Food and Drug Administration considers it a food supplement rather than a bioactive drug. DHEA replacement is still hampered by the lack of formulations produced according to Good Pharmaceutical Practice, and a study that analyzed several over-the-counter preparations that claimed to contain 25 mg of DHEA demonstrated actual DHEA concentrations between 0 and 140 mg per 25-mg tablet.[42]

Currently, replacement doses of 25 to 50 mg once daily are recommended, and replacement should be reserved for patients who complain about significantly impaired well-being (and impaired libido in women) despite optimized conventional corticosteroid replacement. Replacement should be monitored by measuring trough serum DHEA levels, androstenedione, and— in women—testosterone and sex hormone binding globulin levels 24 hours after the ingestion of the preceding morning dose. Treatment should aim at levels around the middle normal range for healthy subjects.

Recently, Miller and colleagues[13,14] investigated the effect of physiologic testosterone replacement over a period of 1 year in premenopausal women with androgen deficiency caused by hypopituitarism ($n = 51$) in a randomized, placebo-controlled study. They observed a positive effect of testosterone on bone density, body composition, and neurobehavioral function.[13] Their data suggested no increase in cardiovascular risk markers and a trend toward lower insulin resistance after 1 year of 300 μg testosterone replacement.[14]

## FUTURE PERSPECTIVE: LONG-ACTING HYDROCORTISONE PREPARATIONS

Quality of life is still reduced even when full replacement therapy of glucocorticoids and mineralocorticoids is optimized with the addition of the DHEA.[5] Hahner and colleagues[5] demonstrated that the higher the glucocorticoid replacement dose, the more severely impaired is quality of life, which most likely reflects the desperate attempts of a caring physician to improve the situation by successive increases in the glucocorticoid dose. No currently available glucocorticoid preparation can reproduce the nocturnal rise in cortisol seen in the physiologic circadian rhythm. This is particularly important with regard to the diurnal variability in glucocorticoid sensitivity. Plat and colleagues[43] demonstrated that the evening administration of a hydrocortisone dose elicits a significantly higher increase in insulin and glucose than a similar morning dose, which suggests that glucocorticoids administered at nighttime have a much more unfavorable metabolic effect than a morning dose. High levels of glucocorticoids disrupt sleep, as shown by the physiologic peak of serum cortisol just before awakening, so late evening hydrocortisone administration should be avoided. A substantial number of patients with chronic adrenal insufficiency suffer from sleep disturbances, which lead to increased early morning fatigue and daytime fatigue.[4,44]

A promising future approach for optimization of replacement therapy in adrenal insufficiency includes modified release formulations of hydrocortisone that permit an oral delayed- and sustained-release of hydrocortisone, thereby closely mimicking the physiologic, diurnal rhythm. Merza and colleagues[45] and Lovas and Husebye[46] demonstrated that variable intravenous infusions of hydrocortisone delivered by a programmable pump allow the reproduction of normal physiologic and circadian levels of cortisol in patients who have adrenal insufficiency. Because this form of therapy is complex and inconvenient, the group of R.J.M. Ross had the goal of designing an oral formulation of hydrocortisone that seems to be able to mimic overnight physiologic levels of cortisol.[47] In a recent first proof-of-principle study in dexamethasone-suppressed healthy volunteers ($n = 11$), the new oral delayed- and sustained-release preparation of hydrocortisone was able to mimic normal circadian rhythm of circulating cortisol.[47] This finding provides a promising perspective for the treatment of patients with adrenal insufficiency because it may provide the basis for physiologic circadian replacement therapy with replication of normal nighttime rise in serum cortisol. This approach lends itself particularly to patients with congenital adrenal hyperplasia, in whom the lack of early morning rise in serum cortisol is particularly detrimental because it elicits increased ACTH drive on adrenal androgen production. Phase II and III studies in patients who have adrenal insufficiency and congenital adrenal hyperplasia with at least two of these new preparations are currently underway. Results are eagerly awaited.

## REFERENCES

1. Addison T. On the constitutional and local effects of diseases of the supra-renal capsules. London: Warrren and Son; 1855.
2. Tomlinson JW, Holden N, Hills RK, et al. Association between premature mortality and hypopituitarism: West Midlands Prospective Hypopituitary Study Group. Lancet 2001;357(9254):425–31.
3. Bergthorsdottir R, Leonsson-Zachrisson M, Oden A, et al. Premature mortality in patients with Addison's disease: a population-based study. J Clin Endocrinol Metab 2006;91(12):4849–53.
4. Lovas K, Loge JH, Husebye ES. Subjective health status in Norwegian patients with Addison's disease. Clin Endocrinol (Oxf) 2002;56(5):581–8.

5. Hahner S, Loeffler M, Fassnacht M, et al. Impaired subjective health status in 256 patients with adrenal insufficiency on standard therapy based on cross-sectional analysis. J Clin Endocrinol Metab 2007;92(10):3912–22.

6. Zelissen PM, Bast EJ, Croughs RJ. Associated autoimmunity in Addison's disease. J Autoimmun 1995;8(1):121–30.

7. Zelissen PM, Croughs RJ, van Rijk PP, et al. Effect of glucocorticoid replacement therapy on bone mineral density in patients with Addison disease. Ann Intern Med 1994;120(3):207–10.

8. Arlt W, Callies F, van Vlijmen JC, et al. Dehydroepiandrosterone replacement in women with adrenal insufficiency. N Engl J Med 1999;341(14):1013–20.

9. Gurnell EM, Hunt PJ, Curran SE, et al. Long-term DHEA replacement in primary adrenal insufficiency: a randomized, controlled trial. J Clin Endocrinol Metab 2008;93(2):400–9.

10. Hunt PJ, Gurnell EM, Huppert FA, et al. Improvement in mood and fatigue after dehydroepiandrosterone replacement in Addison's disease in a randomized, double blind trial. J Clin Endocrinol Metab 2000;85(12):4650–6.

11. Johannsson G, Burman P, Wiren L, et al. Low dose dehydroepiandrosterone affects behavior in hypopituitary androgen-deficient women: a placebo-controlled trial. J Clin Endocrinol Metab 2002;87(5):2046–52.

12. Brooke AM, Kalingag LA, Miraki-Moud F, et al. Dehydroepiandrosterone improves psychological well-being in male and female hypopituitary patients on maintenance growth hormone replacement. J Clin Endocrinol Metab 2006;91(10):3773–9.

13. Miller KK, Biller BM, Beauregard C, et al. Effects of testosterone replacement in androgen-deficient women with hypopituitarism: a randomized, double-blind, placebo-controlled study. J Clin Endocrinol Metab 2006;91(5):1683–90.

14. Miller KK, Biller BM, Schaub A, et al. Effects of testosterone therapy on cardiovascular risk markers in androgen-deficient women with hypopituitarism. J Clin Endocrinol Metab 2007;92(7):2474–9.

15. Esteban NV, Loughlin T, Yergey AL, et al. Daily cortisol production rate in man determined by stable isotope dilution/mass spectrometry. J Clin Endocrinol Metab 1991;72(1):39–45.

16. Kerrigan JR, Veldhuis JD, Leyo SA, et al. Estimation of daily cortisol production and clearance rates in normal pubertal males by deconvolution analysis. J Clin Endocrinol Metab 1993;76(6):1505–10.

17. Charmandari E, Johnston A, Brook CG, et al. Bioavailability of oral hydrocortisone in patients with congenital adrenal hyperplasia due to 21-hydroxylase deficiency. J Endocrinol 2001;169(1):65–70.

18. Mah PM, Jenkins RC, Rostami-Hodjegan A, et al. Weight-related dosing, timing and monitoring hydrocortisone replacement therapy in patients with adrenal insufficiency. Clin Endocrinol (Oxf) 2004;61(3):367–75.

19. Arlt W, Allolio B. Adrenal insufficiency. Lancet 2003;361(9372):1881–93.

20. Groves RW, Toms GC, Houghton BJ, et al. Corticosteroid replacement therapy: twice or thrice daily? J R Soc Med 1988;81(9):514–6.

21. Riedel M, Wiese A, Schurmeyer TH, et al. Quality of life in patients with Addison's disease: effects of different cortisol replacement modes. Exp Clin Endocrinol 1993;101(2):106–11.

22. Braatvedt GD, Joyce M, Evans M, et al. Bone mineral density in patients with treated Addison's disease. Osteoporos Int 1999;10(6):435–40.

23. Arlt W, Rosenthal C, Hahner S, et al. Quality of glucocorticoid replacement in adrenal insufficiency: clinical assessment vs. timed serum cortisol measurements. Clin Endocrinol (Oxf) 2006;64(4):384–9.

24. Allolio B, Winkelmann W, Fricke U, et al. [Cortisol plasma concentration in patients with primary adrenal cortex insufficiency during substitution therapy with cortisone acetate]. Verh Dtsch Ges Inn Med 1978;84:1456–8.
25. Feek CM, Ratcliffe JG, Seth J, et al. Patterns of plasma cortisol and ACTH concentrations in patients with Addison's disease treated with conventional corticosteroid replacement. Clin Endocrinol (Oxf) 1981;14(5):451–8.
26. Scott RS, Donald RA, Espiner EA. Plasma ACTH and cortisol profiles in Addisonian patients receiving conventional substitution therapy. Clin Endocrinol (Oxf) 1978;9(6):571–6.
27. Allolio B, Kaulen DUD, Hipp FX, et al. Comparison between hydrocortisone and cortisone acetate as replacement therapy in adrenocortical insufficiency. Akt Endokr Stoffw 1985;6:35–9.
28. Burch WM. Urine free-cortisol determination: a useful tool in the management of chronic hypoadrenal states. JAMA 1982;247(14):2002–4.
29. Howlett TA. An assessment of optimal hydrocortisone replacement therapy. Clin Endocrinol (Oxf) 1997;46(3):263–8.
30. Oelkers W, Diederich S, Bahr V. Diagnosis and therapy surveillance in Addison's disease: rapid adrenocorticotropin (ACTH) test and measurement of plasma ACTH, renin activity, and aldosterone. J Clin Endocrinol Metab 1992;75(1):259–64.
31. Hahner S, Löffler M, Bleicken B, et al. Adrenal crisis in primary and secondary adrenal insufficiency: frequency and causes. Endocrine Abstracts 2008;16:55.
32. White K, Wass J, Elliott A, et al. Adrenal emergency is a regular event for treated Addison's patients. Endocrine Abstracts 2008;15:308.
33. Flemming TG, Kristensen LO. Quality of self-care in patients on replacement therapy with hydrocortisone. J Intern Med 1999;246(5):497–501.
34. Nicholas JA, Burstein CL, Umberger CJ, et al. Management of adrenocortical insufficiency during surgery. AMA Arch Surg 1955;71(5):737–42.
35. Plumpton FS, Besser GM. The adrenocortical response to surgery and insulin-induced hypoglycaemia in corticosteroid-treated and normal subjects. Br J Surg 1969;56(3):216–9.
36. Arlt W, Hammer F, Sanning P, et al. Dissociation of serum dehydroepiandrosterone and dehydroepiandrosterone sulfate in septic shock. J Clin Endocrinol Metab 2006;91(7):2548–54.
37. Oppert M, Reinicke A, Graf KJ, et al. Plasma cortisol levels before and during "low-dose" hydrocortisone therapy and their relationship to hemodynamic improvement in patients with septic shock. Intensive Care Med 2000;26(12):1747–55.
38. Thomsen AF, Kvist TK, Andersen PK, et al. The risk of affective disorders in patients with adrenocortical insufficiency. Psychoneuroendocrinology 2006;31(5):614–22.
39. Miller KK, Biller BM, Hier J, et al. Androgens and bone density in women with hypopituitarism. J Clin Endocrinol Metab 2002;87(6):2770–6.
40. Arlt W. Androgen therapy in women. Eur J Endocrinol 2006;154(1):1–11.
41. Coles AJ, Thompson S, Cox AL, et al. Dehydroepiandrosterone replacement in patients with Addison's disease has a bimodal effect on regulatory (CD4 + CD25hi and CD4 + FoxP3+) T cells. Eur J Immunol 2005;35(12):3694–703.
42. Parasrampuria J, Schwartz K, Petesch R. Quality control of dehydroepiandrosterone dietary supplement products. JAMA 1998;280(18):1565.
43. Plat L, Leproult R, L'Hermite-Baleriaux M, et al. Metabolic effects of short-term elevations of plasma cortisol are more pronounced in the evening than in the morning. J Clin Endocrinol Metab 1999;84(9):3082–92.

44. Lovas K, Husebye ES, Holsten F, et al. Sleep disturbances in patients with Addison's disease. Eur J Endocrinol 2003;148(4):449–56.

45. Merza Z, Rostami-Hodjegan A, Memmott A, et al. Circadian hydrocortisone infusions in patients with adrenal insufficiency and congenital adrenal hyperplasia. Clin Endocrinol (Oxf) 2006;65(1):45–50.

46. Lovas K, Husebye ES. Continuous subcutaneous hydrocortisone infusion in Addison's disease. Eur J Endocrinol 2007;157(1):109–12.

47. Newell-Price J, Whiteman M, Rostami-Hodjegan A, et al. Modified-release hydrocortisone for circadian therapy: a proof-of-principle study in dexamethasone-suppressed normal volunteers. Clin Endocrinol (Oxf) 2008;68(1):130–5.

# Diagnosis and Management of Polyendocrinopathy Syndromes

Catherine J. Owen, MBBS, MRCP, MRCPCH, PhD*,
Tim D. Cheetham, MB, ChB, MD, MRCP, MRCPCH

---

**KEYWORDS**

• APS2 • APS1 • IPEX

---

The autoimmune polyendocrinopathy syndromes (APS) encompass a wide clinical spectrum of disease with monogenic and complex genetic etiologies. Their presentation is highly variable with the first manifestation occurring anywhere between infancy and late adult life. The commonest group of disorders seen, APS2 and its associated disorders, generally present in adulthood (**Table 1**) and are of complex genetic etiology. The rarer monogenic disorders, APS1 (see **Table 1**) and IPEX, tend to present in childhood or adolescence. In this article, we review the presentation, investigation, and management of these varied conditions.

## AUTOIMMUNE POLYGLANDULAR SYNDROME TYPE 2 AND ASSOCIATED DISORDERS
### APS 2

APS2 is defined by the presence of primary adrenocortical insufficiency with either autoimmune thyroid disease or type 1 diabetes in the same individual. An autoimmune origin of all the major components is necessary for the correct diagnosis of APS2. The association of autoimmune Addison's disease and autoimmune thyroid disease is known as Schmidt syndrome, and the association of Addison's disease with type 1 diabetes is also called Carpenter syndrome. Other endocrine and nonendocrine autoimmune disorders occur with increased frequency in these individuals and their families.[1]

### Clinical features and course

APS2 is rare, with an estimated prevalence of 4 to 5/100,000.[2,3] Clinical presentation can be at any age but is most frequently in early adulthood, with a peak onset in the fourth decade. It affects both sexes, with a female–male ratio of 3:1.[2]

---

Institute of Human Genetics, University of Newcastle, Newcastle upon Tyne, NE1 3BZ, UK
* Corresponding author.
E-mail address: c.j.owen@ncl.ac.uk (C. J. Owen).

Endocrinol Metab Clin N Am 38 (2009) 419–436
doi:10.1016/j.ecl.2009.01.007
0889-8529/09/$ – see front matter © 2009 Elsevier Inc. All rights reserved.

endo.theclinics.com

**Table 1**
**Comparison of the features of APS1 versus APS2**

|  | APS1 | APS2 |
|---|---|---|
| Commonest age of onset | Childhood, 4–10 years | Adults, 16–40 years |
| Female:male ratio | ~1:1 | ~3:1 |
| Main manifestations | Hypoparathyroidism<br>Candidiasis<br>Addison's disease | Addison's disease<br>Hypothyroidism<br>Type 1 diabetes |
| Prevalence | Rare, 3/million | Commoner, 1 in 15,000 |
| Genetics | Autosomal recessive; *AIRE* gene | Complex; *HLA, CTLA4, PTPN22,* others |

## Major manifestations

By definition, Addison's disease is present in 100% of APS2 cases. Autoimmune thyroid disease occurs in 70% to 90% and type 1 diabetes in 20% to 50%.[1,4–6] Only about 10% have the complete triad.[4,6] Adrenal failure is the first endocrine abnormality in around 50%; however, type 1 diabetes already exists in around 20% and autoimmune thyroid disease in around 30%. Autoimmune thyroid disease encompasses a variety of thyroid disorders, including Hashimoto's thyroiditis, atrophic hypothyroidism, and less commonly Graves' disease and postpartum thyroiditis.

Delayed diagnosis and preventable deaths still occur in patients with undiagnosed adrenal failure. Signs and symptoms are often vague and nonspecific until an adrenal crisis ensues. Low morning serum cortisol concentrations and electrolyte abnormalities (hyponatremia and hyperkalemia) represent late changes, occurring at or just before the onset of clinical adrenal insufficiency. Hyperpigmentation may be observed and be a telltale feature.

In those who already have type 1 diabetes, deterioration of glycemic control with recurrent hypoglycemia and a decrease in total insulin requirements can be the presenting sign. The onset of autoimmune hyperthyroidism or thyroxine replacement for newly diagnosed hypothyroidism leads to enhanced cortisol clearance and can precipitate adrenal crisis in subjects with subclinical adrenocortical failure.[7] Clinicians should maintain a high degree of alertness for underlying adrenal failure before initiating thyroid hormone replacement. Conversely, cortisol inhibits thyrotrophin release, so thyroid-stimulating hormone (TSH) levels are often high at the initial diagnosis of adrenal insufficiency (typically 5–10 mU/L) but return to normal after initiation of glucocorticoid replacement in the absence of coexistent thyroid disease. An increasingly recognized component of APS2 is latent autoimmune diabetes in adults – LADA. By definition this is diabetes developing in adulthood with the presence of diabetes-associated autoantibodies but with relatively well-preserved islet cell function.[8] Thus, the clinician needs to remain vigilant for the development of other autoimmune conditions regardless of the age of the patient.

## Minor manifestations

Minor manifestations are listed in **Table 2** together with their frequency. Primary hypogonadism is one of the commonest minor manifestations in APS2 females, with premature ovarian failure leading to secondary amenorrhea in around 10% of women younger than 40 years. Testicular failure is rare in APS2.[9] Pituitary involvement is occasionally seen with lymphocytic hypophysitis leading to empty sella syndrome, panhypopituitarism, or isolated failure of any of the anterior pituitary hormones.[10]

**Table 2**
**Minor manifestations frequently associated with APS2**

|  | Frequency, % |
|---|---|
| Minor manifestation |  |
| Pernicious anemia | 1–25 |
| Gonadal failure |  |
|   Females | 3.5–10 |
|   Males | 1–2 |
| Vitiligo | 4–12 |
| Alopecia | 2–5 |
| Autoimmune hepatitis | 4 |
| Malabsorption (including celiac disease) | 1–2 |
| Sjögren syndrome | 1 |
| Neoplasias | 3 |
| Rarer manifestations |  |
| *Endocrine* | *Neurological* |
| Pituitary involvement | Myositis |
| Hypophysitis | Myasthenia gravis |
| Empty sella syndrome | Neuropathy |
| Late-onset hypoparathyroidism | Stiff man syndrome |
| *Gastrointestinal* | *Other* |
| Ulcerative colitis | Sarcoidosis |
| Primary biliary cirrhosis | Serositis |
| *Dermatological* | Selective IgA deficiency |
| Granuloma annulare | Idiopathic heart block |
| Dermatitis herpetiformis | Idiopathic thrombocytopenia purpura |

*Data from* Refs. [9,40,41,44.]

In contrast to APS1, hypoparathyroidism is rare in APS2 (or APS3). If hypocalcemia does occur then celiac disease is the most likely reason, and the finding of an elevated parathyroid hormone (PTH) concentration in the latter will distinguish between the two.

### Incomplete APS2
Patients with autoimmune thyroid disease or type 1 diabetes and adrenal autoantibodies in the serum or patients with Addison's disease and either thyroid and/or islet cell autoantibodies are sometimes classified as incomplete APS2.[4] Self-evidently, these patients may develop APS2 in the future, particularly those with evidence of subclinical disease such as an elevated TSH or impaired glucose tolerance. About 30% of subjects with positive adrenal antibodies progress to adrenal failure over a 6-year period.[11]

### APS3

APS3 is defined as the association between autoimmune thyroid disease and an additional autoimmune disease other than Addison's disease.[4] Some authors use the term APS4 to encompass an association of autoimmune diseases not falling into the categories APS1 to 3.[4] This includes an extremely heterogeneous group of patients and it is generally more helpful to describe the individual components. Hashimoto's thyroiditis is the commonest form of autoimmune thyroid disease seen in APS3, although

Graves' disease and postpartum thyroiditis are also seen. Autoimmune thyroid disease is most commonly isolated, and polyglandular involvement in the form of APS3 or APS2 is rare (about 5%). Only 1% of patients with isolated autoimmune thyroid disease have adrenal autoantibodies (with risk of APS2), whereas 3% to 5% have evidence of pancreatic islet autoimmunity and/or clinical type 1 diabetes.[12]

Autoimmune thyroid disease is more commonly associated with pernicious anemia, vitiligo, alopecia, myasthenia gravis, and Sjögren syndrome, and autoimmune thyroid disease should be sought prospectively in patients with these conditions. Around 30% of subjects with vitiligo have another autoimmune disorder, with autoimmune thyroid disease and pernicious anemia being the most common. Many patients with vitiligo are asymptomatic, and other autoimmune diseases are diagnosed only by prospective screening, including evaluation of autoantibody status.[9,13] Up to 15% of patients with alopecia and nearly 30% of those with myasthenia gravis have autoimmune thyroid disease.

### Genetics

APS2 is a genetically complex and multifactorial disease. It clusters in families and appears to show an autosomal-dominant pattern of inheritance with incomplete penetrance in some.[14] Susceptibility is determined by multiple genetic loci that interact with environmental factors. Only three genes have shown consistent association with APS2: *HLA, CTLA4,* and *PTPN22.* Of these, *HLA* appears to have the strongest gene effect.[1]

Many of the component disorders in APS2, including autoimmune thyroid disease, type 1 diabetes, Addison's disease, celiac disease, myasthenia gravis, selective IgA deficiency, and dermatitis herpetiformis, are associated with the same extended *HLA* haplotype: *HLA-A1, HLA-B8, HLA DR3, DQA1\*0501, DQB1\*0201 (DQ2).* Thus, unsurprisingly, *HLA DR3, DQB1\*0201* is associated with APS2.[4,15] Other HLA haplotype associations include *HLA DR4* with type 1 diabetes and, to a lesser extent, Addison's disease and *HLA DR5* in patients with a combination of Addison's disease and autoimmune hypothyroidism.[4] Other *HLA* haplotypes appear to be protective such as the *DR2 (DRB1\*1501), DQA1\*0102, DQB1\*0602* haplotype, which appears to provide dominant protection against type 1 diabetes, even in the presence of insulin autoantibodies.[14]

*CTLA4* encodes an important negative regulator of T-cell activation that is expressed on the surface of activated T lymphocytes. Alleles of *CTLA4* have been linked primarily to autoimmune thyroid disease, both Graves' disease and Hashimoto thyroiditis,[16,17] but there is also an effect in type 1 diabetes.[18,19] Less consistent association has been shown in Addison's disease (either isolated or as part of APS2).[18,20]

The *PTPN22* gene encodes lymphoid tyrosine phosphatase (LYP), which plays a key role in early T-cell activation. Association with a functionally significant tryptophan for arginine variant in LYP has been found in a mixed UK cohort of AAD and APS2 subjects[21] and in Norwegian subjects.[22] A recent meta-analysis looking at results from five different European regions, including a German AAD cohort where association was not found, showed that overall there was a significant effect of PTPN22 in AAD.[23]

The association of the component disorders in APS2 is, therefore, in part related to the shared susceptibility alleles of *HLA, CTLA4,* and *PTPN22* conferring risk to the different diseases. It is also likely that there is a complex interaction between these variants, *CYP27B1* (see article by Husebye and Lovas elsewhere in this issue), and other as yet unidentified loci and environmental factors.

## Autoantibodies and Pathogenesis

There are several hypotheses to explain why autoimmunity occurs against multiple organs in individuals with APS. It has been suggested that this may result from a shared epitope(s) between an environmental agent and a common antigen present in several endocrine tissues.[24] More likely, there is a subtle thymic defect of negative selection of autoreactive T cells, caused either by a defect in T-cell apoptosis or by a problem in presentation of self-antigens. Defects in $CD4^+CD25^+$ regulatory T-cell suppressor function[25] and impaired caspase-3 expression by peripheral T cells[26] have also been demonstrated. Thus, loss of peripheral suppression and/or defective peripheral apoptosis could be involved in the pathogenesis of this syndrome.[25,26]

At the onset of autoimmune adrenal failure, anti- 21-hydroxylase (21-OH; anti-P450c21) autoantibodies are detectable in more than 90% of patients with APS2,[3,4] declining to 60% with disease duration over 15 years. These 21-OH autoantibodies are highly specific, being found in only 0.5% of healthy subjects and those with other autoimmune diseases. Some 40% to 50% of patients with such adrenal autoantibodies have abnormal ACTH stimulation tests. Thus, 21-OH autoantibodies have a high predictive value for clinical Addison's disease.[3]

Other steroid-producing cell autoantibodies (SCA), such as those directed against 17$\alpha$-hydroxylase and cholesterol side-chain cleavage enzyme, are present in 20% to 30% of patients with Addison's disease and are more frequent in females than males.[3,27] There is a strong association between the presence of these SCA and ovarian failure in women with APS2/3, but SCA are extremely rare in women with ovarian failure with no signs of adrenal autoimmunity.[3,27]

Autoimmune thyroid disease and type 1 diabetes are frequent components of APS2. In Hashimoto's thyroiditis, thyroid peroxidase autoantibodies are found in 90% to 100% and thyroglobulin autoantibodies in 60% to 70%. They are both also frequently found in Graves' disease, where TSH receptor autoantibodies are found in more than 90% of cases.[9] Many patients with thyroid autoantibodies but normal TSH progress very slowly to clinical disease (about 5% yearly).[28]

Islet cell autoantibodies are found in around 80% of new-onset type 1 diabetes patients.[3] The main islet autoantigens are insulin, GAD65, and the tyrosine phosphatase-related protein IA-2. Among recently diagnosed subjects with type 1 diabetes, the prevalence of antibodies to insulin and IA-2 is dependent on age, being most frequent in children and adolescents with type 1 diabetes, but less than 30% with adult onset or LADA.[8] The frequency of antibodies to GAD65 is 70% to 80% and is not influenced by age; this therefore gives the highest diagnostic sensitivity in LADA.[8,29]

## Diagnosis and Follow-up

Once APS2/3 is suspected, a full assessment of endocrine function is needed. The number of disorders that will develop and the age at which they will present is unpredictable, so long-term follow-up is needed. Presymptomatic recognition of autoimmune disease minimizes associated morbidity and mortality. There is a clear link between the presence of organ-specific autoantibodies and the progression to disease, although there is often an asymptomatic latent period of months or years.

An autoimmune etiology should be sought in all subjects, but the presence of autoimmune disorders in family members is suggestive. In all patients with Addison's disease, there is a need to screen for other endocrine disorders, particularly autoimmune thyroid disease and type 1 diabetes. At diagnosis, screening for TPO and GAD65 autoantibodies is worthwhile. If negative, this should be repeated occasionally, perhaps every 2 to 3 years.

The determination of thyroid function should be carried out at least annually for early recognition of thyroid disease in all subjects with type 1 diabetes and Addison's disease. The determination of 17α-hydroxylase and cholesterol side-chain cleavage enzyme antibodies in females with Addison's disease and APS2 may identify subjects at high risk from primary hypogonadism before gonadotropins become elevated. Such subjects may be suitable for cryopreservation of ovarian material.

The determination of 21-OH autoantibodies should be performed in children presenting with type 1 diabetes, as positive adrenal autoantibodies are highly predictive of future adrenal insufficiency.[3] In subjects with 21-OH autoantibodies, an ACTH stimulation test, determination of electrolytes, and plasma renin activity enables identification of patients with preclinical adrenal dysfunction. If normal, the ACTH stimulation test should be repeated yearly with interval determination of postural blood pressure and electrolytes.

Screening for APS2-associated disorders should also be performed in women with primary or secondary amenorrhea or premature ovarian failure and young patients with vitiligo. As APS2 shows strong familial tendencies, family members should also be checked for features of associated endocrine conditions.

### Management and Prognosis

Hormone replacement or other therapies for the component diseases of APS2 are similar whether the disease occurs in isolation or in association with other conditions, and disorders should be treated as they are diagnosed; however, certain combinations of diseases require specific attention. Thus, to avoid adrenal crisis, clinicians should maintain a high degree of suspicion for coexisting adrenal failure in subjects who are hypothyroid.[7] Hyperthyroidism increases cortisol clearance, so in patients with adrenal insufficiency who have unresolved hyperthyroidism, glucocorticoid replacement should be at least doubled until the patient is euthyroid. Decreasing insulin requirements or increasing occurrence of hypoglycemia in type 1 diabetes can be one of the earliest indications of adrenocortical failure. One of the most important aspects of managing these patients is to be continually alert to the possibility of the development of further endocrinopathies to ensure early diagnosis and treatment.

Mortality in patients with primary adrenal insufficiency is elevated approximately twofold compared with the background population.[30] Life expectancy is often reduced as a consequence of unrecognized adrenal crisis, but infectious disease, cardiovascular disease, and cancer also appear to be increased. Despite adequate hormonal replacement, quality of life is often impaired in these patients, with predominant complaints being unpredictable fatigue, lack of energy, depression, and anxiety (see article by Reisch and Arlt elsewhere in this issue). It has been shown that the number of patients receiving disability pensions is two- to threefold higher than the general population in certain countries.[31]

### Summary

A high index of suspicion needs to be maintained whenever one organ-specific autoimmune disorder is diagnosed in order to prevent morbidity and mortality from the index disease as well as associated diseases. Further definition of susceptibility genes and autoantigens, as well as a better understanding of the pathogenesis, is required to improve the diagnosis and management of these patients.

## AUTOIMMUNE POLYGLANDULAR SYNDROME TYPE I (APS1)
### Definition

APS1, known as the autoimmune polyendocrinopathy–candidiasis–ectodermal dystrophy syndrome (APECED), is a rare and frequently debilitating disorder of childhood. It is inherited as an autosomal-recessive condition and the female–male ratio is close to 1. The clinical diagnosis of APS1 classically requires the presence of two of the three cardinal components: chronic mucocutaneous candidiasis, autoimmune hypoparathyroidism, and autoimmune adrenal failure.[1,32–36] Only one of these manifestations is required if a sibling has the syndrome.[1] There is a spectrum of associated minor components, which include endocrine and nonendocrine manifestations.

Although a rare disorder in most countries (about two or three cases per million in the United Kingdom),[37] it shows a founder effect leading to a much higher prevalence in certain populations: Finns 1:25,000,[32] Iranian Jews 1:9000,[33] and Sardinians 1:14,500.[38] There are also differences in the phenotype between different populations: for example, chronic mucocutaneous candidiasis and adrenal failure are among the commonest manifestations in most patients of European descent but are present in only about 20% of Iranian Jews.[33,36]

### Clinical Features and Course

The first manifestation is typically mucocutaneous candidiasis, which develops in infancy or early childhood. Hypoparathyroidism characteristically develops around the age of 7 years and adrenocortical failure by the age of 13 years.[4,34,37] The complete evolution of the three cardinal features usually occurs in the first 20 years, with additional minor manifestations continuing to appear at least until the fifth decade.[1] Importantly, APS1 can present in other ways, either with one cardinal feature and several minor manifestations or with several minor manifestations and characteristic ectodermal dystrophy. This variability in the early clinical picture can make the diagnosis of APS1 challenging.

The cardinal triad occurs in around 60% of subjects, and the median number of disease components is four, with up to 10 manifestations in some subjects. Patients who present initially with adrenal insufficiency rather than candidiasis tend to develop fewer components than others.[32,36] It has also been reported that the earlier the first component presents, the more likely it is that multiple components will develop.[1,34] **Table 3** lists the cardinal and more common minor manifestations together with their frequency.

### Cardinal Manifestations

#### Chronic mucocutaneous candidiasis (CMC)
Chronic mucocutaneous candidiasis is commonly the first manifestation of the syndrome, occurring as early as 1 month of age, but more typically in the first 2 years of life, and it should alert the clinician to the possibility of APS1. It is the most frequently occurring cardinal manifestation, present in 73% to 100% of patients,[1,32,34–36] and is usually mild or intermittent and responds well to periodic systemic anticandidal treatment. Oral candidiasis is the commonest presentation, but esophagitis is also found, causing substernal pain and odynophagia. Infection of the intestinal mucosa leads to abdominal discomfort and diarrhea. Candidal infection can also affect the vaginal mucosa, nails, and skin.

#### Hypoparathyroidism
This is frequently the first endocrine feature of APS1,[1,32–36,39] with a peak incidence between 2 and 11 years of age. Hypoparathyroidism occurs in around 75% to

**Table 3**
**Frequencies of the major and main minor components of APS1**

| Disease | Frequency, % |
|---|---|
| *Main manifestations* | |
| Chronic mucocutaneous candidiasis | 72–100 |
| Autoimmune hypoparathyroidism | 76–93 |
| Autoimmune adrenal failure | 73–100 |
| *Common minor manifestations* | |
| Autoimmune endocrinopathies | |
|   Hypergonadotrophic hypogonadism | 17–69 |
|   Autoimmune thyroid disease | 4–31 |
|   Type 1 diabetes mellitus | 0–33 |
|   Pituitary defects | 7 |
| Gastrointestinal components | |
|   Pernicious anemia | 13–31 |
|   Malabsorption | 10–22 |
|   Cholelithiasis | 44 |
|   Chronic active hepatitis | 5–31 |
| Skin autoimmune diseases | |
|   Vitiligo | 8–31 |
|   Alopecia | 29–40 |
|   Urticarial-like erythema with fever | 15 |
| Ectodermal dysplasia | |
|   Nail dystrophy | 10–52 |
|   Dental enamel hypoplasia | 40–77 |
|   Tympanic membrane calcification | 33 |
| Other manifestations | |
|   Keratoconjunctivitis | 2–35 |
|   Hypo/Asplenia | 15–40 |

*Data from* European and North American patients.[32,33,35–37,41] Iranian Jews have distinctly different frequencies from the other populations and have been excluded.

95%,[1,4,32,34–36] although there appears to be a slightly reduced penetrance, and later age of onset, in males.[40,41] Hypoparathyroidism may be asymptomatic but presents typically with tetany and grand mal seizures. Presentation may be precipitated by factors such as fasting or low calcium or high phosphate intake. The diagnosis is confirmed by a low or undetectable PTH level in the presence of hypocalcemia. Hyperphosphatemia and hypomagnesemia are common, with low urinary calcium excretion.

### Adrenal failure
Autoimmune adrenal failure (Addison's disease) is typically the third of the cardinal manifestations to present in APS1, with a peak incidence around 13 years.[1,4,32–36] In most populations of APS1 patients, it occurs less frequently than the other major components (72% to 100%).[1,32,34–36] Destruction of the adrenal cortex may develop gradually, and deficiencies of cortisol and aldosterone can appear in either order up to 20 years apart.[36] Diagnosis of adrenal insufficiency is confirmed by a normal or low cortisol concentration with increased adrenocorticotrophic hormone (ACTH) and

a subnormal cortisol response to ACTH stimulation. Deficiency of aldosterone may be heralded by postural hypotension or salt craving, and is confirmed by a raised plasma renin activity even before the development of overt electrolyte disturbance.

## Minor Manifestations

### Autoimmune endocrinopathies
Primary hypogonadism is the commonest minor manifestation of APS1, occurring in 17% to 61% of cases.[1-4,36,42] It is almost invariably accompanied by adrenal failure. About half of APS1 females with hypogonadism present with primary amenorrhea, and the remainder have secondary amenorrhea. Male hypogonadism has been reported from puberty onward.[36] One male patient has been reported with azoospermia and possible antisperm autoimmunity.[36] Other autoimmune endocrinopathies are relatively infrequent and include type 1 diabetes mellitus and destructive autoimmune thyroid diseases (Hashimoto's thyroiditis or primary atrophic thyroiditis). Pituitary defects such as lymphocytic hypophysitis or autoimmune pituitary disease have occasionally been described ($\approx$ 5%) and can induce single or multiple hormonal defects.[4]

### Gastrointestinal components
Chronic atrophic gastritis affects up to a third of patients with APS1 and can lead to a megaloblastic anemia due to vitamin B12 deficiency (pernicious anemia) or a microcytic anemia because of iron deficiency.[1,4,32-36] It can be a characteristic feature of an early "atypical" presentation of APS1 in the first year of life, being an initial manifestation in around 10%. Malabsorption occurs in 10% to 22% of cases [1,4,32-36] and presents with periodic or chronic diarrhea, usually with steatorrhea, but may be associated with constipation. It can be a result of a variety of causes including villous atrophy, exocrine pancreatic insufficiency, intestinal infections (*Giardia lamblia* or *Candida*), defective bile acid reabsorption, intestinal lymphangiectasia, and autoimmune destruction of the enterochromaffin cells of the small intestine.[34,36,43,44] There is a strong association with the hypocalcemia of hypoparathyroidism, as hypocalcemia impairs the secretion of cholecystokinin leading to a failure of normal gall bladder contraction and pancreatic enzyme secretion. Cholelithiasis is present in up to 40% on ultrasonography,[4] but is usually asymptomatic. Chronic active hepatitis develops in 5% to 30% of cases.[1,4,32-36] The clinical course varies from chronic but asymptomatic in most cases to the development of cirrhosis or fulminant hepatic failure with a potentially fatal outcome.[1,45] It may present in early childhood and can be the first manifestation of APS1; however, the risk of hepatitis is low after adolescence.

### Skin autoimmune diseases
Vitiligo and alopecia are well recognized components that can appear at any age and are very variable in severity.[1,4,32-36] Recurrent urticaria with fever has been reported as an unusual manifestation in about 10% of patients during childhood.

## Other Manifestations

Ectodermal dystrophy affects the nails and tooth enamel (**Fig. 1**). The pitted nails are unrelated to candidal infection and can be an important clue to the diagnosis of APS1. Dental enamel hypoplasia has been reported in 40% to 75% of patients,[1,4,32-36] although deciduous teeth are never affected. Keratoconjunctivitis may be the first manifestation of APS1 in some cases, and incidence varies from 10% to 40% between reports.[1,4,32-36,39] The initial symptoms are intense photophobia, blepharospasm, and lacrimation; permanent visual impairment and even blindness is not infrequent.[36] Asplenia or hyposplenism has been documented by ultrasonography or suggested by hematological parameters in up to 15% of APS1 cases.[36] It may be congenital or

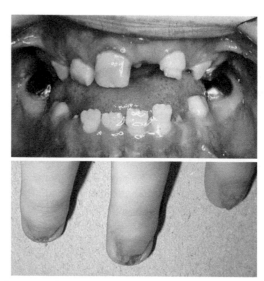

**Fig. 1.** Ectodermal features of APS1 illustrating the nail dystrophy and the dental enamel hypoplasia.

acquired, secondary to progressive autoimmune-mediated destruction or vascular insult to the spleen. It causes an additional secondary immunodeficiency, rendering subjects susceptible to pneumococcal sepsis.

Sudden death is well recognized in established APS1 patients, their siblings, and from postmortem studies of subjects in whom the diagnosis was not suspected.[32,35,37] It is presumed that these deaths are linked to undiagnosed adrenal failure, fulminant sepsis, or hypoparathyroidism.

### Genetics

The gene defective in APS1 was identified by positional cloning in 1997 and is located on chromosome 21q22.3. It is named the autoimmune regulator or *AIRE* gene.[46,47] *AIRE* encodes a putative nuclear protein, containing several motifs suggestive of a transcription factor. It is expressed in a variety of tissues of the immune system but particularly in the medullary epithelial antigen-presenting cells in the thymus, where it is thought to play an important role in the central induction of self-tolerance (see article by Shikama, Nusspaumer, and Hollander, elsewhere in this issue). The molecular mechanism by which the AIRE protein induces central tolerance is still unexplained, however it is thought to be involved in the negative selective of potentially autoreactive thymocytes by regulating expression of self-antigens in the antigen-presenting cells of the thymus.[35,48]

Over 60 different disease-causing mutations have now been described in the *AIRE* gene.[32,34,35,38,46,47,49,50] These include point mutations, insertions, and deletions, and are spread through the whole coding region of the gene. Mutations affecting splice sites have also been reported. The most frequent *AIRE* mutations include the founder Finnish mutation in exon 6 (R257X) [46,47] and the common northern European mutation in exon 8 (964del13).[50] This 13-base pair (bp) deletion is seen frequently in Norwegian patients and in whites from the United States and United Kingdom,[50] where it accounts for more than 70% of all mutant *AIRE* alleles. Additional common mutations are found in isolated populations such as a mutation in exon 3 (R139X) found in

Sardinians[38] and a mutation in exon 2 (Y85C) in the Iranian Jewish population.[32] In several instances, only one mutant allele of the *AIRE* gene has been reported in typical APS1 patients, suggesting that the second mutation might be located in the regulatory regions of the gene.

It is possible that the specific manifestations that develop in a particular APS1 patient may depend on alleles at other loci such as human leukocyte antigens (*HLA*), because the same *AIRE* mutations are associated with varying phenotypes and clinical course even among affected siblings.[41,51] No consistent associations between APS1 manifestations and *HLA* alleles have been found, and no association between HLA type and autoantibodies in APS1 patients is seen.[52] No correlation between cytotoxic T lymphocyte antigen 4 (*CTLA4*) gene polymorphisms and APS1 have been found to date[4]; however, a negative correlation has been shown between an insulin gene polymorphism and the development of T1D in these subjects.[53] The factors determining an individual phenotype are not understood, and it is likely that there are several modifier loci involved.

### Autoantibodies and Pathogenesis

The pathogenesis of many of the manifestations of APS1 is unclear, but autoimmunity is involved in the development of the endocrinopathies, and patients have circulating autoantibodies to a variety of antigens from other affected tissues. One recently identified autoantibody is directed against interferons, in particular interferon (IFN)-$\alpha$ and IFN-$\omega$, and has almost 100% prevalence in APS1 subjects, regardless of the clinical picture or mutation type.[54] These anti-interferon autoantibodies have been found to be present at a very early stage and persist, being present after over 30 years of disease. They have not been found in any subjects with isolated AAD or APS2, so appear to be disease specific.[51,54] This clearly provides an excellent tool to aid in the diagnosis of APS1 in the prodromal stage or in atypical cases, and suggests the intriguing possibility that these autoantibodies may modulate the expression of immune responses directly.

Steroid 21-hydroxylase (P450c21) and cholesterol side-chain cleavage enzyme (P450scc) are the major adrenal autoantigens,[55] and were found in 81% of APS1 patients with and in 21% of those without adrenal failure. The presence of antibodies for at least one of these three enzymes correlates significantly with gonadal failure in female but not male patients.[34,35]

Autoantibodies to the extracellular domain of the calcium-sensing receptor have been reported in idiopathic hypoparathyroidism including up to 86% of subjects with APS1 (see article by Brown elsewhere in this issue).[56,57] This has not been replicated in several other studies,[40,55] and the prognostic significance and pathophysiological role of these autoantibodies remains undetermined. In addition, antibodies against a novel parathyroid-specific antigen, NALP5, have recently been found in about half of APS1 patients with hypoparathyroidism.[58]

Glutamic acid decarboxylase (GAD)-65 autoantibodies have been found in 75% of patients with diabetes up to 8 years before the onset, but these are nonspecific and are also found in 40% of nondiabetic APS1 patients.[59] Antibodies against the IA-2 tyrosine phosphatase-like protein and insulin are less common in these patients but have higher specificity (96% to 100%).[40] Circulating antithyroid antibodies have been found to be a poor marker for predicting hypothyroidism in APS1.[34]

The main autoantigens for hepatitis in APS1 appear to be cytochrome P450 1A2 (CYP1A2), P450 2A6 (CYP2A6), and aromatic L-amino acid decarboxylase (AADC).[60] Tryptophan hydroxylase autoantibodies have also been found to be a sensitive predictor of autoimmune hepatitis in APS1.[55] Although a rise in antibody titers to liver antigens may predate biochemical evidence of liver disease, raised autoantibodies are not found in all APS1 patients with autoimmune hepatitis at biopsy.[45] Antiparietal cell and intrinsic factor autoantibodies precede parietal cell atrophy. Villous atrophy is associated with endomysial and/or tissue transglutaminase (TTG) autoantibodies.[34] Gastrointestinal dysfunction has been associated with autoantibodies to tryptophan hydroxylase (48% cases), histidine decarboxylase, and GAD-65.[55]

Measurement of autoantibodies may be of limited use in patients with APS1 in determining their risk of developing new components because the sensitivity of the antibody test may frequently be less than the patient's preexisting risk of the complication. There are, however, certain autoantibodies that are almost exclusive to APS1, particularly AADC, CYP1A2, tyrosine hydroxylase, tryptophan hydroxylase, IFN-$\alpha$, and IFN-$\omega$. This unique spectrum of autoantibodies can thus help to differentiate APS1 and other autoimmune diseases.[54,55]

## Diagnosis of APS1

Perheentupa[36] found the classic criteria (two out of three cardinal manifestations) to be fulfilled by 5 years of age in only 22.0% cases, by 10 years in 67.0%, by 20 years in 89.0%, and by 30 years in 93.5%. Suspicion should be high in patients younger than 30 years with mucocutaneous candidiasis, hypoparathyroidism, adrenal failure, ectodermal dystrophy, keratoconjunctivitis, prolonged diarrhea, vitiligo, or noninfectious hepatitis. Such patients should be checked for other manifestations, particularly the sometimes subtle nail signs of ectodermal dystrophy, or oral or ophthalmic components. DNA screening for *AIRE* mutations and an autoantibody screen should be considered in subjects with an atypical presentation.

There is often no direct clinical value in DNA analysis in subjects with two or more cardinal features, but the molecular findings in a proband will be of value in counseling and for screening siblings. All patients with established APS1 and those with one or more suspicious features need close follow-up for the development of new components. Their siblings should also be examined, as one of the cardinal manifestations or a definite ectodermal component is diagnostic.

Diagnosis is often delayed, perhaps because of the long interval between development of the first and second manifestation. Up to two thirds of patients are not diagnosed until admission to hospital with acute adrenal insufficiency or hypocalcemic crisis, and nearly half of these already have one major component of APS1 present.[35] Increased awareness of APS1 is essential to prevent fatalities. Mutational analysis has aided the early diagnosis of APS1, but it must be remembered that there are a large number of possible mutations and, in the United Kingdom, only the commonest two are routinely screened. Thus, APS1 is not excluded by negative routine DNA analysis, and the presence of one abnormal allele in a child with a major or minor manifestation makes the diagnosis highly likely. The use of the recently identified anti-interferon autoantibodies may well play an important role in aiding diagnosis in the future.[54] The individual disease components of APS1 should be recognized by the standard endocrine surveillance methods.

## Follow-up

The most important goal is the recognition of new disease components, which is essential, as some manifestations are life threatening. Regular review particularly for oral mucocutaneous candidiasis and signs of evolving adrenal insufficiency, such as postural change in blood pressure, is essential. Blood should be taken for basal hormone, hematological, and biochemical markers, and an occasional antibody screen performed. This, together with a high index of clinical suspicion, allows earlier diagnosis and treatment of additional components as they develop.

The early diagnosis of Addison's disease is of particular importance and individuals at risk need an annual measurement of ACTH until adrenocortical failure develops.[32] Plasma renin activity should be measured at the same time. The patient, immediate family, and primary health care team must be made aware of the signs and symptoms of adrenal failure.[37]

## Treatment

Treatment of the individual disorders is no different from treating patients with the isolated disorders, except that polypharmacy is the rule, and that malabsorption may complicate therapy. The different endocrine failures are managed by conventional hormonal replacement, which may be complex when a patient has several endocrine deficiencies. Immunosuppressive treatment with glucocorticoids (eg, for autoimmune hepatitis) can also complicate matters.

Mucocutaneous candidiasis is treated with local and/or systemic antifungal drugs, dental care, and oral hygiene, with expert oral surgical follow-up for refractory cases. Suppression of oral candidiasis is important because of the risk of oral carcinoma.

The serum calcium levels of APS1 patients appear to be labile compared with non-APS1 hypoparathyroidism. This is presumed to be a result of malabsorption, and the intermittent nature of this can lead to marked hypercalcemia with rapid onset of renal impairment. Standard treatment with vitamin D analogs often leads to hypercalciuria, so serum calcium levels need to be maintained at around the lower end of the normal range (2.0–2.2 mmol/L total serum calcium). The vicious cycle of hypocalcemia and malabsorption can usually be broken by an increased oral dose, but parenteral therapy may be required in severe situations. Hypomagnesemia may contribute to resistance and require treatment. In patients with adrenal insufficiency, alteration of the hydrocortisone dose will lead to an alteration in calcium absorption. Also of note is that unexplained hypercalcemia may be the first sign of the development of adrenal failure.

Autoimmune hepatitis is treated with immunosuppressive therapy, most experience being with the use of prednisolone and/or azathioprine. Liver transplantation has occasionally been reported in APS1-associated hepatitis.[45] Immunosuppressive therapy may increase the risk of *Candida*-related cancer and predispose the patient to generalized candidal infection.[34] Immunosuppressants are occasionally required for severe intestinal dysfunction with diarrhea, and there can be an associated improvement in control of serum calcium levels. Milder diarrhea has been found to respond to gut motility-reducing agents such as loperamide.

Live vaccines must be avoided in view of the underlying immunodeficiency[36] but, as splenic atrophy is a common component, all APS1 patients should receive polyvalent pneumococcal vaccine.[37]

## Prognosis

Many patients feel chronically unwell, and the physical and psychological impact of the multiple problems should not be underestimated. Despite improved survival, mortality rates are still high at 10% to 20% and a recent review in Finland has found the average age of death to be 34 years (range 6.8 to 63 years).[41] Death is from a variety of causes including adrenal crisis, diabetic ketoacidosis, fulminant hepatic failure, oral carcinoma, septicemia, hypocalcemia, generalized candidal infection during immunosuppressive treatment, complications of kidney failure, and alcoholism.[32,34,36] Around 3% die before the diagnosis of APS1 has been made, with adrenal failure the likely cause. Depression and suicide is high among this patient group, as the disease poses a great psychological burden, with the constant risk of developing life-threatening complications, disfiguring disease components, and the requirement for multiple medications. Working capacity may be maintained in subjects with a limited number of manifestations, but many are significantly incapacitated.[36,41]

### Summary

The clinical presentation of APS1 is very variable. Diagnosis can be difficult initially when only one manifestation is present, and it often takes years for others to appear. Increased awareness of the condition, combined with analysis of specific autoantibodies and mutational analysis of the *AIRE* gene, should help to diagnose this condition earlier and prevent serious complications and fatalities.

## IMMUNE DYSREGULATION, POLYENDOCRINOPATHY, AND ENTEROPATHY (X-LINKED) SYNDROME

Immune dysregulation, polyendocrinopathy, and enteropathy (X-linked) syndrome (IPEX) is a rare and devastating X-linked condition of male infants, affecting immune regulation and resulting in multiple autoimmune disorders. The first feature is commonly intractable diarrhea and failure to thrive because of autoimmune enteropathy occurring around 3 to 4 months of age. Type 1 diabetes and autoimmune hypothyroidism develop in the first year of life in around 90% and 50% of males respectively. Additional clinical features include eczema, autoimmune hemolytic anemia, autoimmune thrombocytopenia, recurrent infections, lymphadenopathy, membranous nephropathy, and striking growth retardation. Other autoimmune features are less frequent.[61] Sepsis may result from a primary defect in immune regulation but is exacerbated by autoimmune neutropenia, immunosuppressive drugs, malnutrition, enteropathy, and eczema.

The condition is heterogeneous in its presentation, with the occasional case not presenting until later childhood or adulthood.[62] Diabetes or eczema is a not infrequent initial presentation, but any of the disease components can present first. There are no estimates of incidence, but it is likely to be underdiagnosed because of the clinical variability in presentation and the presence of frequent new mutations. Diagnosis relies on the clinical presentation, family history, and elimination of other diagnoses with similar presentations. Genetic screening has proved useful in some cases. There is a high mortality in these infants, many succumbing to the untreatable diarrhea, malnutrition, and superimposed infections by 24 months of age. Survival into adolescence is occasionally seen with the use of aggressive immunosuppression and parenteral feeding, although symptoms are rarely entirely relieved.[61,63] There are increasing reports of the use of bone marrow transplantation in these infants, but experience is very limited.[61]

IPEX has been shown to be caused by mutations in the *FOXP3* gene, located at Xp11, encoding a transcription factor belonging to the forkhead/winged-helix family.[61] An increasing number of mutations have been reported, mainly in the coding region of *FOXP3*, although one mutation in the regulatory region has also been found.[61,63] *FOXP3* is specifically expressed in naturally arising CD4+CD25+ regulatory T cells and appears to convert naïve T cells to this regulatory phenotype (see article by Chatila elsewhere in this issue). Thus, *FOXP3* is a critical regulator of CD4+CD25+ T-cell development and function.[64] Severe autoimmunity in FOXP3 deficiency may in part therefore be because of aggressive helper T cells that develop from regulatory

T-cell precursors that, because of a lack of FOXP3, cannot mature.[65] In a few cases, no mutation has been identified. Although female carriers of *FOXP3* mutations appear to be healthy, a small number of cases of an IPEX-like syndrome have been reported recently in families with affected girls in whom no mutation was found.[63] It is likely that there may be an autosomal locus accounting for the problem in some families, and mutations in the interleukin (IL)-2 receptor subunit CD25 have been shown to cause a similar syndrome.[66] This genetic heterogeneity may explain some of the clinical variation seen in this syndrome but, as yet, no obvious genotype–phenotype relationship has been identified, and other modifying genes, such as *HLA*, as well as environmental factors, may influence the outcome.

## SUMMARY

Most physicians will be made acutely aware of the diverse nature of the polyglandular syndromes at some point in their career. In the modern era, we should aim to use the powerful combination of clinical skills, autoantibody assays, and molecular genetic investigation, along with basal and dynamic endocrine testing, to institute early diagnosis and therapy for these clustering conditions. In the future, more accurate disease prediction may allow us to counsel individuals and families with greater certainty. Ultimately, when disease pathogenesis is more clearly understood, interventions to prevent an autoimmune endocrinopathy developing in those at high risk may become more than a theoretical possibility.

## REFERENCES

1. Neufeld M, Maclaren NK, et al. Two types of auto-immune Addison's disease associated with different polyglandular autoimmune (PGA) syndromes. Medicine (Baltimore) 1981;60(5):355–62.
2. Laureti S, Vecchi L, et al. Is the prevalence of Addison disease underestimated? J Clin Endocrinol Metab 1999;84(5):1762.
3. Falorni A, Laureti S, et al. Autoantibodies in autoimmune polyendocrine syndrome type II. Endocrinol Metab Clin North Am 2002;31(2):369–89.
4. Betterle C, Dal Pra C, et al. Autoimmune adrenal insufficiency and autoimmune polyendocrine syndromes: autoantibodies, autoantigens, and their applicability in diagnosis and disease prediction. Endocr Rev 2002;23(3):327–64.
5. Betterle C, Volpato M, et al. Type 2 polyglandular autoimmune disease (Schmidt's syndrome). J Pediatr Endocrinol Metab 1996;9(Suppl 1):113–23.
6. Betterle C, Lazzarotto F, et al. Autoimmune polyglandular syndrome type 2: the tip of an iceberg? Clin Exp Immunol 2004;137(2):225–33.
7. Murray JS, Jayarajasingh R, et al. Deterioration of symptoms after start of thyroid hormone replacement. BMJ 2001;323(7308):332–3.
8. Leslie RD, Williams R, et al. Type 1 diabetes and latent autoimmune diabetes in adults: one end of the rainbow. J Clin Endocrinol Metab 2006;91(5):1654–9.
9. Schatz DA, Winter WE. Autoimmune polyglandular syndrome II: clinical syndrome and treatment. Endocrinol Metab Clin North Am 2002;31(2):339–52.
10. Belvisi L, Bombelli F, et al. Organ-specific autoimmunity in patients with premature ovarian failure. J Endocrinol Invest 1993;16(11):889–92.
11. Betterle C, Volpato M, et al. I. Adrenal cortex and steroid 21-hydroxylase autoantibodies in adult patients with organ-specific autoimmune diseases: markers of low progression to clinical Addison disease. J Clin Endocrinol Metab 1997;82(3):932–8.

12. Yamaguchi Y, Chikuba N, et al. Islet cell antibodies in patients with autoimmune thyroid disease. Diabetes 1991;40(3):319–22.
13. Mandry RC, Ortiz LJ, et al. Organ-specific autoantibodies in vitiligo patients and their relatives. Int J Dermatol 1996;35(1):18–21.
14. Robles DT, Fain PR, et al. The genetics of autoimmune polyendocrine syndrome type II. Endocrinol Metab Clin North Am 2002;31(2):353–68.
15. Huang W, Connor E, et al. Although DR3-DQB1*0201 may be associated with multiple component diseases of the autoimmune polyglandular syndromes, the human leukocyte antigen DR4-DQB1*0302 haplotype is implicated only in beta-cell autoimmunity. J Clin Endocrinol Metab 1996;81(7):2259–63.
16. Donner H, Braun J, et al. Codon 17 polymorphism of the cytotoxic T lymphocyte antigen 4 gene in Hashimoto thyroiditis and Addison disease. J Clin Endocrinol Metab 1997;82(12):4130–2.
17. Yanagawa T, Hidaka Y, et al. CTLA-4 gene polymorphism associated with Graves disease in a Caucasian population. J Clin Endocrinol Metab 1995; 80(1):41–5.
18. Vaidya B, Pearce S, et al. Recent advances in the molecular genetics of congenital and acquired primary adrenocortical failure. Clin Endocrinol (Oxf) 2000;53(4): 403–18.
19. Nisticò L, Buzzetti R, et al. The CTLA-4 gene region of chromosome 2q33 is linked to, and associated with, type 1 diabetes. Belgium Diabetes Registry. Hum Mol Genet 1996;5(7):1075–80.
20. De Nanclares GP, Martin-Pagola A, et al. No evidence of association of CTLA4 polymorphisms with Addison's disease. Autoimmunity 2004;37(6–7):453–6.
21. Velaga MR, Wilson V, et al. The codon 620 tryptophan allele of the lymphoid tyrosine phosphatase (LYP) gene is a major determinant of Graves' disease. J Clin Endocrinol Metab 2004;89(11):5862–5.
22. Skinningsrud B, Husebye ES, et al. Mutation screening of PTPN22: association of the 1858T-allele with Addison's disease. Eur J Hum Genet 2008;16(8): 977–82.
23. Roycroft M, Fichna M, et al. The tryptophan 620 allele of the lymphoid tyrosine phosphatase (PTPN22 gene) predisposes to autoimmune Addison's disease. Clin Endocrinol (Oxf) Aug 15, 2008;10.1111/j.1365-2265.2008.03380.x [Epub ahead of print].
24. Kamradt T, Mitchison NA. Tolerance and autoimmunity. N Engl J Med 2001; 344(9):655–64.
25. Kriegel MA, Lohmann T, et al. Defective suppressor function of human CD4+CD25+ regulatory T cells in autoimmune polyglandular syndrome type II. J Exp Med 2004;199(9):1285–91.
26. Vendrame F, Segni M, et al. Impaired caspase-3 expression by peripheral T cells in chronic autoimmune thyroiditis and in autoimmune polyendocrine syndrome-2. J Clin Endocrinol Metab 2006;91(12):5064–8.
27. Betterle C, Volpato M, et al. Adrenal-cortex autoantibodies and steroid-producing cells autoantibodies in patients with Addison disease: comparison of immunofluorescence and immunoprecipitation assays. J Clin Endocrinol Metab 1999;84(2): 618–22.
28. Vanderpump MP, Tunbridge WM, et al. The incidence of thyroid disorders in the community: a twenty-year follow-up of the Wickham Survey. Clin Endocrinol (Oxf) 1995;43(1):55–68.
29. Vandewalle CL, Falorni A, et al. High diagnostic sensitivity of glutamate decarboxylase autoantibodies in insulin-dependent diabetes mellitus with clinical onset

between age 20 and 40 years. The Belgian Diabetes Registry. J Clin Endocrinol Metab 1995;80(3):846–51.

30. Bergthorsdottir R, Leonsson-Zachrisson M, et al. Premature mortality in patients with Addison's disease: a population based study. J Clin Endocrinol Metab 2006;91(12):4849–53.

31. Lovas K, Husebye ES. High prevalence and increasing incidence of Addison disease in western Norway. Clin Endocrinol (Oxf) 2002;56(6):787–91.

32. Ahonen P, Myllärniemi S, et al. Clinical variation of autoimmune polyendocrinop-athy–candidiasis–ectodermal dystrophy (APECED) in a series of 68 patients. N Engl J Med 1990;322(26):1829–36.

33. Zlotogora J, Shapiro MS. Polyglandular autoimmune syndrome type I among Iranian Jews. J Med Genet 1992;29(11):824–6.

34. Betterle C, Greggio NA, et al. Clinical review 93: autoimmune polyglandular syndrome type I. J Clin Endocrinol Metab 1998;83(4):1049–55.

35. Myhre AG, Halonen M, et al. Autoimmune polyendocrine syndrome type I (APS1) in Norway. Clin Endocrinol (Oxf) 2001;54(2):211–7.

36. Perheentupa J. APS-I/APECED: the clinical disease and therapy. Endocrinol Metab Clin North Am 2002;31(2):295–320.

37. Pearce SH, Cheetham TD. Autoimmune polyendocrinopathy syndrome type I: treat with kid gloves. Clin Endocrinol (Oxf) 2001;54(4):433–5.

38. Rosatelli MC, Meloni A, et al. A common mutation in Sardinian autoimmune poly-endocrinopathy–candidiasis–ectodermal dystrophy patients. Hum Genet 1998; 103(4):428–34.

39. Gass JD. The syndrome of keratoconjunctivitis, superficial moniliasis idio-pathic hypoparathyroidism and Addison disease. Am J Ophthalmol 1962;54: 660–74.

40. Gylling M, Kääriäinen E, et al. The hypoparathyroidism of autoimmune polyen-docrinopathy–candidiasis–ectodermal dystrophy protective effect of male sex. J Clin Endocrinol Metab 2003;88(10):4602–8.

41. Perheentupa J. Autoimmune polyendocrinopathy-candidiasis-ectodermal dystrophy. J Clin Endocrinol Metab 2006;91(8):2843–50.

42. Sotsiou F, Bottazzo GF, et al. Immunofluorescence studies on autoantibodies to steroid-producing cells, and to germline cells in endocrine disease and infertility. Clin Exp Immunol 1980;39(1):97–111.

43. Bereket A, Lowenheim M, et al. Intestinal lymphangiectasia in a patient with auto-immune polyglandular disease type I and steatorrhea. J Clin Endocrinol Metab 1995;80(3):933–5.

44. Högenauer C, Meyer RL, et al. Malabsorption due to cholecystokinin deficiency in a patient with autoimmune polyglandular syndrome type 1. N Engl J Med 2001; 344(4):270–4.

45. Smith D, Stringer MD, et al. Orthoptic liver transplantation for acute liver failure secondary to autoimmune hepatitis in a child with autoimmune polyglandular syndrome type 1. Pediatr Transplant 2002;6(2):166–70.

46. Nagamine K, Peterson P, et al. Positional cloning of the APECED gene. Nature Genet 1997;17(4):393–8.

47. The Finnish–German APECED Consortium. An autoimmune disease, APECED, caused by mutations in a novel gene featuring two PHD-type zinc-finger domains. Nature Genet 1997;17(4):399–403.

48. Liston A, Lesage S, et al. AIRE regulates negative selection of organ-specific T cells. Nat Immunol 2003;4(4):350–4.

49. Mathis D, Benoist C. A decade of AIRE. Nat Rev Immunol 2007;7(8):645–50.

50. Pearce SH, Cheetham T, et al. A common and recurrent 13-bp deletion in the autoimmune regulator gene in British kindreds with autoimmune polyendocrinopathy type I. Am J Hum Genet 1998;63(6):1675–84.

51. Wolff AS, Erichsen MM, et al. Autoimmune polyendocrinopathy syndrome type 1 in Norway: phenotypic variation, autoantibodies, and novel mutations in the autoimmune regulator gene. J Clin Endocrinol Metab 2007;92(2):595–603.

52. Halonen M, Eskelin P, et al. AIRE mutations and human leukocyte antigen genotypes as determinants of the autoimmune polyendocrinopathy–candidiasis–ectodermal dystrophy phenotype. J Clin Endocrinol Metab 2002;87(6):2568–74.

53. Adamson KA, Cheetham TD, et al. The role of the IDDM2 locus in the susceptibility of UK APS1 subjects to type 1 diabetes mellitus. Int J Immunogenet 2007;34(1):17–21.

54. Meager A, Visvalingam K, et al. Anti-interferon autoantibodies in autoimmune polyendocrinopathy syndrome type 1. PLoS Med 2006;3(7):1152–64.

55. Söderbergh A, Myhre AG, et al. Prevalence and clinical associations of 10 defined autoantibodies in autoimmune polyendocrine syndrome type 1. J Clin Endocrinol Metab 2004;89(2):557–62.

56. Li Y, Song YH, et al. Autoantibodies to the extracellular domain of the calcium sensing receptor in patients with acquired hypoparathyroidism. J Clin Invest 1996;97(4):910–4.

57. Gavalas NG, Kemp EH, et al. The calcium-sensing receptor is a target of autoantibodies in patients with autoimmune polyendocrine syndrome type 1. J Clin Endocrinol Metab 2007;92(6):2107–14.

58. Alimohammadi M, Björklund P, et al. Autoimmune polyendocrine syndrome type 1 and NALP5, a parathyroid autoantigen. N Engl J Med 2008;358(10):1018–28.

59. Tuomi T, Björses P, et al. Antibodies to glutamic acid decarboxylase and insulin-dependent diabetes in patients with autoimmune polyendocrine syndrome type I. J Clin Endocrinol Metab 1996;81(4):1488–94.

60. Obermayer-Straub P, Perheentupa J, et al. Hepatic autoantigens in patients with autoimmune polyendocrinopathy–candidiasis–ectodermal dystrophy. Gastroenterology 2001;121(3):668–77.

61. Wildin RS, Smyk-Pearson S, et al. Clinical and molecular features of the immunodysregulation, polyendocrinopathy, enteropathy, X linked (IPEX) syndrome. J Med Genet 2002;39(8):537–45.

62. Powell BR, Buist NR, et al. An X-linked syndrome of diarrhea, polyendocrinopathy, and fatal infection in infancy. J Pediatr 1982;100(5):731–7.

63. Owen CJ, Jennings CE, et al. Mutational analysis of the FOXP3 gene and evidence for genetic heterogeneity in the immunodysregulation, polyendocrinopathy, enteropathy syndrome. J Clin Endocrinol Metab 2003;88(12):6034–9.

64. Fontenot JD, Gavin MA, et al. FOXP3 programs the development and function of CD4[+]CD25[+] regulatory T cells. Nat Immunol 2003;4(4):330–6.

65. Gavin MA, Torgerson TR, et al. Single-cell analysis of normal and FOXP3-mutant human T cells: FOXP3 expression without regulatory T cell development. Proc Natl Acad Sci U S A 2006;103(17):6659–64.

66. Caudy AA, Reddy ST, et al. CD25 deficiency causes an immune dysregulation, polyendocrinopathy, enteropathy, X-linked syndrome, and defective IL-10 expression from CD4 lymphocytes. J Allergy Clin Immunol 2007;119(2):482–7.

# Anti-Parathyroid and Anti-Calcium Sensing Receptor Antibodies in Autoimmune Hypoparathyroidism

Edward M. Brown, MD

**KEYWORDS**

- Parathyroid • Calcium-sensing receptor • CaSR
- Autoantibody • Anti-parathyroid antibody
- Anti-CaSR antibody • Autoimmune • Hypoparathyroidism
- Autoimmune hypocalciuric hypercalcemia

Autoimmunity is an important cause of hypoparathyroidism, either as an isolated endocrinopathy or a component of autoimmune polyglandular syndromes (eg, APS1 and 2, discussed elsewhere in this issue).[1,2] In Norway, the prevalence of APS1, comprising candidiasis, hypoparathyroidism, and Addison's disease, which can be accompanied by chronic active hepatitis, alopecia, and primary hypogonadism, is about 1 in 90,000. In some genetically more homogeneous populations it is more common, with a prevalence of 1 in 600 to 1 in 9000 in Iranian Jews and 1 in 25,000 in Finns.[2] The first direct evidence in support of an autoimmune basis for idiopathic hypoparathyroidism (IH) was provided by Blizzard and colleagues[3] in 1966 who identified anti-parathyroid antibodies in patients with presumed autoimmune hypoparathyroidism (AH). The identity of the parathyroid antigens remained uncertain for 30 years. The cloning and characterization of the calcium-sensing receptor (CaSR) in 1993 (**Fig. 1**)[4] as the molecular mechanism by which parathyroid cells recognize and respond to changes in the extracellular calcium concentration ($Ca^{2+}_o$) identified a logical target for anti-parathyroid antibodies.[4] Shortly thereafter, antibodies directed at the extracellular domain (ECD) of the CaSR were found in patients with IH.[5] Several years later, additional studies documented that some anti-CaSR antibodies can stimulate[6] or inhibit[7] the receptor, producing, respectively, hypoparathyroidism or parathyroid hormone (PTH)–dependent hypercalcemia. This article briefly describes the

The author has a financial interest in the calcimimetic cinacalcet HCl (Sensipar). He was supported by NIH grants DK67111 and DK67155.

Division of Endocrinology, Diabetes and Hypertension, Department of Medicine, Brigham and Women's Hospital, EBRC 223A, 221 Longwood Avenue, Boston, MA 02115, USA

*E-mail address:* embrown@partners.org

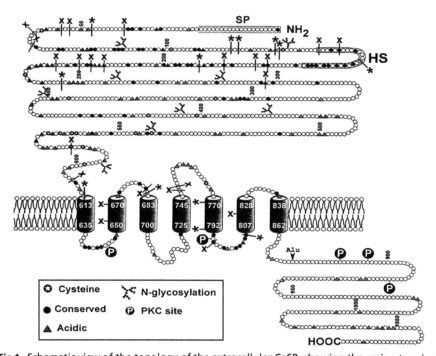

**Fig. 1.** Schematic view of the topology of the extracellular CaSR, showing the amino terminal extracellular domain of the receptor in the upper part of the figure, the seven membrane-spanning domains as barrel-like structures in the middle, and the intracellular C-tail at the bottom right. Also shown are cysteines, which are involved in intra- or intercellular disulfide bonds, N-glycosylation sites, acidic sites that may bind calcium ions, and regulatory protein kinase C (PKC) phosphorylation sites. X denotes inactivating mutations, which, like inactivating antibodies, inhibit activation of the receptor. The asterisk (*) indicates activating mutations, which, similar to activating antibodies, render the receptor more sensitive to extracellular calcium.

role of CaSR in the homeostatic mechanisms that maintain near constancy of $Ca^{2+}_o$ in the blood and other extracellular fluids (ECF). It then reviews the history of anti-parathyroid antibodies and the subsequent elucidation of the CaSR as a target for at least some of these antibodies, including those that can directly activate or inhibit the receptor. It discusses the treatment of the conditions associated with immunity-mediated alterations in parathyroid function.

### ROLE OF THE CaSR IN NORMAL MINERAL ION HOMEOSTASIS

An understanding of the pathophysiology of hypoparathyroidism requires some knowledge of how humans maintain near constancy of $Ca^{2+}_o$.[8,9] The homeostatic mechanism that accomplishes this comprises three key components: (1) kidney, bone, and intestine, which translocate $Ca^{2+}$ into or out of the ECF in response to homeostatic signals; (2) two $Ca^{2+}_o$–elevating hormones, PTH and 1,25-dihdroxyvita-min $D_3$ [1,25$(OH)_2D_3$], and a $Ca^{2+}_o$–lowering hormone, calcitonin (CT), which regulate the fluxes of $Ca^{2+}$ into and out of the ECF; and (3) $Ca^{2+}_o$–sensing cells that regulate the production/secretion of these $Ca^{2+}_o$–regulating hormones and, in some cases, the transport of calcium ions per se. The production of the two $Ca^{2+}_o$–elevating hormones is normally stimulated by hypocalcemia and inhibited by hypercalcemia, whereas that of CT, which lowers $Ca^{2+}_o$ by inhibiting bone resorption, is stimulated by hypercalcemia and inhibited by hypocalcemia, creating homeostatically appropriate negative feedback loops.[8,9] In a hypocalcemic challenge, low $Ca^{2+}_o$ directly stimulates the secretion of PTH by the parathyroid glands and the production of $1,25(OH)_2D_3$ by the proximal tubular cells of the kidney[10] while at the same time inhibiting CT secretion by the thyroidal C cells. PTH increases renal tubular $Ca^{2+}$ reabsorption and enhances $1,25(OH)_2D_3$ synthesis from its precursor, $25(OH)D_3$. Hypocalcemia also directly increases renal tubular reabsorption of $Ca^{2+}$ through a mechanism described later. $1,25(OH)_2D_3$ increases intestinal $Ca^{2+}$ absorption and acts in concert with PTH to enhance net release of $Ca^{2+}$ from bone. The increased fluxes of $Ca^{2+}$ into the ECF from intestine and bone, coupled with renal $Ca^{2+}$ conservation, restore $Ca^{2+}_o$ toward normal, usually within a matter of minutes to hours. In addition to PTH, $1,25(OH)_2D_3$, and CT, another recently identified protein, alpha-klotho, present in kidney and parathyroid in both membrane-bound and secreted forms, likely has a key role in $Ca^{2+}_o$ homeostasis by promoting PTH secretion and renal tubular $Ca^{2+}_o$ reabsorption and inhibiting $1,25(OH)_2D_3$ synthesis.[11,12]

## ROLE OF THE CaSR IN $Ca^{2+}_o$ HOMEOSTASIS

The molecular mechanism through which the parathyroid gland and kidney respond to changes in $Ca^{2+}_o$ was identified in 1993 as the extracellular CaSR,[4] which is a G protein–coupled receptor (GPCR) of the same family (family 3 or C) as those sensing glutamate, gamma-aminobutyric acid, odorants, sweet taste, and pheromones.[13] This family of receptors has large amino terminal ECDs, comprising 612 amino acids in the human CaSR and the seven membrane-spanning helices characteristic of the superfamily of GPCRs. The CaSR is heavily glycosylated and resides on the cell surface as a disulfide-linked dimer. The ECD contains important determinants for binding $Ca^{2+}_o$, the receptor's principal biologically relevant ligand, although there are additional $Ca^{2+}$–binding sites within the seven membrane-spanning domain, because a "headless" receptor entirely lacking the ECD still responds to $Ca^{2+}_o$.[13] In addition to $Ca^{2+}_o$, the CaSR also responds to $Mg^{2+}_o$, polycations (eg, spermine and aminoglycoside antibiotics), aromatic and other amino acids, and pharmacologic activators ("calcimimetics") and antagonists ("calcilytics").[14] Of the naturally occurring CaSR agonists/activators, $Ca^{2+}_o$, $Mg^{2+}_o$, spermine, and amino acids can be present in biologic fluids at concentrations appropriate to serve as biologically relevant ligands of the receptor, although $Ca^{2+}_o$ is by far the best characterized regulator of the CaSR. The CaSR controls cellular functions via numerous intracellular signaling pathways. It activates phospholipases $A_2$ ($PLA_2$), C (PLC), and D (PLD) and mitogen-activated protein kinases (MAPK) and inhibits adenylate cyclase.[15] These effector systems enable it to regulate numerous biologic processes, including hormonal and other secretory processes, ion transporters and channels, and chemotaxis, and cellular proliferation, differentiation, and death, to name a few.[16]

The best established roles of the CaSR in $Ca^{2+}_o$ homeostasis are to inhibit parathyroid cellular proliferation, PTH secretion, and PTH gene expression, to stimulate CT secretion, and to directly inhibit renal tubular $Ca^{2+}$ reabsorption.[17] Less well-documented actions are promoting proliferation, chemotaxis, and differentiation of osteoblasts and their mineralization of bone, as well as inhibiting osteoclastic differentiation and activity.[16] Some anti-CaSR antibodies exert functional effects on the CaSR, stimulating or inhibiting PTH secretion as well as CaSR-regulated second messenger pathways.

## ANTI-PARATHYROID ANTIBODIES IN HYPOPARATHYROIDISM

In 1966, Blizzard and colleagues[3] first reported the presence of anti-parathyroid anti-bodies in 38% of 75 patients with IH, 26% of 92 patients with idiopathic Addison's disease, 12% of 49 patients with Hashimoto's thyroiditis, and 6% of 245 normal controls using indirect immunofluorescence. Sections of parathyroid adenomas or normal human parathyroid glands were incubated with the patient's sera and then with a fluorescein-conjugated anti-human immunoglobulin antibody. The antibodies appeared to be specific for parathyroid, because it was blocked by preabsorption with parathyroid extracts but not those from gastric, thyroid, adrenal, liver, or kidney tissue. Several subsequent studies raised the possibility that at least some anti-para-thyroid antibodies were not, in fact, specific for parathyroid tissue but reacted with mitochondrial[18,19] or endomyseal[20] (eg, in celiac sprue) antigens. Brandi and colleagues[21] in two publications in the late 1980s further investigated the potential role of anti-parathyroid antibodies in the pathogenesis of AH. They first identified anti-bodies that reacted with bovine parathyroid cells and elicited complement-dependent cytotoxicity. In a second study, these antibodies were shown to be directed predom-inantly at bovine parathyroid endothelial cells, raising the possibility of a novel para-digm whereby damage to parathyroid endothelial cells serves as the basis for parathyroid gland damage and destruction.[22] There have been no follow-up investiga-tions related to these two studies.

## DOCUMENTATION OF ANTI-CaSR ANTIBODIES IN AUTOIMMUNE HYPOPARATHYROIDISM

Li and colleagues[5] first identified anti-CaSR antibodies in patients with AH. They studied 25 patients with IH, 17 with APS1, and 8 with coexistent AH but no other en-docrinopathies. By immunoblotting of human parathyroid gland extracts, sera from 5 of the 25 patients (25%) had immunoreactivity with proteins of a size consistent with the CaSR. They then used membrane fractions from HEK293 cells transfected with the human CaSR, which express more CaSR protein than parathyroid glands, to show that eight sera were positive, including the five serum samples identified previously using parathyroid extracts. No reactivity was observed with membranes prepared from non-transfected HEK cells, documenting that the sera reacted with the CaSR per se. When the sera were tested for their capacity to immunoprecipitate in vitro translated CaSR ECD, 14 (56%) were positive [6 (35%) with APS1 and 8 (100%) with adult onset IH], whereas no anti-CaSR antibodies were detected in sera from 22 normal controls and 50 patients with other autoimmune disorders who did not have hypoparathyroidism. Patients with AH for less than 5 years were more likely to harbor anti-CaSR antibodies (72%) than those with the condition for more than 5 years (14%), presumably because of loss of the antigen with ongoing destruction of the parathyroid glands. Although the antibodies did not change the intracellular $Ca^{2+}$ level of CaSR-transfected HEK293 cells, slow binding of antibody to the CaSR might preclude observing the transient release of $Ca^{2+}$ from intracellular stores due to anti-body-evoked, CaSR-mediated PLC activation in this assay.

Several subsequent studies using a variety of techniques to identify anti-CaSR anti-bodies have yielded generally similar results but with varying rates of positivity. Gos-wami and colleagues[23] documented the presence of anti-CaSR antibodies in 49% of 51 patients with sporadic IH and 13.3% of healthy controls as assessed by immuno-blotting of membrane preparations of parathyroid adenomas shown to express robust CaSR levels. Six of the patients with IH had other forms of autoimmunity, including three with hypothyroidism and one with type 1 diabetes. In contrast to the results of Li and colleagues,[5] a study of 90 patients with APS1 failed to identify anti-CaSR antibodies using immunoprecipitation of in vitro translated CaSR.[24] The basis for the difference between the results of these two studies is not known; however, the methodologies differed. Although the reactivity of a commercial anti-CaSR antiserum with its peptide antigen was used as a positive control, there were no positive controls using patient sera in the latter study. Another study[25] published the same year investigated 17 patients with acquired IH and 14 with either APS1 or APS2 for the presence of anti-CaSR antibodies using immunoblotting with in vitro translated CaSR ECD, similar to Li and colleagues.[5] Five (29%) of the patients with IH and two (14%) of those with APS (one with APS1 and one with APS2) harbored anti-CaSR antibodies. A recent study by Gavalas and colleagues[26] used three techniques—immunoprecipitate of CaSR expressed by CaSR-transfected HEK293 cells, a flow cytometry assay, and a radiobinding assay—to identify anti-CaSR antibodies in 14 patients with APS1 and 28 patients with Graves' disease but without AH. The first technique was most sensitive and identified anti-CaSR antibodies in 12 (86%) of the patients with APS1 and 2 (7%) of those with Graves' disease. The variety of techniques used in these studies to identify anti-CaSR antibodies makes it difficult to compare the results directly, and some techniques likely underestimate the prevalence of anti-CaSR antibodies. Nevertheless, it appears that a substantial proportion of patients with either APS1 or adult onset IH harbor anti-CaSR antibodies. Based on the studies reviewed to this point, it is not possible to determine whether the antibodies had any direct role in the pathogenesis of the disorder or were simply a marker of the disease process, perhaps owing to destruction of the parathyroid glands and associated production of antibodies to self-antigen.

## HYPOPARATHYROIDISM DUE TO ACTIVATING ANTIBODIES TO THE CaSR

Kifor and colleagues[6] reported in 2004 that anti-CaSR antibodies occurring in AH could exert direct functional actions on the CaSR and, in turn, the parathyroid gland. They described two patients with IH. In one, transient hypoparathyroidism developed in a patient with Addison's disease, as manifested by hypocalcemia with an inappropriately low-normal PTH level. Over several weeks, the serum calcium and PTH levels normalized, and long-term therapy was not needed to maintain normocalcemia. The second patient had coexistent hypoparathyroidism causing seizures and requiring therapy with oral calcium and vitamin D and difficult-to-treat Graves' disease that eventually necessitated subtotal thyroidectomy. During surgery, a parathyroid gland normal by both size and histologic criteria was identified, demonstrating that the patient's AH had not destroyed the parathyroid glands. Both patients harbored anti-CaSR antibodies as assessed by immunoblotting of CaSR extracted from parathyroid glands or CaSR-transfected HEK cells, by immunoprecipitation using the patients' sera, and by an ELISA using peptides from within the CaSR's ECD. In the first case, the antibody titer decreased as the hypoparathyroidism remitted. Furthermore, the anti-CaSR antibodies in both patients activated the CaSR, as documented by stimulation of PLC and MAPK in CaSR-transfected HEK293 cells and inhibition of PTH release from dispersed cells from parathyroid adenomas. In both cases, the hypoparathyroidism may have resulted from a functional effect of the antibodies on the CaSR in the parathyroid glands and not from irreversible parathyroid damage.[6] In retrospect, the patient described by Posillico and colleagues[27] with hypoparathyroidism that fluctuated in its severity may have harbored activating antibodies that varied in their titer. It is also noteworthy that polyclonal or monoclonal antibodies raised to the CaSR have been shown to either activate [28,29] or inhibit the receptor.[7,28] In addition, the impact of activating antibodies to the CaSR on calcium homeostasis and the functions of parathyroid and kidney is conceptually equivalent to the bio-chemically similar syndrome arising from activating mutations of the CaSR, autosomal dominant hypoparathyroidism, or hypocalcemia [17]

## PTH-DEPENDENT HYPERCALCEMIA DUE TO INACTIVATING ANTIBODIES TO THE CaSR

In contrast to the AH due to activating antibodies to the CaSR, Kifor and colleagues[7] described four patients, two sisters as well as a mother and her daughter, with PTH-dependent hypercalcemia, three of whom exhibited hypocalciuria. The mother had coexistent celiac sprue, whereas her daughter and the two sisters had Hashimoto's thyroiditis. A genetic cause of PTH-dependent, hypocalciuric hypercalcemia is the autosomal dominant syndrome familial hypocalciuric hypercalcemia (FHH), which results from heterozygous inactivating CaSR mutations[17]; however, Kifor and colleagues[7] ruled out FHH in these patients. Nevertheless, their autoimmune manifes-tations prompted a search for an autoimmune basis for the hypocalciuric hypercal-cemia. All four patients, in fact, harbored inactivating CaSR antibodies that mitigated high $Ca^{2+}{}_o$–stimulated activation of PLC and MAPK and stimulated PTH secretion. This condition has been termed acquired or autoimmune hypocalciuric hypercalcemia (AHH).[30]

A subsequent report from the same group[31] described a 66-year-old hypercalcemic woman with multiple autoimmune manifestations (psoriasis, adult onset asthma, Coomb's positive hemolytic anemia, rheumatoid arthritis, uveitis, bullous pemphigoid, sclerosing pancreatitis, and autoimmune hypophysitis with hypothyroidism and dia-betes insipidus). Her hypercalcemia (as high as 13.4 mg/dL) was accompanied by elevated intact PTH levels (75–175 pg/mL) and hypocalciuria. A diagnosis of primary hyperparathyroidism had been made earlier, but a subtotal parathyroidectomy was followed within 3 weeks by recrudescence of the hypercalcemia. Remarkably, the hypercalcemia subsequently resolved during treatment with glucocorticoids given for the bullous pemphigoid, and the intact PTH level decreased concomitantly to the upper limit of normal. While hypercalcemic, the patient's serum harbored anti-CaSR antibodies, but there was a substantial drop in the titer of these antibodies during glucocorticoid therapy. To date, therapy with glucocorticoids has only been undertaken in this AHH patient and might be expected to be associated with long-term complications (eg, osteoporosis and diabetes) if used chronically. As in the earlier four cases of AHH,[7] the persistence of PTH-dependent hypercalcemia proves unequivocally that the anti-CaSR antibodies had not destroyed the patients' parathy-roid glands.

Another study [30] described a 74-year-old male patient who developed AHH and was found to harbor anti-CaSR antibodies. Interestingly, in this case the antibodies miti-gated the stimulatory effect of high $Ca^{2+}{}_o$ on MAPK activation in CaSR-transfected HEK293 cells while at the same time sensitizing the HEK cells to the activation of PLC by high $Ca^{2+}{}_o$. These findings were interpreted as evidence that the anti-CaSR antibodies stabilized a novel conformation of the receptor that activates one heterotri-meric G protein, $G_q$, which is responsible for activating PLC, while at the same time reducing the coupling of the CaSR to $G_i$, the G protein responsible for activating MAPK in this experimental system. Such a mechanism may make it possible for phys-iologic agonists of the CaSR and other GPCRs to couple preferentially to one or another G protein and, in turn, the signaling pathway. A provocative finding worthy of follow-up was the identification of anti-parathyroid antibodies in a substantial proportion of patients with parathyroid adenomas,[32] raising the possibility that autoimmunity to the parathyroid, and perhaps the CaSR, could participate in the pathogenesis of primary hyperparathyroidism.

Additional antigens in the parathyroid gland can also be the target of autoantibodies. Autoantibodies to NALP5 (NACHT leucine-rich-repeat protein 5) have recently been identified in 49% of patients with APS1 and hypoparathyroidism but not in any patients with APS1 without hypoparathyroidism,[33] suggesting that it might be a major autoantibody in the hypoparathyroidism of APS1. NALP5 is expressed in the parathyroid in men and women as well as in the ovary in the latter. Although its function is unknown, it has some of the structural characteristics of an intracellular signaling molecule.

### TREATMENT OF HYPO- AND HYPERPARATHYROIDISM ARISING FROM AUTOIMMUNE HYPOPARATHYROIDISM

The usual treatment of hypoparathyroidism of any etiology is to administer active metabolites of vitamin D, such as $1,25(OH)_2D_3$ (Rocaltrol), ranging from 0.5 to 1.5 µg/day, as well as calcium supplementation of about 1 to 3 g of elemental calcium in two to four divided doses.[2,8] The desired therapeutic result is to maintain the serum calcium close to the lower limit of normal (8–8.5 mg/dL; 2.0–2.3 mmol/L) while at the same time avoiding the hypercalciuria (>4 mg/kg/day) that results from increased gastrointestinal absorption of calcium in the absence of the renal $Ca^{2+}$ conservation normally promoted by PTH. If the desired serum calcium concentration cannot be achieved without overt hypercalciuria, treatment with a thiazide diuretic may reduce renal calcium excretion to an acceptable level. Another approach to the problem of excessive renal calcium excretion during treatment with calcium and vitamin D is once, or preferably twice, daily subcutaneous injection of PTH(1-34), which uses the renal calcium-conserving action of PTH to achieve the desired level of serum calcium without excessive hypercalciuria.[34]

The identification of patients with activating or inactivating antibodies to the CaSR raises the possibility of treatment with pharmacologic antagonists (calcilytics) or activators (calcimimetics) of the receptor,[35] respectively, in these two clinical settings. In the former situation, antagonizing the antibody-mediated activation of the CaSR could stimulate PTH secretion and promote renal calcium conservation due to the actions of the drug in parathyroid and kidney, respectively, thereby returning serum calcium toward normal. Even in patients with AH and irreversible loss of parathyroid function, it might be possible to develop a calcilytic agent that would increase renal tubular reabsorption at any given level of serum calcium by antagonizing the renal CaSR, thereby facilitating maintenance of the desired level of serum calcium without hypercalciuria. Conversely, in patients with inactivating antibodies causing AHH, activation of the CaSR in parathyroid and kidney with a calcimimetic agent might reverse or ameliorate the PTH-dependent hypercalcemia and hypocalciuria.

### REFERENCES

1. Betterle C. Parathyroid and autoimmunity. Ann Endocrinol (Paris) 2006;67: 147–54.
2. Whyte MP. Autoimmune hypoparathyroidism. In: Bilezikian JP, Marcus R, Levine MA, editors. The parathyroids. 2nd edition. San Diego (CA): Academic Press; 2001. p. 791–805.
3. Blizzard RM, Chee D, Davis W. The incidence of parathyroid and other antibodies in the sera of patients with idiopathic hypoparathyroidism. Clin Exp Immunol 1966;1:119–28.

4. Brown EM, Gamba G, Riccardi D, et al. Cloning and characterization of an extracellular Ca(2+)-sensing receptor from bovine parathyroid. Nature 1993;366: 575–80.

5. Li Y, Song YH, Rais N, et al. Autoantibodies to the extracellular domain of the calcium sensing receptor in patients with acquired hypoparathyroidism. J Clin Invest 1996;97:910–4.

6. Kifor O, McElduff A, LeBoff MS, et al. Activating antibodies to the calcium-sensing receptor in two patients with autoimmune hypoparathyroidism. J Clin Endocrinol Metab 2004;89:548–56.

7. Kifor O, Moore FD Jr, Delaney M, et al. A syndrome of hypocalciuric hypercalcemia caused by autoantibodies directed at the calcium-sensing receptor. J Clin Endocrinol Metab 2003;88:60–72.

8. Bringhurst FR, Demay MB, Kronenberg HM. Hormones and disorders of mineral metabolism. In: Wilson JD, Foster DW, Kronenberg HM, et al, editors. Williams textbook of endocrinology. 9th edition. Philadelphia: W.B. Saunders; 1998. p. 1155–209.

9. Brown EM. Physiology of calcium homeostasis. In: Biliezikian JP, Raisz LG, Rodan G, editors. The parathyroids. 2nd edition. San Diego (CA): Academic Press; 2001. p. 167–81.

10. Weisinger JR, Favus MJ, Langman CB, et al. Regulation of 1,25-dihydroxyvitamin D3 by calcium in the parathyroidectomized, parathyroid hormone–replete rat. J Bone Miner Res 1989;4:929–35.

11. Nabeshima YI, Imura H. Alpha-klotho: a regulator that integrates calcium homeostasis. Am J Nephrol 2007;28:455–64.

12. Renkema KY, Alexander RT, Bindels RJ, et al. Calcium and phosphate homeostasis: concerted interplay of new regulators. Ann Med 2008;40:82–91.

13. Brauner-Osborne H, Wellendorph P, Jensen AA. Structure, pharmacology and therapeutic prospects of family C G-protein coupled receptors. Curr Drug Targets 2007;8:169–84.

14. Conigrave AD, Quinn SJ, Brown EM. Cooperative multi-modal sensing and therapeutic implications of the extracellular Ca(2+) sensing receptor. Trends Pharmacol Sci 2000;21:401–7.

15. Ward DT. Calcium receptor-mediated intracellular signalling. Cell Calcium 2004; 35:217–28.

16. Brown EM, MacLeod RJ. Extracellular calcium sensing and extracellular calcium signaling. Physiol Rev 2001;81:239–97.

17. Hauache OM. Extracellular calcium-sensing receptor: structural and functional features and association with diseases. Braz J Med Biol Res 2001;34: 577–84.

18. Swana GT, Swana MR, Bottazzo GF, et al. A human-specific mitochondrial antibody: its importance in the identification of organ-specific reactions. Clin Exp Immunol 1977;28:517–25.

19. Betterle C, Caretto A, Zeviani M, et al. Demonstration and characterization of antihuman mitochondria autoantibodies in idiopathic hypoparathyroidism and in other conditions. Clin Exp Immunol 1985;62:353–60.

20. Kumar V, Valeski JE, Wortsman J. Celiac disease and hypoparathyroidism: crossreaction of endomysial antibodies with parathyroid tissue. Clin Diagn Lab Immunol 1996;3:143–6.

21. Brandi ML, Aurbach GD, Fattorossi A, et al. Antibodies cytotoxic to bovine parathyroid cells in autoimmune hypoparathyroidism. Proc Natl Acad Sci U S A 1986; 83:8366–9.

22. Fattorossi A, Aurbach GD, Sakaguchi K, et al. Anti-endothelial cell antibodies: detection and characterization in sera from patients with autoimmune hypoparathyroidism. Proc Natl Acad Sci U S A 1988;85:4015–9.
23. Goswami R, Brown EM, Kochupillai N, et al. Prevalence of calcium sensing receptor autoantibodies in patients with sporadic idiopathic hypoparathyroidism. Eur J Endocrinol 2004;150:9–18.
24. Soderbergh A, Myhre AG, Ekwall O, et al. Prevalence and clinical associations of 10 defined autoantibodies in autoimmune polyendocrine syndrome type I. J Clin Endocrinol Metab 2004;89:557–62.
25. Mayer A, Ploix C, Orgiazzi J, et al. Calcium-sensing receptor autoantibodies are relevant markers of acquired hypoparathyroidism. J Clin Endocrinol Metab 2004; 89:4484–8.
26. Gavalas NG, Kemp EH, Krohn KJ, et al. The calcium-sensing receptor is a target of autoantibodies in patients with autoimmune polyendocrine syndrome type 1. J Clin Endocrinol Metab 2007;92:2107–14.
27. Posillico JT, Wortsman J, Srikanta S, et al. Parathyroid cell surface autoantibodies that inhibit parathyroid hormone secretion from dispersed human parathyroid cells. J Bone Miner Res 1986;1:475–83.
28. Hu J, Reyes-Cruz G, Goldsmith PK, et al. Functional effects of monoclonal antibodies to the purified amino-terminal extracellular domain of the human Ca(2+) receptor. J Bone Miner Res 2007;22:601–8.
29. Roussanne MC, Gogusev J, Hory B, et al. Persistence of Ca(2+)-sensing receptor expression in functionally active, long-term human parathyroid cell cultures. J Bone Miner Res 1998;13:354–62.
30. Makita N, Sato J, Manaka K, et al. An acquired hypocalciuric hypercalcemia autoantibody induces allosteric transition among active human Ca-sensing receptor conformations. Proc Natl Acad Sci U S A 2007;104:5443–8.
31. Pallais JC, Kifor O, Chen YB, et al. Acquired hypocalciuric hypercalcemia due to autoantibodies against the calcium-sensing receptor. N Engl J Med 2004;351: 362–9.
32. Bjerneroth G, Juhlin C, Gudmundsson S, et al. Major histocompatibility complex class II expression and parathyroid autoantibodies in primary hyperparathyroidism. Surgery 1998;124:503–9.
33. Alimohammadi M, Bjorklund P, Hallgren A, et al. Autoimmune polyendocrine syndrome type 1 and NALP5, a parathyroid autoantigen. N Engl J Med 2008; 358:1018–28.
34. Winer KK, Ko CW, Reynolds JC, et al. Long-term treatment of hypoparathyroidism: a randomized controlled study comparing parathyroid hormone-(1-34) versus calcitriol and calcium. J Clin Endocrinol Metab 2003;88:4214–20.
35. Nemeth EF. Calcimimetic and calcilytic drugs: just for parathyroid cells? Cell Calcium 2004;35:283–9.

# Index

*Note:* Page numbers of article titles are in **boldface** type.

### A

Acquired hypercalcemia, 442
ACTH stimulation test, for autoimmune polyglandular syndromes, 423–424, 427, 431
Addison's disease, autoimmune polyglandular syndrome type 1 with, 275, 426–427, 431
  autoimmune thyroid disease with, 419–421
  disability with, 413–414
  immunology of, **389–405**
    autoimmune ovarian failure and, 396–398
    cellular autoimmunity in, 391–392
    clinical features in, 389–390
    genes associated with, 392–395
    historical evaluations of, 390–391
    humoral autoimmunity in, 391
    in dogs, 395
    mouse model of, 395–396
    onset of, 390
    prevalence of, 390
    standard replacement therapy in, 390
    summary overview of, 389, 398
  mortality issues with, 413–414
  21st century approach to, **407–418**
    adrenal crisis and, 412–413
    corticosteroid replacement as, 407–412
      DHEA in, 408, 411, 414–415
      glucocorticoids in, 408–411
      long-acting hydrocortisone in, 409, 415
      mineralocorticoids in, 410–412
      monitoring guidelines for, 411
      optimization of, 407–408
    future perspectives on, 415
    historical treatments vs., 407
    quality of life issues with, 413–415
  type 1 diabetes with, 419–421
Adenovirus vectors, for DNA, in Graves' disease models, 343, 345–347
Adenylate cyclase (AC)/cAMP cascade, in thyroid-stimulating hormone receptor signaling
  pathway, 328
Adipocytes, thyroid-stimulating hormone receptor role, 321
Adrenal crisis, in Addison's disease, prevention and management of, 412–413
Adrenal failure, in autoimmune polyglandular syndrome type 1, 426–427
β-Adrenergic antagonists, for Graves' disease, 360–361

Endocrinol Metab Clin N Am 38 (2009) 447–470
doi:10.1016/S0889-8529(09)00040-1
0889-8529/09/$ – see front matter © 2009 Elsevier Inc. All rights reserved.

endo.theclinics.com

# Moving?

## Make sure your subscription moves with you!

To notify us of your new address, find your **Clinics Account Number** (located on your mailing label above your name), and contact customer service at:

**E-mail: elspcs@elsevier.com**

**800-654-2452 (subscribers in the U.S. & Canada)**
**314-453-7041 (subscribers outside of the U.S. & Canada)**

**Fax number: 314-523-5170**

**Elsevier Periodicals Customer Service**
11830 Westline Industrial Drive
St. Louis, MO 63146

*To ensure uninterrupted delivery of your subscription, please notify us at least 4 weeks in advance of move.

Printed and bound by CPI Group (UK) Ltd, Croydon, CR0 4YY

03/10/2024

01040453-0002